Transient Receptor Potential (TRP) Channels in Drug Discovery: Old Concepts & New Thoughts

Special Issue Editor

Arpad Szallasi

Susan M. Huang

MDPI • Basel • Beijing • Wuhan • Barcelona • Belgrade

MDPI

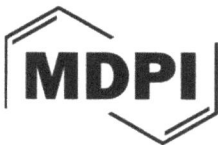

Special Issue Editors
Arpad Szallasi
Baptist-MD Anderson Cancer Center
USA

Susan M. Huang
AbbVie Inc.
USA

Editorial Office
MDPI AG
St. Alban-Anlage 66
Basel, Switzerland

This edition is a reprint of the Special Issue published online in the open access journal *Pharmaceuticals* (ISSN 1424-8247) from 2016–2017 (available at: http://www.mdpi.com/journal/pharmaceuticals/special_issues/old_concepts_new_thoughts).

For citation purposes, cite each article independently as indicated on the article page online and as indicated below:

Author 1; Author 2. Article title. *Journal Name* **Year**, *Article number*, page range.

First Edition 2017

ISBN 978-3-03842-638-7 (Pbk)
ISBN 978-3-03842-639-4 (PDF)

Table of Contents

About the Special Issue Editors

Arpad Szallasi is a Diplomate of the American Board of Pathology. At present, he is the Medical Director of Hematopathology at Baptist Medical Center and Baptist-MD Anderson Cancer Center, Jacksonville, Florida, USA. He received his MD degree Summa cum Laude from the University Medical School of Debrecen, Hungary. He also holds a PhD degree in Pharmacology from the Karolinska Institute. In the past, he held research positions in both academia and the pharma industry. He has published over a hundred peer-reviewed papers, invited reviews and book chapters on the roles of TRP channels in health and disease. Moreover, he is the editor of four books and several thematic journal issues on TRP channels. He is an Associate Editor to Pharmaceuticals and Temperature, and he has sat on the scientific advisory board of several biotech companies with an active TRP channel research program.

pharmaceuticals

MDPI

Editorial

Transient Receptor Potential (TRP) Channels in Drug Discovery: Old Concepts & New Thoughts

Susan Huang [1] and Arpad Szallasi [2,*]

[1] AbbVie Inc, 1 North Waukegan Road, North Chicago, IL 60064, USA; susan.huang@abbvie.com
[2] Baptist Medical Center, 800 Prudential Drive, Jacksonville, FL 32207, USA
* Correspondence: Arpad.Szallasi@BMCJAX.com

Received: 25 June 2017; Accepted: 26 June 2017; Published: 6 July 2017

2017 marks the 20th anniversary of the molecular cloning by David Julius and colleagues (1997) of the long sought-after capsaicin receptor, now known as TRPV1 (Transient Receptor Potential Vanilloid 1) [1]. This seminal discovery has opened up a "hot" new field of basic research and launched drug discovery efforts into the large family (by the latest count 28 mammalian members, 27 in humans) of TRP ion channels [2]. Indeed, it took less than a decade for the first potent, small molecule TRPV1 antagonists to enter phase 1 clinical trials [3]. Yet, despite the large amount of resources that has been invested in TRPV1 research, there are currently no TRPV1-targeted drugs in phase 3 clinical trials. In this special issue of Pharmaceuticals, we aim to capture the progress in the TRP channel field over the past twenty years, with 15 articles covering a variety of TRP channels and potential relevant disease states and applications.

Fitting to the root of TRP channel discovery, Mickle and colleagues provide a comprehensive review of the nociceptive TRP ion channels, including TRPV1 [4]. TRP channel activation by specific physical-chemical stimuli, expression in the nociceptive system, and involvement in various types of pain are discussed. They argue that inhibition of TRP channels expressed on nociceptive neurons represents a viable therapeutic pain target. Small molecule modulators of TRP channels that have already progressed into clinical development for the treatment of pain are also discussed.

Natural products offer a rich source of chemical diversity to identify novel drug candidates. Indeed, one in three new medicines approved by the FDA is derived from natural products. In sensory pharmacology, capsaicin (the pungent principle in hot chili peppers) and its ultrapotent analog, resiniferatoxin, are useful tools to dissect the pain pathway. Drs. Man-Kyo Chung and James Campbell summarize the sensory and physiological effects of capsaicin (a natural TRPV1 agonist) and the rationale of its therapeutic use [5]. They describe how the short-term excitatory effects of capsaicin (characterized by pungency or pain) are followed by a lasting refractory state in which the previously excited neurons are unresponsive to various unrelated stimuli. Mechanisms underlying capsaicin-induced analgesia both in the form of desensitization and denervation are discussed, along with potential clinical implications.

Dr. Dorothy Cimino-Brown continues the theme of TRPV1 agonism by discussing the therapeutic potential of the ultrapotent TRPV1 agonist, resiniferatoxin, as a "molecular scalpel" to achieve permanent pain relief [6]. The review recounts both preclinical studies (including bone cancer in companion dogs) and clinical trials in patients with advanced cancer pain. The pain relief and the improvement of quality of life observed in these limited studies warrant further exploration in more patients.

Capsaicin and resiniferatoxin are natural products. Existing TRPV1 antagonists have come from mass-screening of compound libraries. Drs. Carnevale and Rohacs suggest an alternative approach: rational, structure-based drug design [7]. They discuss the advances in elucidating the structure of TRPV1, and how these led to a better understanding of the mechanisms underlying agonist binding and channel function. Rational drug design based on structural information and computational modeling may generate libraries of compounds that hold promise as potent TRPV1 modulators.

TRPV3 is a cousin of TRPV1 [2]. Indeed, TRPV3 can form hetero-tetrameric channels with TRPV1, hence TRPV3 can reasonably be expected to potentially serve similar roles or impact TRPV1 function in some circumstances. Dr. Broad and colleagues review our current understanding of TRPV3 expression and function, as well as their potential clinical relevance [8]. In their paper, drug development efforts centered on TRPV3 by various pharmaceutical companies are summarized.

Exemplified by TRPV3, which is expressed in keratinocytes (where its gain-of-function mutation has been linked to Olmsted syndrome [9], a pruritic skin disorder), various TRP channels are found in different cell types in the skin. Drs. Caterina and Pang provide a comprehensive review of cutaneous TRP channel expression [10]. They summarize the growing body of evidence suggesting that these channels play an important role in skin physiology, from sensation through keratinocyte differentiation and barrier function to hair growth. Malfunction of these channels has been implicated in various disease states, including pruritus, dermatitis, hirsutism/alopecia, and cancer.

Unlike TRPV1 and TRPV3, that respond to heat, TRPM8 is a cold-activated channel expressed on nociceptive neurons. Drs. Weyer and Lehto discuss the on-going efforts to develop TRPM8 antagonists for the treatment of chronic pain and migraine [11]. The role of TRPM8 in mechanical and heat analgesia, cold hyperalgesia, bladder pain, and migraine is discussed. They note that TRPM8 appears to be analgesic in some cases but nociceptive in others—a challenging feature for the clinical development of TRPM8 antagonists.

Drs. Kumamoto and Fujita report the differential activation of TRPV1, TRPA1, and TRPM8 channels in rat spinal cord slices by stereoisomers using whole-cell patch clamp recording [12]. They show that carvacrol and thymol (from the essential oil of thyme), carvone (from caraway), and cineole (from eucalyptol) increase the frequency of spontaneous excitatory postsynaptic currents; however, these presynaptic activities differ when activated by different stereoisomers, suggesting potential additional consideration for modulating these channels.

Inhaled capsaicin has been used clinically to identify a subset of chronic cough patients. Dr. Eva Millqvist discusses the putative role of TRPV1 and TRPM8 in chronic idiopathic cough and cough hypersensitivity syndrome [13]. Indeed, chronic cough was a potential clinical indication for TRPV1 antagonism. Disappointingly, TRPV1 antagonists failed to show any antitussive effect in clinical trials. Thus, the role of TRPV1 in the pathogenesis of chronic cough remains speculative.

TRPA1 is another channel that is expressed in the respiratory tract. Mukhopadhyay and colleagues summarize the state of our understanding of the role of TRPA1 in chronic cough, asthma, chronic obstructive pulmonary disease, allergic rhinitis, and cystic fibrosis [14]. They describe the preclinical and clinical progress achieved so far with selected TRPA1 antagonists.

Another area of active TRP channel research is the area of cancer biology. Dr. Nelson Yee reviews the expression and role of TRPM7 in human malignancies, such as pancreatic, gastric, and breast carcinomas [15]. The potential of modulating TRPM7 as an anti-cancer therapy is discussed.

Drs. Grolez and Gkika focus on another member of the TRPM family, TRPM8, in prostate cancer [16]. They describe the androgen-dependent characteristics of TRMP8, and discuss the data implying a role for TRPM8 in prostate cancer cell proliferation, survival, and migration. They also note the promise of TRPM8 as a diagnostic marker in the clinic.

Drs. Zsombok and Derbenev discuss the emerging role of TRP channels in obesity and diabetes [17]. They review laboratory data on the regulation of hormonal release, energy expenditure, pancreatic function, and neurotransmitter release, and describe the effects of capsaicin in human subjects. Obesity is a world-wide epidemic. It is an attractive hypothesis that such an inexpensive and readily available dietary substance as capsaicin may be used for weight control.

Drs. Yamamoto and Shimizu review the role of another TRPM family member, TRPM2, in reactive oxygen species (ROS)-coupled diseases [18]. TRPM2 can be activated by ROS in an ADP-ribose-mediated manner to function as a transducer that converts oxidative stress into calcium signaling. The relevance to conditions such as inflammation, infection, ischemia-reperfusion, and Alzheimer's disease is discussed.

Staying with the non-ligand mode of activation, Drs. Nagarajan and colleagues describe the ability of hydroxylation enzymes to regulate the channel activity of TRPA1 and TRPV3 [19]. The potential of targeting these enzymes as a means of modulating TRP channel activity is discussed.

The literature on TRP channels is immense. TRPV1 alone is a keyword in over 5000 publications searchable in PubMed. It is not possible to capture the entire literature in a single thematic issue. Consequently, the selection of articles presented in this issue represents a sampling of the literature, and is admittedly subjective. We tried to survey the wide range of human diseases in which TRP channels have been implicated, ranging from chronic pain through asthma and diabetes, to cancer, and highlight the channels that appear to hold the greatest promise for therapeutic targeting, in our opinion. Unfortunately, promising results obtained in laboratory species do not always yield equivalent results in clinical trials. Yet, from the richness of the investigations over the last 20 years, and the wide range of human conditions that have been implicated, it is fair to say that TRP channels constitute a formidable family of potential therapeutic targets that will likely continue to demand attention.

Acknowledgments: We thank the authors for their hard work to produce an up-to-date and fairly comprehensive issue on TRP channels as therapeutic targets in a timely fashion. We also thank the Editor-in-Chief of Pharmaceuticals, Vanden Eynde, for giving us the opportunity of editing this special issue. Last but not least, the editorial help of Changzhen Fu and Flora Li is much appreciated.

Conflicts of Interest: The authors declare no conflict of interest.

References

1. Caterina, M.J.; Schumacher, M.A.; Tominaga, M.; Rosen, T.A.; Levine, J.D.; Julius, D. The capsaicin receptor: A heat-activated ion channel in the pain pathway. *Nature* **1997**, *389*, 816–824. [PubMed]
2. Nilius, B.; Szallasi, A. Transient Receptor Potential channels as drug targets: From the science of basic science to the art of medicine. *Pharmacol. Rev.* **2014**, *66*, 676–814. [CrossRef] [PubMed]
3. Szallasi, A.; Cortright, D.N.; Blum, C.A.; Eid, S.R. The vanilloid receptor TRPV1: 10 years from channel cloning to antagonist proof-of-concept. *Nat. Rev. Drug Discov.* **2007**, *6*, 357–372. [CrossRef] [PubMed]
4. Mickle, A.D.; Shephens, A.J.; Mohapatra, D.P. Nociceptive TRP channels: Sensory detectors and transducers in multiple pain pathologies. *Pharmaceuticals* **2016**, *9*, 72–76. [CrossRef] [PubMed]
5. Chung, M.-K.; Campbell, J.N. Use of capsaicin to treat pain: Mechanistic and therapeutic considerations. *Pharmaceuticals* **2016**, *9*, 66. [CrossRef] [PubMed]
6. Cimino, B.D. Resiniferatoxin: The evolution of the "molecular scalpel" for chronic pain relief. *Pharmaceuticals* **2016**, *9*, 47.
7. Carnevale, V.; Rohacs, T. TRPV1: A target for rational drug design. *Pharmaceuticals* **2016**, *9*, 52. [CrossRef] [PubMed]
8. Broad, L.M.; Mogg, A.J.; Eberle, E.; Tolley, M.; Li, D.L.; Knopp, K.L. TRPV3 in drug development. *Pharmaceuticals* **2016**, *9*, 55. [CrossRef] [PubMed]
9. Lin, Z.; Chen, Q.; Lee, M.; Cao, X.; Zhang, J.; Ma, D.; Chen, L.; Hu, X.; Wang, H.; Wang, X.; et al. Exome sequencing reveals mutations in TRPV3 as a cause of Olmsted syndrome. *Am. J. Hum. Genet.* **2012**, *90*, 558–564. [CrossRef] [PubMed]
10. Caterina, M.J.; Pang, Z. TRP channels in skin biology and pathophysiology. *Pharmaceuticals* **2016**, *9*, 77. [CrossRef] [PubMed]
11. Weyer, A.D.; Lehto, S. Development of TRPM8 antagonists to treat chronic pain and migraine. *Pharmaceuticals* **2017**, *10*, 37. [CrossRef] [PubMed]
12. Kumamoto, E.; Fujita, T. Differential activation of TRP channels in the adult rat spinal substantia gelatinosa by stereoisomers of plant-derived chemicals. *Pharmaceuticals* **2016**, *9*, 46. [CrossRef] [PubMed]
13. Millqvist, E. TRPV1 and TRPM8 in the treatment of chronic cough. *Pharmaceuticals* **2016**, *9*, 45. [CrossRef] [PubMed]
14. Mukhopadhyay, I.; Kulkarni, A.; Khairatkar-Joshi, N. Blocking TRPA1 in respiratory disorders: Does it hold a promise? *Pharmaceuticals* **2016**, *9*, 70. [CrossRef] [PubMed]

15. Yee, N.S. Role of TRPM7 in cancer: Potential as molecular biomarker and therapeutic target. *Pharmaceuticals* **2017**, *10*, 39. [CrossRef] [PubMed]

16. Grolez, G.P.; Gkika, D. TRPM8 puts the chill on prostate cancer. *Pharmaceuticals* **2016**, *9*, 44. [CrossRef] [PubMed]

17. Zsombok, A.; Derrbenev, A.V. TRP channels as therapeutic targets in diabetes and obesity. *Pharmaceuticals* **2016**, *9*, 50. [CrossRef] [PubMed]

18. Yamamoto, S.; Shimizu, S. Targeting TRPM2 in ROS-coupled diseases. *Pharmaceuticals* **2016**, *9*, 57. [CrossRef] [PubMed]

19. Nagarajan, Y.; Rychkov, G.Y.; Peet, D.J. Modulation of TRP channel activity by hydroxylation and its therapeutic potential. *Pharmaceuticals* **2017**, *10*, 35. [CrossRef] [PubMed]

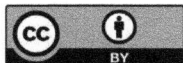

pharmaceuticals

MDPI

Review

Use of Capsaicin to Treat Pain: Mechanistic and Therapeutic Considerations

Man-Kyo Chung [1],* and James N. Campbell [2],*

[1] Department of Neural and Pain Sciences, University of Maryland, School of Dentistry,
Program in Neuroscience, Center to Advance Chronic Pain Research, Baltimore, MD 21201, USA
[2] Centrexion Therapeutics, Baltimore, MD 21202, USA
* Correspondence: mchung@umaryland.edu (M.-K.C.); jcampbel@jhmi.edu (J.N.C.);
Tel.: +1-410-706-4452 (M.-K.C.); +1-410-369-2201(J.N.C.)

Academic Editors: Arpad Szallasi and Susan M. Huang
Received: 7 September 2016; Accepted: 27 October 2016; Published: 1 November 2016

Abstract: Capsaicin is the pungent ingredient of chili peppers and is approved as a topical treatment of neuropathic pain. The analgesia lasts for several months after a single treatment. Capsaicin selectively activates TRPV1, a Ca^{2+}-permeable cationic ion channel that is enriched in the terminals of certain nociceptors. Activation is followed by a prolonged decreased response to noxious stimuli. Interest also exists in the use of injectable capsaicin as a treatment for focal pain conditions, such as arthritis and other musculoskeletal conditions. Recently injection of capsaicin showed therapeutic efficacy in patients with Morton's neuroma, a painful foot condition associated with compression of one of the digital nerves. The relief of pain was associated with no change in tactile sensibility. Though injection evokes short term pain, the brief systemic exposure and potential to establish long term analgesia without other sensory changes creates an attractive clinical profile. Short-term and long-term effects arise from both functional and structural changes in nociceptive terminals. In this review, we discuss how local administration of capsaicin may induce ablation of nociceptive terminals and the clinical implications.

Keywords: capsaicin; pain; nociceptors; TRPV1 receptors

1. Introduction

Anyone who has eaten a hot pepper knows about the pungency of capsaicin. Capsaicin's pro-nociceptive effects are not confined to the mouth, as this molecule evokes pain in multiple other tissues, including the cornea, skin, joints, and muscles. The discovery of the neural receptor, TRPV1 [1], established the basis for this effect, and represented a major advance in understanding how nociceptors (primary afferents that signal pain) are activated.

The capacity of capsaicin to evoke pain is of value commercially. Of course capsaicin is a staple of many diets and in many cuisines, the capsaicin content is very high [2]. Why capsaicin is such a popular spice remains unclear, given that it essentially evokes a burning sensation in the mouth when eaten. Capsaicin is the active agent in "pepper spray," a deterrent used for riot control and to ward off assailants [3]. As a repellent, capsaicin is used to discourage intrusions by bears, deer, and other mammals [4]. Bird enthusiasts use capsaicin in their feeders to fend off squirrels, given that the TRPV1 receptor in birds is capsaicin-insensitive [5].

The activation of nociceptors is ordinarily linked with at least the threat of tissue harm. This imposes limits on the use of heat, chemical, and mechanical stimuli to study pain particularly in human studies [6–8]. Histological studies of the areas where capsaicin is applied reveal no enduring pathological findings, however. Therefore elicitation of pain without tissue harm makes the use of capsaicin attractive in pain studies.

TRPV1 acts as a transduction channel in nociceptors not only for capsaicin analogues, but also for heat, and acid as well. It has been logical therefore to pursue small molecule antagonists as potential new candidates to treat pain. Unfortunately, antagonists also induce hyperthermia due to the critical contribution of TRPV1 to body temperature regulation. Whether these effects can be avoided ultimately has yet to be seen. Antagonists can also block heat sensibility to the extent that patients may be susceptible to burn injury [9].

Paradoxically, however, capsaicin, and its ultra-potent naturally occurring analogue, resiniferatoxin (RTX), have yet a further property—they act as "excitotoxins". In other words, these molecules have the capacity to both activate and destroy nociceptive terminals [10]. The selective neurotoxic action of capsaicin was first reported in newborn animals [11], which opened research on capsaicin-sensitive neurons in primary afferents. A single systemic injection of high dose of capsaicin into neonatal rats or mice causes loss of a large proportion of primarily small diameter neurons and unmyelinated afferent fibers. In adult rats, systemic administration of capsaicin at extremely high doses may also induce degeneration of DRG neurons and unmyelinated axons although the extent is less than that in neonatal animals [12].

In a sense, a common observation supports the idea that capsaicin is an excitotoxin. People unaccustomed to eating this spice can tolerate only small amounts. However, a regular habit of eating capsaicin leads to tolerability. Higher and higher doses can be consumed without burning pain. This eventual tolerability reflects the ablative effects of the capsaicin on the nociceptive terminals. This capacity to ablate nociceptive afferents specifically has many implications with regard to therapy.

Perhaps the clearest demonstration of the relative specificity of capsaicin in terms of ablative effects was in an experiment by Simone et al. [13]. Up to 20 µg was injected into the skin in normal human volunteers. Psychophysical testing done on subsequent days revealed a selective loss of heat pain sensibility with sparing of touch sensation. Skin biopsies at the site of injection stained with the pan-axonal marker, PGP 9.5, revealed nearly complete ablation of the C fibers in the epidermis days after the capsaicin injection. Further biopsies weeks after the initial injection revealed restoration of innervation consistent with the regeneration of the afferents. Other studies demonstrated similar findings as discussed below [14,15].

With the demonstration of selective but reversible ablative effects, the stage was set to determine the therapeutic effects of capsaicin administration. Could this pungent spice be used to treat pain?

2. Therapeutic Uses of Capsaicin

Low concentrations of topical capsaicin have been available "over the counter" for decades for treatment of pain. Daily application is associated with burning pain and trials have shown varying results in terms of efficacy. The daily application discomfort affects compliance and repeated application over a period of weeks may be necessary to get a therapeutic effect. Given the striking effects of intradermal capsaicin, the idea arose that it might be best to begin with a high dose of topical capsaicin such that the acute pain would be circumscribed in duration, and with the expectation that therapeutic effects would follow within days and last weeks to months. The initial open label report of use of this technique suggested efficacy [16]. Trials with topical 8% capsaicin were conducted subsequently in patients with post-herpetic neuralgia which demonstrated both safety and efficacy, leading to US Food and Drug Administration approval (Qutenza®, Acorda Therapeutics, Ardsley, NY, USA). The European Medicines Agency has approved Qutenza® for the more general label, neuropathic pain, based on additional clinical data indicating safety and efficacy in painful diabetic neuropathy, and AIDS related neuropathic pain [17,18].

Pre-clinical data supports additional clinical indications. TRPV1-expressing afferents are known to contribute to spontaneous pain in rodents. Intraplantar injection of capsaicin or RTX attenuates development of guarding behavior following incision of hindpaw skin or carrageenan injection [19,20]. Systemic administration of RTX abolishes spontaneous pain following spinal nerve ligation or complete Freund's adjuvant (CFA) injection evaluated by conditioned place preference in rats [21,22].

Focal injection of vanilloids (referring to capsaicin and other analogues) also attenuates hyperalgesia in the knee joint. TRPV1 and TRPV1-expressing afferents contribute to mechanical hyperalgesia in knee joints. Pharmacological inhibition or genetic ablation of TRPV1 attenuates arthritis-induced hyperalgesia, such as weight-bearing imbalance, in rodent models [23–25]. Intraarticular administration of a TRPV1 antagonist suppressed monosodium iodoacetate (MIA)-induced sensitization of knee joint afferents to mechanical stimuli [26]. This is similar to the situations in other deep tissues such as muscle or visceral organs [27–29]. Consistently, intraarticular injection of RTX or capsaicin improves weight-distribution behavior in carrageenan or MIA-induced arthritis in rats and mice [30–32]. Therefore, focal injection of capsaicin or RTX can be used to provide relief of mechanical hyperalgesia from deep tissues such as muscle or joints.

Application of capsaicin onto nerve trunks produces a selective and long-lasting increase in the threshold for pain from heat stimuli. This change is confined to the skin region served by the treated nerves [33]. Perineural application of RTX also induces a reduction of inflammation-related thermal hyperalgesia in rats [34,35]. Pre-emptive perineural injection of capsaicin or RTX prevents development of post-incisional pain in rats [20,36]. Local injection of capsaicin into an incision site also has analgesic effects [6,14,15].

Lumbar epidural or intrathecal injection of vanilloids produces long-lasting heat hypoalgesia confined to an area innervated by the cauda equina [37–39]. Intrathecal RTX also attenuates inflammatory hyperalgesia [40]. In canines, intrathecal RTX decreases bone cancer-related pain behaviors, and improves functions [41,42], suggesting the promising clinical application of this approach.

Limited data are available from double blind randomized trials regarding the use of injected capsaicin to treat pain [43]. One study has suggested the use of instilled capsaicin to treat post-operative pain [44]. Another condition where this strategy has been pursued relates to Morton's neuroma, a painful condition that affects the foot. The most common location is between the third and fourth metatarsal bones. A focal swelling of the common digital nerve to the third and fourth toes is evident on imaging studies. Orthotics and other conservative measures often fail in helping the patients. Capsaicin injected into the area of the neuroma significantly relieved pain in comparison to placebo [45]. There were no effects on tactile sensibility consistent with the relatively selective effects on nociceptive afferents. No safety concerns were raised. If supported by further trials this approach has the promise of relieving pain with a single injection. Topical high dose capsaicin typically relieves pain for an average time of five months before re-dosing is necessary [46]. The duration of benefit of injected capsaicin has not yet been determined.

3. Functional and Histological Effects

Focal injection or topical administration of capsaicin activates TRPV1 receptors in TRPV1-expressing nociceptors. This activation is followed by multiple events resulting in functional and potentially histological changes in nerve terminals as summarized in Figure 1.

3.1. TRPV1-Expressing Nociceptors

TRPV1, the receptor for capsaicin, is localized primarily in the plasma membrane of Aδ and C fiber primary afferents [1]. TRPV1 is a homo-tetrameric non-selective cationic channel that opens with exposure to agonists. Activation of TRPV1 leads to depolarization associated with the influx of Na^+ and Ca^{2+} ions. Depolarization is associated with the firing of action potentials in nociceptive fibers which accounts for the capacity of capsaicin to induce burning pain. Since capsaicin-induced nocifensive behavior is ablated in mice lacking TRPV1 expression, capsaicin-induced pain likely depends on activation of TRPV1 [47].

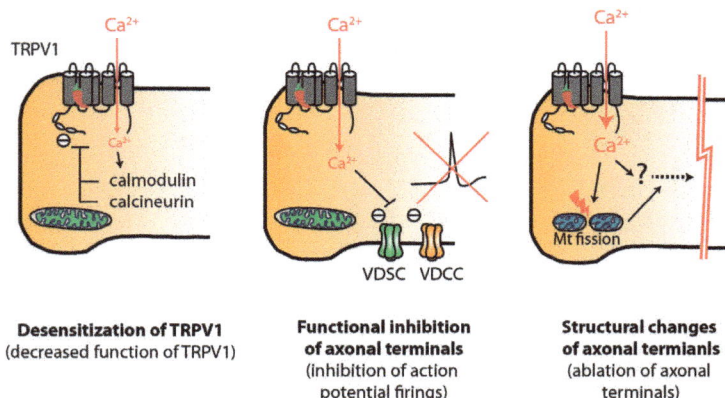

Figure 1. Responses of peripheral terminals of TRPV1-expressing nociceptors following focal injection or topical application of vanilloids. Locally administered capsaicin or RTX induces functional and, potentially, structural changes in nociceptive terminals. With therapeutic doses of capsaicin, these changes are reversible through regenerative mechanisms, and are likely localized to the nerve terminals without affecting the soma. Structural ablation of axonal terminals might play major roles in long-lasting analgesia. TRPV1, transient receptor potential vanilloid subtype 1; VDSC, voltage-dependent sodium channels; VDCC, voltage-dependent calcium channels; Mt, mitochondria.

What types of nociceptors signal the pain associated with capsaicin? Different schemes have been used to classify nociceptors and detailed information regarding properties and types of nociceptors has been reviewed elsewhere [48]. One method relates to conduction velocity. Accordingly, there are both Aδ and C fibers. When a heat stimulus is applied to the forearm, there is a double pain sensation. The first, is a sharp pricking sensation and relates to signaling from a type of Aδ nociceptors, and the second is a slow burning sensation, which relates to the discharge of a type of C fiber nociceptors [48,49].

The response to natural stimuli can also be used to classify nociceptors. Nociceptors responsive to heat and mechanical stimuli are referred to AMHs or CMHs depending on whether they are A fibers or C fibers. There are also C and Aδ fibers which are primarily chemically sensitive, and are relatively insensitive to mechanical and heat stimuli. These nociceptors are referred to as CMiHi fibers. As one may infer from the multiple classification systems, nociceptors do not fall neatly into clear discrete categories [48]. Especially confusing is the response to capsaicin. One microneurography study in humans suggested that CMHs account for the magnitude and duration of pain [50]. Further study suggests that capsaicin-induced burning pain in humans is correlated with firings of mechano-insensitive heat-insensitive C fibers (CMiHi) [51]. Intracutaneous injection of capsaicin leads to marked pain during the first 30 s followed by a gradual decrease over the next 5–10 min. Capsaicin induces firing of CMiHi for ~170 s, whereas CMHs discharge only for several seconds, suggesting that capsaicin-induced burning pain maintained for minutes must involve signaling from CMiHi. Furthermore, mechano-insensitive C units become responsive to heat and mechanical stimuli following capsaicin injection, suggesting their role in primary hyperalgesia. Therefore, procedural pain and hyperalgesia following capsaicin injection apparently depends on the sustained discharge of CMiHi units.

A-fiber nociceptors likely also contribute to capsaicin-induced pain. Type I AMHs have a delayed response to heat which increases over time with sustained stimulation. Type II AMHs respond in similar fashion to CMHs and have an immediate response to heat. In primate skin, cutaneous type II AMHs are activated by capsaicin [52]. Upon intradermal injection, the afferent shows strong responses with a high frequency for approximately 15 s, which is followed by low frequency ongoing discharge for approximately 10 min. In contrast, most type I heat-insensitive afferents show only brief high frequency discharge for approximately 5 s without further response. Interestingly, a further subpopulation of heat-insensitive A fiber nociceptors show a vigorous response to capsaicin (>100 action potentials per 10 min).

Nociceptors are also classified based on neurochemical properties. One group expresses neuropeptides such as substance P or calcitonin gene related peptide, and demonstrate a dependency on nerve growth factor. The other class binds isolectin B4 (IB4), and is sensitive to glial cell line-derived neurotrophic factor [53]. TRPV1 is highly enriched in nociceptors containing neuropeptides and approximately 85% of substance P-containing afferents express TRPV1 [54]. IB4-positive neurons also express TRPV1, but to a lesser extent. It is well known that topical application or intradermal injection of capsaicin not only induces burning pain, but also causes flare in human skin [55,56]. Capsaicin induces release and depletion of neuropeptides from afferent terminals, which may lead to attenuation of neurogenic inflammation caused by injury [57]. Capsaicin-induced release of neuropeptides from afferent terminals is primarily due to Ca^{2+} influx through the TRPV1 channel, rather than involving action potential firing since lidocaine, tetrodotoxin, and inhibitors of voltage-gated Ca^{2+} channels do not affect capsaicin-induced release [58,59].

3.2. Variations in Acute Pungency of Capsaicin

Injection of capsaicin into peripheral tissues can produce not only spontaneous pain but thermal and mechanical hyperalgesia [60]. In addition to acute pain, injection of capsaicin into the skin induces hyperalgesia to heat stimuli at the site of injection, and stroking pain (allodynia) in the surrounding area. These phenomena again wane within 1–2 h. Hyperalgesia to punctuate stimuli develops in a larger area of skin than thermal or stroking hyperalgesia and lasts up to 24 h. Hyperalgesia that occurs over the skin area outside the injected site is termed secondary hyperalgesia. Secondary hyperalgesia has been determined to result primarily from central sensitization of spinothalamic tract neurons rather than sensitization of the peripheral terminals of nociceptors [61,62].

The above paints the general picture of what happens with acute administration of capsaicin to the skin. However, the extent and duration of acute pain from delivery of capsaicin shows striking variation in humans and animals. This may derive from multiple sources. To begin one has to consider the source of capsaicin. There may be batch to batch variation in the amount of capsaicin and other vanilloids in agriculturally sourced supplies. The formulation used to dissolve capsaicin varies from laboratory to laboratory and this could make a difference. In the case of topical or intradermal delivery, skin temperature can profoundly affect the pain. Where capsaicin is applied on the body clearly matters, though this variable has not received very much attention. Of interest however, is that despite having adequate controls for each of these variables there continues to be considerable inter-individual differences.

In one study polymorphisms of the enzyme, GTP cyclohydrolase, accounted for a surprisingly high (35%) degree of the inter-individual variance in pain ratings from high concentration topical capsaicin [63]. Polymorphisms of catechol-*O*-methyltransferase (COMT) were also associated with nociception following topical application of capsaicin [64]. In another study, other psychological factors were found to account for variations in response to capsaicin [65].

Undoubtedly, a myriad of other factors involved in nociceptive processing will continue to be uncovered. However, one of the particularly compelling variables to consider is the extent to which individual differences in TRPV1 variants account for differences in acute pain. The most common genetic defect in a rare disease known as cystinosis involves a 57k base pair homozygous deletion on chromosome 17, that extends from the cystinosis gene into the early non-coding area for the TRPV1 gene (intron 2). There is a knock down of TRPV1 expression [66] and there was found to be a corresponding decrease in ratings of pain from topical capsaicin [67]. No hyperthermia or inadvertent burns were noted, though there were other possible minor indications of thermoregulatory disturbances and a documented increase in the threshold to warmth stimuli.

Other polymorphisms of TRPV1 are associated with multiple pathological pain conditions such as neuropathic pain, painful osteoarthritis, and dyspepsia. Some genetic variations of TRPV1 occurring in exons alter amino acid sequence of the protein, which affect functional properties of TRPV1 [68,69]. Therefore, genetic variation of TRPV1 may contribute to the variability of pain associated with capsaicin administration [70].

3.3. Pungency and Therapeutic Effect?

If capsaicin is to be viewed as an excitotoxin, then one would presume that the "toxic" effects should be correlated with the "excito" effects. As noted above, evidence exists to indicate that injection of capsaicin decreases pain associated with the painful foot condition, Morton's neuroma. In this study, however, "procedural pain" (acute pain induced by capsaicin administration) was not correlated with therapeutic efficacy [45]. Subjects who reported low levels of procedure pain were just as likely to benefit, and vice versa.

If procedure pain is not a necessary component to the therapeutic effects of capsaicin, then perhaps pungency can be controlled without interfering with analgesic effects. Suppression of procedure pain upon capsaicin injection could also decrease post-procedural discomfort due to mechanical hyperalgesia. One way to cut down on procedural pain is to apply an anesthetic such as lidocaine to the tissue prior to applying capsaicin. Pre-emptive application of lidocaine prior to the application of RTX attenuates acute nociception without affecting analgesic effects in rat cornea [71]. This approach has been tried in an attempt to control the pain associated with Qutenza® application. It is not clear however, that the topically applied lidocaine is of any benefit [72]. A nerve block upstream from the capsaicin blocks all conduction in the nerve and therefore will block all pain from capsaicin applied distally. So why does locally applied lidocaine not have a clear benefit? It is worth noting that lidocaine blocks voltage-gated sodium channels, whereas activation of the TRPV1 channel is associated with an inward current related both to a sodium and calcium ion influx. The failure of lidocaine to be locally effective could relate to the length constant of the sodium current arising from activation of voltage-gated sodium channels relative to the length constant associated with inward current that arises from opening of the TRPV1 channel. If the length constant associated with TRPV1 activation is longer, then the passive current could jump ahead (that is further upstream) and activate voltage-gated sodium channels beyond the point of blockade of the local lidocaine, and thus initiate action potentials that would propagate centrally to produce pain. Though probably not a factor, it is of interest that lidocaine robustly activates TRPV1 over the therapeutic dose range [73].

Interestingly, cold temperature helps to attenuate capsaicin-induced burning pain associated with topical administration [72]. Cold temperature slows down the kinetics of TRPV1 activation by capsaicin [74]. In addition, voltage-gated sodium channels, such as Nav1.7, are largely inactivated at cold temperature, which may reduce the conduction of action potentials [75]. Activation of the cold receptor, TRPM8, could also contribute to analgesia [76]. Despite its benefit, one potential concern is whether maintaining the cold temperature affects the therapeutic effects of capsaicin, since TRPV1 activation by capsaicin is counteracted at temperatures below 15 °C [74]. However, degeneration of epidermal nerve fibers by topical capsaicin was not affected by pretreatment with cooling (20 °C) in humans [72]. As a caveat, more substantial cooling could aggravate pain symptoms by inducing cold hyperalgesia through activation of another nociceptive cold receptor, TRPA1 [77].

Recently, a novel mechanism amplifying capsaicin-induced pungency was suggested. TRPV1 mediated Ca^{2+} influx activates anoctamine 1 (ANO1), Ca^{2+}-activated Cl^- channels in nociceptive terminals, which leads to further depolarization [78]. Indeed, pharmacological inhibition of ANO1 attenuates capsaicin-mediated acute nocifensive behaviors in rodents [78,79].

3.4. Transient Analgesia and Decreased Function of TRPV1 Mechanisms

There are acute effects of capsaicin that could be associated with a component of analgesia, independent of any enduring overt morphological changes. These effects may or may not be of clinical significance. Capsaicin-induced excitation of nociceptors is followed by a refractory state characterized by an insensitivity to subsequent application of capsaicin or other noxious insults such as heat, mechanical or chemical stimuli. To complicate matters, sensitization and desensitization mechanisms are involved since it is observed that topical capsaicin in humans initially decreases heat threshold followed by an increase in threshold [57,80]. The area of skin directly exposed to capsaicin following intradermal injection shows hyposensitivity to pinprick stimuli, which starts as early as 15 min after injection [60]. In rodents, intraplantar injection of RTX immediately induces heat hyperalgesia reflected by a decrease in paw withdrawal latency. This heat hyperalgesia, however, converts to heat hypoalgesia after approximately 2.5 h following injection [34,81]. This quickly developing hypoalgesia may be evident in terms of responses to chemical stimuli and spontaneous pain as well. Formalin-evoked nocifensive behaviors in mice were attenuated by intraplantar injection of capsaicin (100 µg) after two hours. CFA-induced mechanical hyperalgesia was modestly attenuated after 2 h following capsaicin injection (100 µg), which was documented for 24 h [82].

TRPV1 receptor desensitization to vanilloids needs to be distinguished from analgesic effects. The extent of receptor desensitization does not necessarily correlate with the impairment of other nociceptor functions. For example, RTX produces analgesia in vivo but does not induce desensitization of the TRPV1 receptor in in vitro voltage clamp recordings [1]. However, the contribution of TRPV1 receptor desensitization to capsaicin-induced analgesia is unknown. Capsaicin is known to suppress action potential firing in nerve preparations from various species [62,83,84]. In humans, capsaicin suppressed impulse conduction in CMHs, but not cold fibers for example. The conduction block started shortly after application of capsaicin and lasted longer than 2 h [85]. Capsaicin-induced desensitization of nociceptors should involve both Aδ as well as CMH units since Aδ nociceptors mediate first heat pain in humans [49] and topical capsaicin induces heat hypoalgesia mediated by both Aδ and C fiber nociceptors in humans [86]. Indeed, it was shown that subcutaneous injection of RTX attenuates responses of both CMHs and AMHs in rats [87]. Different concentrations of capsaicin result in differential impairment in responses to various stimuli [88]. Dray et al. used a rat spinal cord-tail in vitro preparation to study chemical and thermal stimuli after exposure to low concentration (0.5–2 µM) capsaicin [88], and noted impaired responses to capsaicin but not bradykinin or heat. Function normalized after several hours. In contrast, when the skin was pretreated with a higher concentration of capsaicin (20–50 µM), responses to a broad range of stimuli were impaired irreversibly. These apparently two different types of impairment of responsiveness induced by different concentrations of capsaicin suggest different mechanisms; desensitization of the TRPV1 receptor by low doses of capsaicin versus inhibition of overall nociceptor function by high doses of capsaicin. Exposure of sensory neurons to capsaicin induces ionic currents, whose size decreases during sustained or repeat exposure or by following application of capsaicin. This process is defined as desensitization or tachyphylaxis and is similar to the desensitization that occurs as a result of heat and mechanical stimuli [89–91]. TRPV1 is desensitized not only by capsaicin but also heat. The mechanisms are apparently distinct [92]. Capsaicin-induced desensitization of the TRPV1 receptor requires influx of Ca^{2+} through TRPV1, and depends on subsequent Ca^{2+}-dependent signaling such as activation of calmodulin and calcineurin, or degradation of PIP_2 [93]. Capsaicin-induced desensitization of the TRPV1 receptor can be reversible [93]. Desensitization or tachyphylaxis may underlie the selective impairment of the response following exposures to low concentrations of capsaicin.

Studies in dissociated sensory neurons suggest effects of capsaicin on voltage-gated Na^+ and Ca^{2+} channels. Capsaicin (1 µM) inhibited action potential firing in dissociated sensory neurons from rodents [82,94]. This effect was absent in TRPV1 knockout neurons and depended on Ca^{2+} influx [82]. In capsaicin sensitive rat DRG neurons, a 1 µM concentration inhibited voltage-dependent Na^+ currents without changing the voltage dependence of activation or markedly changing channel inactivation and use-dependent block [94]. In colon sensory neurons from the rat dorsal root ganglia (DRG), capsaicin inhibited both tetrodotoxin (TTX)-sensitive and TTX-resistant Na^+ currents. The inhibitory effects were prevented by capsazepine [95] or a specific antagonist of TRPV1, SB366791 [96], suggesting that TRPV1 activation by capsaicin is necessary for the inhibition. Capsaicin also decreased high voltage-activated Ca^{2+} currents through Ca^{2+}-dependent calcineurin. This inhibition was prevented by iodoresiniferatoxin, a specific TRPV1 antagonist [97]. Thus several reports support the idea that capsaicin-induced activation of TRPV1 leads to the inhibition of voltage-dependent Na^+ and Ca^{2+} currents, which in turn suppresses action potential firing in nociceptors. Alternatively, vanilloid-induced membrane reorganization could produce functional suppression of nociceptors. For example, capsaicin and RTX rapidly decrease membrane capacitance of TRPV1-expressing neurons in a Ca^{2+}-dependent manner [98]. This effect might involve endocytosis of TRPV1 [99] as well as other ion channels in TRPV1-expressing nociceptive membranes.

Very high doses of capsaicin could potentially affect nociception through effects at the level of the spinal cord [100]. Subcutaneous systemic application of capsaicin at a high dose (20 μmol/kg = 6 mg/kg = 150 μg/mouse) into the scruff of the neck inhibited C-fiber responses in wide dynamic range lumbar dorsal horn neurons activated by transcutaneous electrical stimulation to the hindpaw. The inhibitory effects were suppressed by intrathecal capsazepine [101], suggesting an effect on the central terminals of nociceptive afferents.

Anti-nociceptive or analgesic effects following capsaicin administration might be also derived from the effects of capsaicin on neuropeptide release from primary afferents. Administration of capsaicin decreased substance P from central and peripheral terminals of primary afferents [39,102]. However, the causal relationship between depletion of substance P and capsaicin-induced anti-nociception is unclear [103]. In contrast, capsaicin-induced release of somatostatin, an antinociceptive neuropeptide, could contribute to analgesia. Somatostatin is released from capsaicin-sensitive peptidergic afferents into the circulation and exerts anti-inflammatory and anti-nociceptive effects [104]. An agonist of somatostatin receptor attenuated the responses to formalin, increased the heat threshold, and diminished mechanical allodynia in a diabetic pain model [105]. Carrageenan-induced mechanical hyperalgesia was greater in mice lacking the somatostatin 4 receptor compared to wild-type [106]. Similarly, antinociceptive effects of galanin were also suggested [107]. These reports are consistent with the possibility that capsaicin or RTX administration can induce release of anti-nociceptive peptides, which attenuate hyperalgesia.

The prevailing evidence suggests that capsaicin-induced analgesia mediated by alteration of the functions of nociceptors or release of anti-nociceptive peptides could account for short term effects. Many studies conflate short term and long term effects. Of note, peripheral administration of RTX or capsaicin may induce degeneration of nerve fiber terminals as early as 1 day [13,81]. Therefore, analgesia lasting longer than 1 day may be attributable entirely to the structural ablation. Possibly, acute loss of function following capsaicin injection may be a bodily defense mechanism for reducing acute pungency. A better understanding underlying capsaicin-induced loss of function may help develop methods for reducing capsaicin-induced pungency and procedural pain.

3.5. Long Acting Effects of Capsaicin

Focal injection of vanilloids induces long-lasting localized analgesia for weeks to months. Intraplantar injection of RTX was found to induce unilateral hypoalgesia to radiant heat for several weeks in rats [108], likely mediated by effects on Aδ and C-fibers [52]. Intraplantar injection of RTX decreased capsaicin-induced nocifensive behaviors for approximately 40 days and increased latency to hot plate for longer than 60 days in mice [109].

In humans, the topical capsaicin patch (Qutenza®) provides pain relief in post-herpetic neuralgia patients for on average five months [110]. Focal injection of capsaicin in Morton's neuroma patients provides pain relief for at least four weeks (the longest interval studied) [45]. The likelihood is that analgesia lasting more than a day following localized injection of capsaicin is derived from structural changes. Intradermal injection of capsaicin in humans begins to ablate intraepidermal fibers within one day [13,14]. In rodents, subcutaneous injection of RTX also induced ablation of skin afferent terminals as early as 1–2 days [81,109]. Nerve terminal ablation following local administration of vanilloids is reversible over the time course that correlates with behavioral changes. In mice, TRPV1-positive fibers in skin recover two months following injection of capsaicin [109]. In humans, the number of TRPV1-positive fibers was partially recovered after eight weeks following intradermal capsaicin injection [14]. In another study, regeneration of nerve fibers in humans was demonstrated after 100 days following capsaicin administration [15].

Systemic injection of high doses of RTX or capsaicin degenerates not only peripheral terminals but may also induce substantial ablation of soma in sensory ganglia [12,111]. Systemic injection of >50 mg/kg of capsaicin or >50 ng of RTX are necessary to induce degeneration of ganglia neurons. In contrast, topical application or peripheral injection of a limited dose of capsaicin or RTX ablates nociceptive terminals focally. Local injection of capsaicin or RTX produced ablation of TRPV1-positive afferent terminals in the hindpaw but did not ablate TRPV1-positive afferents in sensory ganglia [108,109]. In humans, therapeutic effects of focally applied capsaicin are reversible, whereas effects on the sensory ganglia are would be expected to be permanent [15]. Intraplantar injection of RTX (~0.5 μg/kg) induced reversible ablation of intraepidermal nerve fibers without degeneration of DRG neurons [108]. In humans, 20 μg of intradermal capsaicin (~0.33 μg/kg) ablated epidermal nerve fibers after 1 day [13]. Of note, at a distance only 1–2 mm from the injection site, the afferents were normal. This makes a more proximal site of action highly unlikely. In Morton's neuroma patients, pain relief is obtained by injection of 0.1 mg of capsaicin [45], which is almost 30,000 fold lower than the systemic dose for inducing ganglia neuronal degeneration. Therefore, the therapeutic dosage of capsaicin for focal injection is orders of magnitude lower than the dosage resulting in toxicity within sensory ganglia. Even with systemic application, effects may be seen at the level of the peripheral terminals at doses that have no effect on the neurons in the ganglia [112]. In other words, the primary afferent terminals (compared to the soma) are most vulnerable to systemic capsaicin, further evidence that the therapeutic effects of focally applied capsaicin are mediated through local effects.

Although the anti-hyperalgesic effects of perineural application of RTX is apparently reversible [34], perineural application of a high concentration of capsaicin or RTX has been argued to induce a selective but delayed permanent loss of unmyelinated axons and small-diameter DRG neurons or TRPV1-positive DRG neurons [34,113]. It is unclear what mechanisms are involved in transganglionic degeneration following perineural application of capsaicin if indeed it occurs. It is speculated that the extent of axonal injury in a nerve bundle might be great enough to cause a "dying-back" pattern of degeneration, where loss of axonal integrity and transport leads to somatic cell death [114,115]. Regeneration of nociceptor innervation after topical or injected capsaicin argues for intact function at the level of the DRG.

4. Potential Mechanisms of Vanilloid-Induced Chemical Ablation of Nociceptor Terminals

The mechanism of vanilloid effects on the nerve terminals may be different than the effects at the ganglion level. Early studies showed that systemic injection of capsaicin to neonatal or adult rat induces irreversible loss of primarily small neurons in sensory ganglia [11]. A single systemic injection of capsaicin into neonatal rats or mice causes a loss of approximately half of the entire DRG neurons and 70%–80% of small diameter DRG neurons. Injection of capsaicin to neonatal rats resulted in losses of ~90% of unmyelinated and ~35% of myelinated fibers from L3 and L4 DRG [116]. In adult rats, high-dose systemic administration of capsaicin also induces degeneration of 17% of small and medium sized DRG neurons, and a 45% decrease in the number of unmyelinated axons in the saphenous nerve [12]. Light and electron microscopy revealed clear degenerative changes of axons and sensory ganglia neurons following the systemic application of capsaicin [12]. Neuronal cell death was suggested to be due to an apoptotic or necrotic mechanism [117,118]. Activation of caspase and DNA fragmentation in DRG neurons following capsaicin administration suggests apoptotic mechanisms [119]. Earlier events following capsaicin administration occurs in cytoplasmic organelles. Dilation of endoplasmic reticulum and swelling of mitochondria was seen following capsaicin treatment [120], which is reminiscent of excitotoxic neuronal death triggered by activation of glutamate receptors [121]. Excessive activation by glutamate mediates death of central neurons through Ca^{2+} overload. Indeed, capsaicin and glutamate both induce accumulation of Ca^{2+} predominantly in mitochondria of the damaged ganglion neurons, suggesting Ca^{2+}-dependent neurotoxic effects of capsaicin [122]. In vagal sensory neurons, capsaicin increased permeability to Ca^{2+}, and capsaicin-induced ultrastructural changes were attenuated by removing extracellular Ca^{2+} [123]. In dissociated sensory neurons, capsaicin and RTX induced Ca^{2+} uptake in a subpopulation of neurons [124]. Again, capsaicin induced Ca^{2+} entry in dissociated sensory neurons and capsaicin-induced death of DRG neurons was prevented by removing extracellular Ca^{2+} [125]. Of note, heterologous expression of recombinant TRPV1 in non-neuronal cell line confers a liability for capsaicin toxicity [1]. In non-neuronal cell lines with heterologous expression of TRPV1 [126], RTX induced Ca^{2+} influx followed by vesiculation of the mitochondria and the endoplasmic reticulum ($\sim$1 min), nuclear membrane disruption (5–10 min), and cell lysis (1–2 h). RTX also induced Ca^{2+} influx and fragmentation of mitochondria (<20 s) restricted to small size DRG neurons with sparing of glia. In aggregate these reports strongly suggest that capsaicin-mediated neurotoxic effects on sensory ganglia neurons are initiated by Ca^{2+}-influx following the activation of TRPV1 in a subset of TRPV1-expressing neurons.

Cytosolic Ca^{2+} can derive also from intracellular sources. TRPV1 receptors are found on the endoplasmic reticulum (ER) [127,128]. Ca^{2+} influx-induced Ca^{2+} release from, in part, the thapsigargin-sensitive Ca^{2+} pool caused cytosolic Ca^{2+} increase [127]. It is not known whether Ca^{2+} released from ER contributes to cell death of sensory neurons following the application of capsaicin or RTX. However, the ER is reported to play a role in cell death of tumor cells through the ER stress pathway involving activation of transcription factor-3 (ATF3) [129] or the mitochondria-mediated death pathway [130]. Since capsaicin induces TRPV1-dependent activation of ATF-3 in sensory ganglia [87,131], it is possible that ER stress following TRPV1 activation might contribute to cell death of sensory neurons.

Intracellular Ca^{2+} homeostasis is critical for physiological functions of nociceptors [97]. In sensory neurons, several mechanisms for controlling Ca^{2+} clearance and homeostasis are known. Ca^{2+} extrusion through plasma membrane Ca^{2+} ATPase, and sequestration of Ca^{2+} into mitochondria, predominantly determine the rate of Ca^{2+} clearance in sensory neurons [132,133]. Increased cytosolic Ca^{2+} mediated by mild electrical stimulation is rapidly cleared by the function of the Ca^{2+} uniporter in the mitochondria membrane, leading to increased mitochondrial Ca^{2+} [134]. However, when Ca^{2+} influx is excessive due for example to intense stimuli, the sequestration capacity by mitochondria proves inadequate, leading to a prolonged elevation of the cytosolic Ca^{2+} level. This happens in sensory neurons following capsaicin application [135].

Excessive Ca^{2+} accumulation in mitochondria is a well-established cause of neuronal excitotoxicity [136]. Ca^{2+} accumulation also leads to the opening of the mitochondrial permeability transition pore (mPTP), a large conductance pore in the mitochondrial membrane that is associated with neuronal apoptosis and necrotic death [137]. Indeed, capsaicin induced death of mesencephalic neurons may result from mitochondrial release of cytochrome c followed by caspase-3 activation leading to apoptosis [138]. Furthermore, pharmacological inhibitors of mPTP attenuated capsaicin-induced death of sensory neurons [139]. Mitochondrial Ca^{2+} accumulation also generates reactive oxygen species (ROS) [140], and mitochondrial Ca^{2+}-uptake induces ROS generation in the spinal cord, which contributes to central neuronal plasticity and persistent pain [141,142]. As part of a vicious cycle, mPTP opening is further enhanced by ROS [143]. Clearly, mitochondria could contribute to vanilloid-induced sensory neuronal toxicity due to Ca^{2+} overloading associated with opening of mPTP and ROS generation. Further evidence supports the hypothesis that capsaicin toxic effects are mediated through mitochondrial mechanisms [144]. In sensory neurons, 50 µM capsaicin dissipates the mitochondrial membrane potential as effectively as carbonyl cyanide *p*-trifluoro-methoxyphenylhydrazone (FCCP), a mitochondrial uncoupler. Capsaicin-mediated mitochondrial depolarization is attenuated, but not eliminated, by removing extracellular Ca^{2+}. It is not settled, however, whether the effects of capsaicin on mitochondria effects are due entirely to TRPV1-mediated phenomena, and whether these effects fully account for capsaicin toxicity.

Capsaicin-induced cell death is also dependent on calpain. Calpains are Ca^{2+}-dependent cysteine proteases associated with multiple neuronal and non-neuronal pathologies [145]. In dissociated DRG neurons, calpain inhibitors attenuated capsaicin-induced cell death independent of a capsaicin-induced cytosolic Ca^{2+} increase [125]. Capsaicin increased breakdown products of α-spectrin, a cytoskeletal target of calpain, which was prevented by a calpain inhibitor. These results suggest that capsaicin-induced activation of calpains contributes to cytotoxicity by perturbing the cytoskeleton. Alternatively, calpain activation may lead to apoptosis. In a breast cell line, capsaicin-induced ER stress elevated intracellular Ca^{2+} leading in turn to calpain activation, and apoptosis related to mitochondrial effects [130].

Since capsaicin-induced cell death involves multiple Ca^{2+}-dependent processes, it is likely that these contributors may also mediate capsaicin-induced ablation of axonal terminals. Studies of mitochondrial fission support the role of mitochondria [146]. In dissociated DRG neurons, capsaicin induced axonal swelling, which was accompanied by reduction in the length of the mitochondria and motility within axons. These changes in mitochondria were attenuated by Ca^{2+} chelators and capsazepine. Transfection with a dominant negative mutant Drp1, a mitochondrial protein responsible for mitochondrial fission, attenuated the capsaicin-induced decrease in mitochondrial length as well as axonal swelling and degeneration. Prevention of mitochondrial fission also prevented capsaicin-induced loss of the mitochondrial membrane potential. Overall this study strongly supports the contribution of mitochondrial mechanisms as an explanation of capsaicin effects.

5. Clinical Correlates

The capacity of capsaicin to ablate nociceptive terminals that express TRPV1 has many therapeutic implications. The agonist effects of capsaicin are not to be confused with the effects of TRPV1 antagonism. A putative TRPV1 antagonist in principle works only on TRPV1 mediated transduction, leaving intact other transduction mechanisms. Capsaicin, as a TRPV1 *agonist*, and as an excitotoxin, by ablating the terminals of nociceptors blocks other transduction mechanisms that may be co-expressed in the nociceptors. For example, TRPA1 is co-expressed with TRPV1 [147]. Thus capsaicin would be expected to block TRPA1 to the extent that TRPA1 is co-expressed with TRPV1. This expands the therapeutic window of an agonist, such as capsaicin, in terms of long term therapeutic effects. One injection is expected to be analgesic for weeks to months, despite a half-life in the blood that lasts for minutes to hours. The additional upside is that all of the functions of the nociceptor are affected. The TRPV1 receptor, in some ways, is simply the Trojan horse.

Capsaicin effects are highly localized to the area of injection. In work of Simone et al. [13], at a distance of only 1–2 mm from the site of intradermal injection, no effects of the capsaicin were seen. Therefore, a pain problem that is widespread would be impractical to treat with topical or injected capsaicin. Another consideration is that TRPV1 is not expressed in all nociceptors. The efficacy of capsaicin will depend on the extent to which the signaling nociceptors that produce the pain express TRPV1. To that point, the predominant long term sensory effect of injected capsaicin in the skin is on heat sensibility with a much lesser effect on pain from mechanical stimuli [13]. Other evidence indicates that mechanical pain in muscle does involve TRPV1 [28,29].

Another important consideration regards the involvement of peripheral and central mechanisms. This is best understood with injury to the skin. Treede and colleagues [61] used electrical stimuli to induce local pain, allodynia, and hyperalgesia. High concentration topical capsaicin (8%) was used to knock out innervation of nociceptors that expressed TRPV1. Pain to the electrical stimuli itself was dropped by about half. The secondary hyperalgesia and the allodynia, both likely due to central mechanisms (central sensitization), were almost entirely eliminated. Secondary hyperalgesia is characterized by heightened mechanical pain (not heat) and results from the initial sensitization of nociceptors at the point of injury. Blocking the input of nociceptors at the point of injury probably accounts for the elimination of abnormal mechanical pain in the secondary zone. This means that capsaicin may affect abnormal mechanical pain indirectly by blocking central sensitization via effects on the primary afferents and peripheral sensitization [61]. Given the likely importance of central mechanisms in most clinical pain problems, these data suggest that a knockout of TRPV1 expressing nociceptors by capsaicin has favorable prospects as a useful therapy. Likewise, the therapeutic application of RTX targeting TRPV1 expressing nociceptors has been advocated [148].

Further support relates to the evidence that indicates up-regulation of the expression and function of TRPV1 receptors in different disease states such as cancer, visceral inflammation, and neuropathic pain [27,149–153]. Therefore, the role of TRPV1 in nociception may evolve to be of greater importance in disease. Heat sensitization may be argued to have little importance with regard to deeper tissues. However, sensitization to the point that nociceptors are activated by the ambient core temperature or locally produced endogenous ligands, indicates a means by which TRPV1 bearing nociceptors may play an pivotal role in "ongoing" or spontaneous pain associated with clinical pain states.

Beneficial effects of ablation of nociceptive terminals are likely maintained for weeks to months, as regeneration of nociceptive fibers reestablishes innervation of the target tissues. Patients might be reinjected in order to extend the therapeutic effects. The mechanisms underlying regeneration following capsaicin-induced ablation may be similar to the regeneration mechanisms that follow axotomy. A subpopulation of skin nerve fibers showed immunoreactivity to GAP43, a marker of regenerating nerves, following topical administration of capsaicin in humans, suggesting regeneration of primary afferents [14]. The intraplantar injection of RTX increases ATF3 and galanin, markers of nerve regeneration, within DRG for up to 10 days suggesting that regeneration processes follow terminal ablation [87]. Since the duration of therapeutic effects of vanilloid-induced analgesia may be correlated with the time course associated with regeneration, better understanding of the mechanisms of regeneration could help to determine ways to extend the duration of effects.

6. Conclusions

The cloning of the TRPV1 receptor ignited a new era of pain research by opening the gateway to understanding how nociceptors are activated. In this same timeframe the study of ligands, such as capsaicin and RTX, also intensified. Capsaicin was recognized as a molecule that could be used as an experimental stimulus to evoke pain. Appreciation also grew that capsaicin was not only powerfully algesic, but that it also led to focal degeneration of nociceptors. High concentration topical capsaicin was approved to treat post-herpetic neuralgia and, in Europe, other neuropathic pain conditions. In focal pain conditions there is appreciation that capsaicin may be given by injection to knockout nociceptors and achieve pain control. Studies in Morton's neuroma, a painful neuropathic pain condition, have shown promise. Injection may also be useful for direct delivery into a joint to control arthritis pain. Other uses for many other pain conditions may evolve.

The major impediment to the clinical use of capsaicin is the immediate pungency. However, with the high dosing associated with topical use or injection to treat Morton's neuroma, for example, the immediate application pain is quite circumscribed, lasting in the order of minutes to hours in exchange for months of therapeutic benefit.

A future challenge for TRPV1 excitotoxins is to mitigate the "excite", and accentuate the "toxin" aspect of the effects. Further understanding the cellular mechanisms of action may very well help fulfill this promise.

Acknowledgments: The authors thank John Joseph for reading of the manuscript and helpful suggestions. This study was supported by the National Institutes of Health grant R01 DE023846 (M.K.C.) and Maryland Industrial Partnership grant #5403 (M.K.C.).

Author Contributions: Man-Kyo Chung and James N. Campbell conceived, structured, and wrote the paper.

Conflicts of Interest: The authors declare no conflict of interest.

References

1. Caterina, M.J.; Schumacher, M.A.; Tominaga, M.; Rosen, T.A.; Levine, J.D.; Julius, D. The capsaicin receptor: A heat-activated ion channel in the pain pathway. *Nature* **1997**, *389*, 816–824. [PubMed]
2. Chaiyasit, K.; Khovidhunkit, W.; Wittayalertpanya, S. Pharmacokinetic and the effect of capsaicin in capsicum frutescens on decreasing plasma glucose level. *J. Med. Assoc. Thai.* **2009**, *92*, 108–113. [PubMed]
3. Kearney, T.; Hiatt, P.; Birdsall, E.; Smollin, C. Pepper spray injury severity: Ten-year case experience of a poison control system. *Prehosp. Emerg. Care* **2014**, *18*, 381–386. [CrossRef] [PubMed]
4. Schulze, B.; Spiteller, D. Capsaicin: Tailored chemical defence against unwanted "frugivores". *Chembiochem* **2009**, *10*, 428–429. [CrossRef] [PubMed]
5. Szolcsanyi, J.; Sann, H.; Pierau, F.K. Nociception in pigeons is not impaired by capsaicin. *Pain* **1986**, *27*, 247–260. [CrossRef]
6. Andersson, J.L.; Lilja, A.; Hartvig, P.; Langstrom, B.; Gordh, T.; Handwerker, H.; Torebjork, E. Somatotopic organization along the central sulcus, for pain localization in humans, as revealed by positron emission tomography. *Exp. Brain Res.* **1997**, *117*, 192–199. [CrossRef] [PubMed]
7. Iadarola, M.J.; Berman, K.F.; Zeffiro, T.A.; Byas-Smith, M.G.; Gracely, R.H.; Max, M.B.; Bennett, G.J. Neural activation during acute capsaicin-evoked pain and allodynia assessed with pet. *Brain* **1998**, *121 Pt 5*, 931–947. [CrossRef] [PubMed]
8. Baron, R.; Baron, Y.; Disbrow, E.; Roberts, T.P. Brain processing of capsaicin-induced secondary hyperalgesia: A functional mri study. *Neurology* **1999**, *53*, 548–557. [CrossRef] [PubMed]
9. Szolcsanyi, J.; Pinter, E. Transient receptor potential vanilloid 1 as a therapeutic target in analgesia. *Expert Opin. Ther. Targets* **2013**, *17*, 641–657. [CrossRef] [PubMed]
10. Szallasi, A.; Blumberg, P.M. Vanilloid (capsaicin) receptors and mechanisms. *Pharmacol. Rev.* **1999**, *51*, 159–212. [PubMed]
11. Jancso, G.; Kiraly, E.; Jancso-Gabor, A. Pharmacologically induced selective degeneration of chemosensitive primary sensory neurones. *Nature* **1977**, *270*, 741–743. [CrossRef] [PubMed]
12. Jancso, G.; Kiraly, E.; Joo, F.; Such, G.; Nagy, A. Selective degeneration by capsaicin of a subpopulation of primary sensory neurons in the adult rat. *Neurosci. Lett.* **1985**, *59*, 209–214. [CrossRef]
13. Simone, D.A.; Nolano, M.; Johnson, T.; Wendelschafer-Crabb, G.; Kennedy, W.R. Intradermal injection of capsaicin in humans produces degeneration and subsequent reinnervation of epidermal nerve fibers: Correlation with sensory function. *J. Neurosci.* **1998**, *18*, 8947–8959. [PubMed]
14. Rage, M.; Van Acker, N.; Facer, P.; Shenoy, R.; Knaapen, M.W.; Timmers, M.; Streffer, J.; Anand, P.; Meert, T.; Plaghki, L. The time course of CO_2 laser-evoked responses and of skin nerve fibre markers after topical capsaicin in human volunteers. *Clin. Neurophysiol.* **2010**, *121*, 1256–1266. [CrossRef] [PubMed]
15. Polydefkis, M.; Hauer, P.; Sheth, S.; Sirdofsky, M.; Griffin, J.W.; McArthur, J.C. The time course of epidermal nerve fibre regeneration: Studies in normal controls and in people with diabetes, with and without neuropathy. *Brain* **2004**, *127*, 1606–1615. [CrossRef] [PubMed]
16. Robbins, W.R.; Staats, P.S.; Levine, J.; Fields, H.L.; Allen, R.W.; Campbell, J.N.; Pappagallo, M. Treatment of intractable pain with topical large-dose capsaicin: Preliminary report. *Anesth. Analg.* **1998**, *86*, 579–583. [CrossRef] [PubMed]
17. Anand, P.; Bley, K. Topical capsaicin for pain management: Therapeutic potential and mechanisms of action of the new high-concentration capsaicin 8% patch. *Br. J. Anaesth.* **2011**, *107*, 490–502. [CrossRef] [PubMed]
18. Derry, S.; Sven-Rice, A.; Cole, P.; Tan, T.; Moore, R.A. Topical capsaicin (high concentration) for chronic neuropathic pain in adults. *Cochrane Database Syst. Rev.* **2013**, *28*, CD007393.
19. Mitchell, K.; Lebovitz, E.E.; Keller, J.M.; Mannes, A.J.; Nemenov, M.I.; Iadarola, M.J. Nociception and inflammatory hyperalgesia evaluated in rodents using infrared laser stimulation after TRPV1 gene knockout or resiniferatoxin lesion. *Pain* **2014**, *155*, 733–745. [CrossRef] [PubMed]
20. Hamalainen, M.M.; Subieta, A.; Arpey, C.; Brennan, T.J. Differential effect of capsaicin treatment on pain-related behaviors after plantar incision. *J. Pain* **2009**, *10*, 637–645. [CrossRef] [PubMed]
21. King, T.; Qu, C.; Okun, A.; Mercado, R.; Ren, J.; Brion, T.; Lai, J.; Porreca, F. Contribution of afferent pathways to nerve injury-induced spontaneous pain and evoked hypersensitivity. *Pain* **2011**, *152*, 1997–2005. [CrossRef] [PubMed]

22. Okun, A.; DeFelice, M.; Eyde, N.; Ren, J.; Mercado, R.; King, T.; Porreca, F. Transient inflammation-induced ongoing pain is driven by TRPV1 sensitive afferents. *Mol. Pain* **2011**, *7*, 4. [CrossRef] [PubMed]
23. Helyes, Z.; Sandor, K.; Borbely, E.; Tekus, V.; Pinter, E.; Elekes, K.; Toth, D.M.; Szolcsanyi, J.; McDougall, J.J. Involvement of transient receptor potential vanilloid 1 receptors in protease-activated receptor-2-induced joint inflammation and nociception. *Eur. J. Pain* **2010**, *14*, 351–358. [CrossRef] [PubMed]
24. Honore, P.; Chandran, P.; Hernandez, G.; Gauvin, D.M.; Mikusa, J.P.; Zhong, C.; Joshi, S.K.; Ghilardi, J.R.; Sevcik, M.A.; Fryer, R.M.; et al. Repeated dosing of ABT-102, a potent and selective TRPV1 antagonist, enhances TRPV1-mediated analgesic activity in rodents, but attenuates antagonist-induced hyperthermia. *Pain* **2009**, *142*, 27–35. [CrossRef] [PubMed]
25. Barton, N.J.; McQueen, D.S.; Thomson, D.; Gauldie, S.D.; Wilson, A.W.; Salter, D.M.; Chessell, I.P. Attenuation of experimental arthritis in TRPV1R knockout mice. *Exp. Mol. Pathol.* **2006**, *81*, 166–170. [CrossRef] [PubMed]
26. Kelly, S.; Chapman, R.J.; Woodhams, S.; Sagar, D.R.; Turner, J.; Burston, J.J.; Bullock, C.; Paton, K.; Huang, J.; Wong, A.; et al. Increased function of pronociceptive TRPV1 at the level of the joint in a rat model of osteoarthritis pain. *Ann. Rheum. Dis.* **2015**, *74*, 252–259. [CrossRef] [PubMed]
27. Jones, R.C., 3rd; Xu, L.; Gebhart, G.F. The mechanosensitivity of mouse colon afferent fibers and their sensitization by inflammatory mediators require transient receptor potential vanilloid 1 and acid-sensing ion channel 3. *J. Neurosci.* **2005**, *25*, 10981–10989. [CrossRef] [PubMed]
28. Lee, J.; Saloman, J.L.; Weiland, G.; Auh, Q.S.; Chung, M.K.; Ro, J.Y. Functional interactions between NMDA receptors and TRPV1 in trigeminal sensory neurons mediate mechanical hyperalgesia in the rat masseter muscle. *Pain* **2012**, *153*, 1514–1524. [CrossRef] [PubMed]
29. Ota, H.; Katanosaka, K.; Murase, S.; Kashio, M.; Tominaga, M.; Mizumura, K. TRPV1 and TRPV4 play pivotal roles in delayed onset muscle soreness. *PLoS ONE* **2013**, *8*, e65751. [CrossRef] [PubMed]
30. Kissin, E.Y.; Freitas, C.F.; Kissin, I. The effects of intraarticular resiniferatoxin in experimental knee-joint arthritis. *Anesth. Analg.* **2005**, *101*, 1433–1439. [CrossRef] [PubMed]
31. Kim, Y.; Kim, E.H.; Lee, K.S.; Lee, K.; Park, S.H.; Na, S.H.; Ko, C.; Kim, J.; Yooon, Y.W. The effects of intra-articular resiniferatoxin on monosodium iodoacetate-induced osteoarthritic pain in rats. *Korean J. Physiol. Pharmacol.* **2016**, *20*, 129–136. [CrossRef] [PubMed]
32. Abdullah, M.; Mahowald, M.L.; Frizelle, S.P.; Dorman, C.W.; Funkenbusch, S.C.; Krug, H.E. The effect of intra-articular vanilloid receptor agonists on pain behavior measures in a murine model of acute monoarthritis. *J. Pain Res.* **2016**, *9*, 563–570. [CrossRef] [PubMed]
33. Jancso, G.; Kiraly, E.; Jancso-Gabor, A. Direct evidence for an axonal site of action of capsaicin. *Naunyn Schmiedebergs Arch. Pharmacol.* **1980**, *313*, 91–94. [CrossRef] [PubMed]
34. Neubert, J.K.; Mannes, A.J.; Karai, L.J.; Jenkins, A.C.; Zawatski, L.; Abu-Asab, M.; Iadarola, M.J. Perineural resiniferatoxin selectively inhibits inflammatory hyperalgesia. *Mol. Pain* **2008**, *4*, 3. [CrossRef] [PubMed]
35. Kissin, I.; Bright, C.A.; Bradley, E.L., Jr. Selective and long-lasting neural blockade with resiniferatoxin prevents inflammatory pain hypersensitivity. *Anesth. Analg.* **2002**, *94*, 1253–1258. [CrossRef] [PubMed]
36. Kissin, I.; Davison, N.; Bradley, E.L., Jr. Perineural resiniferatoxin prevents hyperalgesia in a rat model of postoperative pain. *Anesth. Analg.* **2005**, *100*, 774–780. [CrossRef] [PubMed]
37. Szabo, T.; Olah, Z.; Iadarola, M.J.; Blumberg, P.M. Epidural resiniferatoxin induced prolonged regional analgesia to pain. *Brain Res.* **1999**, *840*, 92–98. [CrossRef]
38. Eimerl, D.; Papir-Kricheli, D. Epidural capsaicin produces prolonged segmental analgesia in the rat. *Exp. Neurol.* **1987**, *97*, 169–178. [CrossRef]
39. Yaksh, T.L.; Farb, D.H.; Leeman, S.E.; Jessell, T.M. Intrathecal capsaicin depletes substance P in the rat spinal cord and produces prolonged thermal analgesia. *Science* **1979**, *206*, 481–483. [CrossRef] [PubMed]
40. Bishnoi, M.; Bosgraaf, C.A.; Premkumar, L.S. Preservation of acute pain and efferent functions following intrathecal resiniferatoxin-induced analgesia in rats. *J. Pain* **2011**, *12*, 991–1003. [CrossRef] [PubMed]
41. Brown, D.C.; Agnello, K.; Iadarola, M.J. Intrathecal resiniferatoxin in a dog model: Efficacy in bone cancer pain. *Pain* **2015**, *156*, 1018–1024. [CrossRef] [PubMed]
42. Brown, D.C.; Iadarola, M.J.; Perkowski, S.Z.; Erin, H.; Shofer, F.; Laszlo, K.J.; Olah, Z.; Mannes, A.J. Physiologic and antinociceptive effects of intrathecal resiniferatoxin in a canine bone cancer model. *Anesthesiology* **2005**, *103*, 1052–1059. [CrossRef] [PubMed]
43. Brederson, J.D.; Kym, P.R.; Szallasi, A. Targeting TRP channels for pain relief. *Eur. J. Pharmacol.* **2013**, *716*, 61–76. [CrossRef] [PubMed]

44. Aasvang, E.K.; Hansen, J.B.; Malmstrom, J.; Asmussen, T.; Gennevois, D.; Struys, M.M.; Kehlet, H. The effect of wound instillation of a novel purified capsaicin formulation on postherniotomy pain: A double-blind, randomized, placebo-controlled study. *Anesth. Analg.* **2008**, *107*, 282–291. [CrossRef] [PubMed]

45. Campbell, C.M.; Diamond, E.; Schmidt, W.K.; Kelly, M.; Allen, R.; Houghton, W.; Brady, K.L.; Campbell, J.N. A randomized, double blind, placebo controlled trial of injected capsaicin for pain in morton's neuroma. *Pain* **2016**, *157*, 1297–1304. [CrossRef] [PubMed]

46. Mou, J.; Paillard, F.; Turnbull, B.; Trudeau, J.; Stoker, M.; Katz, N.P. Efficacy of qutenza®(capsaicin) 8% patch for neuropathic pain: A meta-analysis of the qutenza clinical trials database. *Pain* **2013**, *154*, 1632–1639. [CrossRef] [PubMed]

47. Caterina, M.J.; Leffler, A.; Malmberg, A.B.; Martin, W.J.; Trafton, J.; Petersen-Zeitz, K.R.; Koltzenburg, M.; Basbaum, A.I.; Julius, D. Impaired nociception and pain sensation in mice lacking the capsaicin receptor. *Science* **2000**, *288*, 306–313. [CrossRef] [PubMed]

48. Ringkamp, M.; Raja, S.N.; Campbell, J.N.; Meyer, R.A. Peripheral mechanisms of cutaneous nociception. In *Wall & Melzack's Textbook of Pain*, 6th ed.; McMahon, S.B., Koltzenburg, M., Tracey, I., Turk, D.C., Eds.; Elsevier Health Sciences: Philadelphia, PA, USA, 2013; pp. 1–30.

49. Campbell, J.N.; LaMotte, R.H. Latency to detection of first pain. *Brain Res.* **1983**, *266*, 203–208. [CrossRef]

50. LaMotte, R.H.; Lundberg, L.E.; Torebjork, H.E. Pain, hyperalgesia and activity in nociceptive C units in humans after intradermal injection of capsaicin. *J. Physiol.* **1992**, *448*, 749–764. [CrossRef] [PubMed]

51. Schmelz, M.; Schmid, R.; Handwerker, H.O.; Torebjork, H.E. Encoding of burning pain from capsaicin-treated human skin in two categories of unmyelinated nerve fibres. *Brain* **2000**, *123 Pt 3*, 560–571. [CrossRef] [PubMed]

52. Ringkamp, M.; Peng, Y.B.; Wu, G.; Hartke, T.V.; Campbell, J.N.; Meyer, R.A. Capsaicin responses in heat-sensitive and heat-insensitive A-fiber nociceptors. *J. Neurosci.* **2001**, *21*, 4460–4468. [PubMed]

53. Snider, W.D.; McMahon, S.B. Tackling pain at the source: New ideas about nociceptors. *Neuron* **1998**, *20*, 629–632. [CrossRef]

54. Tominaga, M.; Caterina, M.J.; Malmberg, A.B.; Rosen, T.A.; Gilbert, H.; Skinner, K.; Raumann, B.E.; Basbaum, A.I.; Julius, D. The cloned capsaicin receptor integrates multiple pain-producing stimuli. *Neuron* **1998**, *21*, 531–543. [CrossRef]

55. Helme, R.D.; McKernan, S. Neurogenic flare responses following topical application of capsaicin in humans. *Ann. Neurol.* **1985**, *18*, 505–509. [CrossRef] [PubMed]

56. Simone, D.A.; Baumann, T.K.; LaMotte, R.H. Dose-dependent pain and mechanical hyperalgesia in humans after intradermal injection of capsaicin. *Pain* **1989**, *38*, 99–107. [CrossRef]

57. Carpenter, S.E.; Lynn, B. Vascular and sensory responses of human skin to mild injury after topical treatment with capsaicin. *Br. J. Pharmacol.* **1981**, *73*, 755–758. [CrossRef] [PubMed]

58. Evans, A.R.; Nicol, G.D.; Vasko, M.R. Differential regulation of evoked peptide release by voltage-sensitive calcium channels in rat sensory neurons. *Brain Res.* **1996**, *712*, 265–273. [CrossRef]

59. Nemeth, J.; Helyes, Z.; Oroszi, G.; Jakab, B.; Pinter, E.; Szilvassy, Z.; Szolcsanyi, J. Role of voltage-gated cation channels and axon reflexes in the release of sensory neuropeptides by capsaicin from isolated rat trachea. *Eur. J. Pharmacol.* **2003**, *458*, 313–318. [CrossRef]

60. LaMotte, R.H.; Shain, C.N.; Simone, D.A.; Tsai, E.F. Neurogenic hyperalgesia: Psychophysical studies of underlying mechanisms. *J. Neurophysiol.* **1991**, *66*, 190–211. [PubMed]

61. Henrich, F.; Magerl, W.; Klein, T.; Greffrath, W.; Treede, R.D. Capsaicin-sensitive C- and A-fibre nociceptors control long-term potentiation-like pain amplification in humans. *Brain* **2015**, *138 Pt 9*, 2505–2520. [CrossRef] [PubMed]

62. Baumann, T.K.; Simone, D.A.; Shain, C.N.; LaMotte, R.H. Neurogenic hyperalgesia: The search for the primary cutaneous afferent fibers that contribute to capsaicin-induced pain and hyperalgesia. *J. Neurophysiol.* **1991**, *66*, 212–227. [PubMed]

63. Campbell, C.M.; Edwards, R.R.; Carmona, C.; Uhart, M.; Wand, G.; Carteret, A.; Kim, Y.K.; Frost, J.; Campbell, J.N. Polymorphisms in the GTP cyclohydrolase gene (GCH1) are associated with ratings of capsaicin pain. *Pain* **2009**, *141*, 114–118. [CrossRef] [PubMed]

64. Belfer, I.; Segall, S.K.; Lariviere, W.R.; Smith, S.B.; Dai, F.; Slade, G.D.; Rashid, N.U.; Mogil, J.S.; Campbell, C.M.; Edwards, R.R.; et al. Pain modality- and sex-specific effects of comt genetic functional variants. *Pain* **2013**, *154*, 1368–1376. [CrossRef] [PubMed]

65. Dimova, V.; Oertel, B.G.; Kabakci, G.; Zimmermann, M.; Hermens, H.; Lautenbacher, S.; Ultsch, A.; Lotsch, J. A more pessimistic life orientation is associated with experimental inducibility of a neuropathy-like pain pattern in healthy individuals. *J. Pain* **2015**, *16*, 791–800. [CrossRef] [PubMed]

66. Freed, K.A.; Blangero, J.; Howard, T.; Johnson, M.P.; Curran, J.E.; Garcia, Y.R.; Lan, H.C.; Abboud, H.E.; Moses, E.K. The 57 kb deletion in cystinosis patients extends into TRPV1 causing dysregulation of transcription in peripheral blood mononuclear cells. *J. Med. Genet.* **2011**, *48*, 563–566. [CrossRef] [PubMed]

67. Buntinx, L.; Voets, T.; Morlion, B.; Vangeel, L.; Janssen, M.; Cornelissen, E.; Vriens, J.; de Hoon, J.; Levtchenko, E. TRPV1 dysfunction in cystinosis patients harboring the homozygous 57 kb deletion. *Sci. Rep.* **2016**, *6*, 35395. [CrossRef] [PubMed]

68. Xu, H.; Tian, W.; Fu, Y.; Oyama, T.T.; Anderson, S.; Cohen, D.M. Functional effects of nonsynonymous polymorphisms in the human TRPV1 gene. *Am. J. Physiol. Renal. Physiol.* **2007**, *293*, F1865–F1876. [CrossRef] [PubMed]

69. Wang, S.; Joseph, J.; Diatchenko, L.; Ro, J.Y.; Chung, M.K. Agonist-dependence of functional properties for common nonsynonymous variants of human transient receptor potential vanilloid 1. *Pain* **2016**, *157*, 1515–1524. [CrossRef] [PubMed]

70. Khairatkar-Joshi, N.; Szallasi, A. TRPV1 antagonists: The challenges for therapeutic targeting. *Trends Mol. Med.* **2009**, *15*, 14–22. [CrossRef] [PubMed]

71. Bates, B.D.; Mitchell, K.; Keller, J.M.; Chan, C.C.; Swaim, W.D.; Yaskovich, R.; Mannes, A.J.; Iadarola, M.J. Prolonged analgesic response of cornea to topical resiniferatoxin, a potent TRPV1 agonist. *Pain* **2010**, *149*, 522–528. [CrossRef] [PubMed]

72. Knolle, E.; Zadrazil, M.; Kovacs, G.G.; Medwed, S.; Scharbert, G.; Schemper, M. Comparison of cooling and emla to reduce the burning pain during capsaicin 8% patch application: A randomized, double-blind, placebo-controlled study. *Pain* **2013**, *154*, 2729–2736. [CrossRef] [PubMed]

73. Leffler, A.; Fischer, M.J.; Rehner, D.; Kienel, S.; Kistner, K.; Sauer, S.K.; Gavva, N.R.; Reeh, P.W.; Nau, C. The vanilloid receptor TRPV1 is activated and sensitized by local anesthetics in rodent sensory neurons. *J. Clin. Investig.* **2008**, *118*, 763–776. [CrossRef] [PubMed]

74. Chung, M.K.; Wang, S. Cold suppresses agonist-induced activation of TRPV1. *J. Dent. Res.* **2011**, *90*, 1098–1102. [CrossRef] [PubMed]

75. Zimmermann, K.; Leffler, A.; Babes, A.; Cendan, C.M.; Carr, R.W.; Kobayashi, J.; Nau, C.; Wood, J.N.; Reeh, P.W. Sensory neuron sodium channel Nav1.8 is essential for pain at low temperatures. *Nature* **2007**, *447*, 855–858. [CrossRef] [PubMed]

76. Dhaka, A.; Murray, A.N.; Mathur, J.; Earley, T.J.; Petrus, M.J.; Patapoutian, A. TRPM8 is required for cold sensation in mice. *Neuron* **2007**, *54*, 371–378. [CrossRef] [PubMed]

77. Del Camino, D.; Murphy, S.; Heiry, M.; Barrett, L.B.; Earley, T.J.; Cook, C.A.; Petrus, M.J.; Zhao, M.; D'Amours, M.; Deering, N.; et al. TRPA1 contributes to cold hypersensitivity. *J. Neurosci.* **2010**, *30*, 15165–15174. [CrossRef] [PubMed]

78. Takayama, Y.; Uta, D.; Furue, H.; Tominaga, M. Pain-enhancing mechanism through interaction between TRPV1 and anoctamin 1 in sensory neurons. *Proc. Natl. Acad. Sci. USA* **2015**, *112*, 5213–5218. [CrossRef] [PubMed]

79. Deba, F.; Bessac, B.F. Anoctamin-1 Cl⁻ channels in nociception: Activation by an *N*-aroylaminothiazole and capsaicin and inhibition by T16A[inh]-A01. *Mol. Pain* **2015**, *11*, 55. [CrossRef] [PubMed]

80. Simone, D.A.; Ochoa, J. Early and late effects of prolonged topical capsaicin on cutaneous sensibility and neurogenic vasodilatation in humans. *Pain* **1991**, *47*, 285–294. [CrossRef]

81. Neubert, J.K.; Karai, L.; Jun, J.H.; Kim, H.S.; Olah, Z.; Iadarola, M.J. Peripherally induced resiniferatoxin analgesia. *Pain* **2003**, *104*, 219–228. [CrossRef]

82. Ma, X.L.; Zhang, F.X.; Dong, F.; Bao, L.; Zhang, X. Experimental evidence for alleviating nociceptive hypersensitivity by single application of capsaicin. *Mol. Pain* **2015**, *11*, 22. [CrossRef] [PubMed]

83. Baranowski, R.; Lynn, B.; Pini, A. The effects of locally applied capsaicin on conduction in cutaneous nerves in four mammalian species. *Br. J. Pharmacol.* **1986**, *89*, 267–276. [CrossRef] [PubMed]

84. Chung, J.M.; Lee, K.H.; Hori, Y.; Willis, W.D. Effects of capsaicin applied to a peripheral nerve on the responses of primate spinothalamic tract cells. *Brain Res.* **1985**, *329*, 27–38. [CrossRef]

85.   Petsche, U.; Fleischer, E.; Lembeck, F.; Handwerker, H.O. The effect of capsaicin application to a peripheral nerve on impulse conduction in functionally identified afferent nerve fibres. *Brain Res.* **1983**, *265*, 233–240. [CrossRef]

86.   Beydoun, A.; Dyke, D.B.; Morrow, T.J.; Casey, K.L. Topical capsaicin selectively attenuates heat pain and A delta fiber-mediated laser-evoked potentials. *Pain* **1996**, *65*, 189–196. [CrossRef]

87.   Mitchell, K.; Bates, B.D.; Keller, J.M.; Lopez, M.; Scholl, L.; Navarro, J.; Madian, N.; Haspel, G.; Nemenov, M.I.; Iadarola, M.J. Ablation of rat TRPV1-expressing Adelta/C-fibers with resiniferatoxin: Analysis of withdrawal behaviors, recovery of function and molecular correlates. *Mol. Pain* **2010**, *6*, 94. [CrossRef] [PubMed]

88.   Dray, A.; Bettaney, J.; Forster, P. Actions of capsaicin on peripheral nociceptors of the neonatal rat spinal cord-tail in vitro: Dependence of extracellular ions and independence of second messengers. *Br. J. Pharmacol.* **1990**, *101*, 727–733. [CrossRef] [PubMed]

89.   Peng, Y.B.; Ringkamp, M.; Meyer, R.A.; Campbell, J.N. Fatigue and paradoxical enhancement of heat response in C-fiber nociceptors from cross-modal excitation. *J. Neurosci.* **2003**, *23*, 4766–4774. [PubMed]

90.   LaMotte, R.H.; Campbell, J.N. Comparison of responses of warm and nociceptive C-fiber afferents in monkey with human judgments of thermal pain. *J. Neurophysiol.* **1978**, *41*, 509–528. [PubMed]

91.   Slugg, R.M.; Meyer, R.A.; Campbell, J.N. Response of cutaneous A- and C-fiber nociceptors in the monkey to controlled-force stimuli. *J. Neurophysiol.* **2000**, *83*, 2179–2191. [PubMed]

92.   Joseph, J.; Wang, S.; Lee, J.; Ro, J.Y.; Chung, M.K. Carboxyl-terminal domain of transient receptor potential vanilloid 1 contains distinct segments differentially involved in capsaicin- and heat-induced desensitization. *J. Biol. Chem.* **2013**, *288*, 35690–35702. [CrossRef] [PubMed]

93.   Vyklicky, L.; Novakova-Tousova, K.; Benedikt, J.; Samad, A.; Touska, F.; Vlachova, V. Calcium-dependent desensitization of vanilloid receptor TRPV1: A mechanism possibly involved in analgesia induced by topical application of capsaicin. *Physiol. Res.* **2008**, *57* (Suppl. S3), 59–68.

94.   Liu, L.; Oortgiesen, M.; Li, L.; Simon, S.A. Capsaicin inhibits activation of voltage-gated sodium currents in capsaicin-sensitive trigeminal ganglion neurons. *J. Neurophysiol.* **2001**, *85*, 745–758. [PubMed]

95.   Su, X.; Wachtel, R.E.; Gebhart, G.F. Capsaicin sensitivity and voltage-gated sodium currents in colon sensory neurons from rat dorsal root ganglia. *Am. J. Physiol.* **1999**, *277*, G1180–G1188. [PubMed]

96.   Onizuka, S.; Yonaha, T.; Tamura, R.; Hosokawa, N.; Kawasaki, Y.; Kashiwada, M.; Shirasaka, T.; Tsuneyoshi, I. Capsaicin indirectly suppresses voltage-gated Na^+ currents through TRPV1 in rat dorsal root ganglion neurons. *Anesth. Analg.* **2011**, *112*, 703–709. [CrossRef] [PubMed]

97.   Wu, Z.Z.; Chen, S.R.; Pan, H.L. Transient receptor potential vanilloid type 1 activation down-regulates voltage-gated calcium channels through calcium-dependent calcineurin in sensory neurons. *J. Biol. Chem.* **2005**, *280*, 18142–18151. [CrossRef] [PubMed]

98.   Caudle, R.M.; Karai, L.; Mena, N.; Cooper, B.Y.; Mannes, A.J.; Perez, F.M.; Iadarola, M.J.; Olah, Z. Resiniferatoxin-induced loss of plasma membrane in vanilloid receptor expressing cells. *Neurotoxicology* **2003**, *24*, 895–908. [CrossRef]

99.   Sanz-Salvador, L.; Andres-Borderia, A.; Ferrer-Montiel, A.; Planells-Cases, R. Agonist- and Ca^{2+}-dependent desensitization of TRPV1 channel targets the receptor to lysosomes for degradation. *J. Biol. Chem.* **2012**, *287*, 19462–19471. [CrossRef] [PubMed]

100. Dickenson, A.; Ashwood, N.; Sullivan, A.F.; James, I.; Dray, A. Antinociception produced by capsaicin: Spinal or peripheral mechanism? *Eur. J. Pharmacol.* **1990**, *187*, 225–233. [CrossRef]

101. Dickenson, A.H.; Dray, A. Selective antagonism of capsaicin by capsazepine: Evidence for a spinal receptor site in capsaicin-induced antinociception. *Br. J. Pharmacol.* **1991**, *104*, 1045–1049. [CrossRef] [PubMed]

102. Micevych, P.E.; Yaksh, T.L.; Szolcsanyi, J. Effect of intrathecal capsaicin analogues on the immunofluorescence of peptides and serotonin in the dorsal horn in rats. *Neuroscience* **1983**, *8*, 123–131. [CrossRef]

103. Miller, M.S.; Buck, S.H.; Sipes, I.G.; Burks, T.F. Capsaicinoid-induced local and systemic antinociception without substance P depletion. *Brain Res.* **1982**, *244*, 193–197. [CrossRef]

104. Pinter, E.; Helyes, Z.; Szolcsanyi, J. Inhibitory effect of somatostatin on inflammation and nociception. *Pharmacol. Ther.* **2006**, *112*, 440–456. [CrossRef] [PubMed]

105. Szolcsanyi, J.; Bolcskei, K.; Szabo, A.; Pinter, E.; Petho, G.; Elekes, K.; Borzsei, R.; Almasi, R.; Szuts, T.; Keri, G.; et al. Analgesic effect of TT-232, a heptapeptide somatostatin analogue, in acute pain models of the rat and the mouse and in streptozotocin-induced diabetic mechanical allodynia. *Eur. J. Pharmacol.* **2004**, *498*, 103–109. [CrossRef] [PubMed]

106. Helyes, Z.; Pinter, E.; Sandor, K.; Elekes, K.; Banvolgyi, A.; Keszthelyi, D.; Szoke, E.; Toth, D.M.; Sandor, Z.; Kereskai, L.; et al. Impaired defense mechanism against inflammation, hyperalgesia, and airway hyperreactivity in somatostatin 4 receptor gene-deleted mice. *Proc. Natl. Acad. Sci. USA* **2009**, *106*, 13088–13093. [CrossRef] [PubMed]

107. Xu, X.J.; Farkas-Szallasi, T.; Lundberg, J.M.; Hokfelt, T.; Wiesenfeld-Hallin, Z.; Szallasi, A. Effects of the capsaicin analogue resiniferatoxin on spinal nociceptive mechanisms in the rat: Behavioral, electrophysiological and in situ hybridization studies. *Brain Res.* **1997**, *752*, 52–60. [CrossRef]

108. Karai, L.; Brown, D.C.; Mannes, A.J.; Connelly, S.T.; Brown, J.; Gandal, M.; Wellisch, O.M.; Neubert, J.K.; Olah, Z.; Iadarola, M.J. Deletion of vanilloid receptor 1-expressing primary afferent neurons for pain control. *J. Clin. Investig.* **2004**, *113*, 1344–1352. [CrossRef] [PubMed]

109. Yu, S.; Premkumar, L.S. Ablation and regeneration of peripheral and central TRPV1 expressing nerve terminals and the consequence of nociception. *Open Pain J.* **2015**, *8*, 1–9. [CrossRef]

110. Mou, J.; Paillard, F.; Turnbull, B.; Trudeau, J.; Stoker, M.; Katz, N.P. Qutenza (capsaicin) 8% patch onset and duration of response and effects of multiple treatments in neuropathic pain patients. *Clin. J. Pain* **2014**, *30*, 286–294. [CrossRef] [PubMed]

111. Szolcsanyi, J.; Jancso-Gabor, A.; Joo, F. Functional and fine structural characteristics of the sensory neuron blocking effect of capsaicin. *Naunyn Schmiedebergs Arch. Pharmacol.* **1975**, *287*, 157–169. [CrossRef] [PubMed]

112. Chung, K.; Klein, C.M.; Coggeshall, R.E. The receptive part of the primary afferent axon is most vulnerable to systemic capsaicin in adult rats. *Brain Res.* **1990**, *511*, 222–226. [CrossRef]

113. Jancso, G.; Lawson, S.N. Transganglionic degeneration of capsaicin-sensitive C-fiber primary afferent terminals. *Neuroscience* **1990**, *39*, 501–511. [CrossRef]

114. Otten, U.; Lorez, H.P.; Businger, F. Nerve growth factor antagonizes the neurotoxic action of capsaicin on primary sensory neurones. *Nature* **1983**, *301*, 515–517. [CrossRef] [PubMed]

115. Kawakami, T.; Hikawa, N.; Kusakabe, T.; Kano, M.; Bandou, Y.; Gotoh, H.; Takenaka, T. Mechanism of inhibitory action of capsaicin on particulate axoplasmic transport in sensory neurons in culture. *J. Neurobiol.* **1993**, *24*, 545–551. [CrossRef] [PubMed]

116. Lawson, S.N. The morphological consequences of neonatal treatment with capsaicin on primary afferent neurones in adult rats. *Acta Physiol. Hung.* **1987**, *69*, 315–321. [PubMed]

117. Sugimoto, T.; Xiao, C.; Ichikawa, H. Neonatal primary neuronal death induced by capsaicin and axotomy involves an apoptotic mechanism. *Brain Res.* **1998**, *807*, 147–154. [CrossRef]

118. Hiura, A.; Nakae, Y.; Nakagawa, H. Cell death of primary afferent nerve cells in neonatal mice treated with capsaicin. *Anat. Sci. Int.* **2002**, *77*, 47–50. [CrossRef] [PubMed]

119. Jin, H.W.; Ichikawa, H.; Fujita, M.; Yamaai, T.; Mukae, K.; Nomura, K.; Sugimoto, T. Involvement of caspase cascade in capsaicin-induced apoptosis of dorsal root ganglion neurons. *Brain Res.* **2005**, *1056*, 139–144. [CrossRef] [PubMed]

120. Hiura, A.; Ishizuka, H. Changes in features of degenerating primary sensory neurons with time after capsaicin treatment. *Acta Neuropathol.* **1989**, *78*, 35–46. [CrossRef] [PubMed]

121. Regan, R.F.; Panter, S.S.; Witz, A.; Tilly, J.L.; Giffard, R.G. Ultrastructure of excitotoxic neuronal death in murine cortical culture. *Brain Res.* **1995**, *705*, 188–198. [CrossRef]

122. Jancso, G.; Karcsu, S.; Kiraly, E.; Szebeni, A.; Toth, L.; Bacsy, E.; Joo, F.; Parducz, A. Neurotoxin induced nerve cell degeneration: Possible involvement of calcium. *Brain Res.* **1984**, *295*, 211–216. [CrossRef]

123. Marsh, S.J.; Stansfeld, C.E.; Brown, D.A.; Davey, R.; McCarthy, D. The mechanism of action of capsaicin on sensory C-type neurons and their axons in vitro. *Neuroscience* **1987**, *23*, 275–289. [CrossRef]

124. Wood, J.N.; Winter, J.; James, I.F.; Rang, H.P.; Yeats, J.; Bevan, S. Capsaicin-induced ion fluxes in dorsal root ganglion cells in culture. *J. Neurosci.* **1988**, *8*, 3208–3220. [PubMed]

125. Chard, P.S.; Bleakman, D.; Savidge, J.R.; Miller, R.J. Capsaicin-induced neurotoxicity in cultured dorsal root ganglion neurons: Involvement of calcium-activated proteases. *Neuroscience* **1995**, *65*, 1099–1108. [CrossRef]

126. Olah, Z.; Szabo, T.; Karai, L.; Hough, C.; Fields, R.D.; Caudle, R.M.; Blumberg, P.M.; Iadarola, M.J. Ligand-induced dynamic membrane changes and cell deletion conferred by vanilloid receptor 1. *J. Biol. Chem.* **2001**, *276*, 11021–11030. [CrossRef] [PubMed]

127. Karai, L.J.; Russell, J.T.; Iadarola, M.J.; Olah, Z. Vanilloid receptor 1 regulates multiple calcium compartments and contributes to Ca^{2+}-induced Ca^{2+} release in sensory neurons. *J. Biol. Chem.* **2004**, *279*, 16377–16387. [CrossRef] [PubMed]

128. Gallego-Sandin, S.; Rodriguez-Garcia, A.; Alonso, M.T.; Garcia-Sancho, J. The endoplasmic reticulum of dorsal root ganglion neurons contains functional TRPV1 channels. *J. Biol. Chem.* **2009**, *284*, 32591–32601. [CrossRef] [PubMed]

129. Stock, K.; Kumar, J.; Synowitz, M.; Petrosino, S.; Imperatore, R.; Smith, E.S.; Wend, P.; Purfurst, B.; Nuber, U.A.; Gurok, U.; et al. Neural precursor cells induce cell death of high-grade astrocytomas through stimulation of TRPV1. *Nat. Med.* **2012**, *18*, 1232–1238. [CrossRef] [PubMed]

130. Lee, M.J.; Kee, K.H.; Suh, C.H.; Lim, S.C.; Oh, S.H. Capsaicin-induced apoptosis is regulated by endoplasmic reticulum stress- and calpain-mediated mitochondrial cell death pathways. *Toxicology* **2009**, *264*, 205–214. [CrossRef] [PubMed]

131. Braz, J.M.; Basbaum, A.I. Differential ATF3 expression in dorsal root ganglion neurons reveals the profile of primary afferents engaged by diverse noxious chemical stimuli. *Pain* **2010**, *150*, 290–301. [CrossRef] [PubMed]

132. Usachev, Y.M.; DeMarco, S.J.; Campbell, C.; Strehler, E.E.; Thayer, S.A. Bradykinin and ATP accelerate Ca^{2+} efflux from rat sensory neurons via protein kinase C and the plasma membrane Ca^{2+} pump isoform 4. *Neuron* **2002**, *33*, 113–122. [CrossRef]

133. Gover, T.D.; Moreira, T.H.; Kao, J.P.; Weinreich, D. Calcium homeostasis in trigeminal ganglion cell bodies. *Cell Calcium* **2007**, *41*, 389–396. [CrossRef] [PubMed]

134. Shutov, L.P.; Kim, M.S.; Houlihan, P.R.; Medvedeva, Y.V.; Usachev, Y.M. Mitochondria and plasma membrane Ca^{2+}-ATPase control presynaptic Ca^{2+} clearance in capsaicin-sensitive rat sensory neurons. *J. Physiol.* **2013**, *591*, 2443–2462. [CrossRef] [PubMed]

135. Medvedeva, Y.V.; Kim, M.S.; Usachev, Y.M. Mechanisms of prolonged presynaptic Ca^{2+} signaling and glutamate release induced by TRPV1 activation in rat sensory neurons. *J. Neurosci.* **2008**, *28*, 5295–5311. [CrossRef] [PubMed]

136. Stout, A.K.; Raphael, H.M.; Kanterewicz, B.I.; Klann, E.; Reynolds, I.J. Glutamate-induced neuron death requires mitochondrial calcium uptake. *Nat. Neurosci.* **1998**, *1*, 366–373. [PubMed]

137. Halestrap, A.P. What is the mitochondrial permeability transition pore? *J. Mol. Cell. Cardiol.* **2009**, *46*, 821–831. [CrossRef] [PubMed]

138. Kim, S.R.; Lee, D.Y.; Chung, E.S.; Oh, U.T.; Kim, S.U.; Jin, B.K. Transient receptor potential vanilloid subtype 1 mediates cell death of mesencephalic dopaminergic neurons in vivo and in vitro. *J. Neurosci.* **2005**, *25*, 662–671. [CrossRef] [PubMed]

139. Shin, C.Y.; Shin, J.; Kim, B.M.; Wang, M.H.; Jang, J.H.; Surh, Y.J.; Oh, U. Essential role of mitochondrial permeability transition in vanilloid receptor 1-dependent cell death of sensory neurons. *Mol. Cell. Neurosci.* **2003**, *24*, 57–68. [CrossRef]

140. Hongpaisan, J.; Winters, C.A.; Andrews, S.B. Strong calcium entry activates mitochondrial superoxide generation, upregulating kinase signaling in hippocampal neurons. *J. Neurosci.* **2004**, *24*, 10878–10887. [CrossRef] [PubMed]

141. Kim, H.Y.; Lee, K.Y.; Lu, Y.; Wang, J.; Cui, L.; Kim, S.J.; Chung, J.M.; Chung, K. Mitochondrial Ca^{2+} uptake is essential for synaptic plasticity in pain. *J. Neurosci.* **2011**, *31*, 12982–12991. [CrossRef] [PubMed]

142. Schwartz, E.S.; Kim, H.Y.; Wang, J.; Lee, I.; Klann, E.; Chung, J.M.; Chung, K. Persistent pain is dependent on spinal mitochondrial antioxidant levels. *J. Neurosci.* **2009**, *29*, 159–168. [CrossRef] [PubMed]

143. Duchen, M.R. Roles of mitochondria in health and disease. *Diabetes* **2004**, *53* (Suppl. S1), 96–102. [CrossRef]

144. Dedov, V.N.; Mandadi, S.; Armati, P.J.; Verkhratsky, A. Capsaicin-induced depolarisation of mitochondria in dorsal root ganglion neurons is enhanced by vanilloid receptors. *Neuroscience* **2001**, *103*, 219–226. [CrossRef]

145. Goll, D.E.; Thompson, V.F.; Li, H.; Wei, W.; Cong, J. The calpain system. *Physiol. Rev.* **2003**, *83*, 731–801. [CrossRef] [PubMed]

146. Chiang, H.; Ohno, N.; Hsieh, Y.L.; Mahad, D.J.; Kikuchi, S.; Komuro, H.; Hsieh, S.T.; Trapp, B.D. Mitochondrial fission augments capsaicin-induced axonal degeneration. *Acta Neuropathol.* **2015**, *129*, 81–96. [CrossRef] [PubMed]

147. Bautista, D.M.; Movahed, P.; Hinman, A.; Axelsson, H.E.; Sterner, O.; Högestätt, E.D.; Julius, D.; Jordt, S.E.; Zygmunt, P.M. Pungent products from garlic activate the sensory ion channel TRPA1. *Proc. Natl. Acad. Sci. USA* **2005**, *102*, 12248–12252. [CrossRef] [PubMed]

148. Iadarola, M.J.; Gonnella, G.L. Resiniferatoxin for pain treatment: An interventional approach to personalized pain medicine. *Open Pain J.* **2013**, *6*, 95–107. [CrossRef] [PubMed]

149. Ghilardi, J.R.; Rohrich, H.; Lindsay, T.H.; Sevcik, M.A.; Schwei, M.J.; Kubota, K.; Halvorson, K.G.; Poblete, J.; Chaplan, S.R.; Dubin, A.E.; et al. Selective blockade of the capsaicin receptor TRPV1 attenuates bone cancer pain. *J. Neurosci.* **2005**, *25*, 3126–3131. [CrossRef] [PubMed]

150. Chen, J.; Winston, J.H.; Sarna, S.K. Neurological and cellular regulation of visceral hypersensitivity induced by chronic stress and colonic inflammation in rats. *Neuroscience* **2013**, *248*, 469–478. [CrossRef] [PubMed]

151. Li, Y.; Cai, J.; Han, Y.; Xiao, X.; Meng, X.L.; Su, L.; Liu, F.Y.; Xing, G.G.; Wan, Y. Enhanced function of TRPV1 via up-regulation by insulin-like growth factor-1 in a rat model of bone cancer pain. *Eur. J. Pain* **2014**, *18*, 774–784. [CrossRef] [PubMed]

152. Hudson, L.J.; Bevan, S.; Wotherspoon, G.; Gentry, C.; Fox, A.; Winter, J. VR1 protein expression increases in undamaged DRG neurons after partial nerve injury. *Eur. J. Neurosci.* **2001**, *13*, 2105–2114. [CrossRef] [PubMed]

153. Kim, Y.S.; Chu, Y.; Han, L.; Li, M.; Li, Z.; Lavinka, P.C.; Sun, S.; Tang, Z.; Park, K.; Caterina, M.J.; et al. Central terminal sensitization of TRPV1 by descending serotonergic facilitation modulates chronic pain. *Neuron* **2014**, *81*, 873–887. [CrossRef] [PubMed]

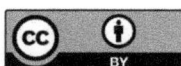

pharmaceuticals

MDPI

Review

Resiniferatoxin: The Evolution of the "Molecular Scalpel" for Chronic Pain Relief

Dorothy Cimino Brown

Department of Clinical Studies—Philadelphia, School of Veterinary Medicine, University of Pennsylvania, Philadelphia, PA 19104, USA; dottie@vet.upenn.edu; Tel.: +1-215-898-0030

Academic Editor: Arpad Szallasi
Received: 1 June 2016; Accepted: 9 August 2016; Published: 11 August 2016

Abstract: Control of chronic pain is frequently inadequate or can be associated with debilitating side effects. Ablation of certain nociceptive neurons, while retaining all other sensory modalities and motor function, represents a new therapeutic approach to controlling severe pain while avoiding off-target side effects. transient receptor potential cation channel subfamily V member 1 (TRPV1) is a calcium permeable nonselective cation channel expressed on the peripheral and central terminals of small-diameter sensory neurons. Highly selective chemoablation of TRPV1-containing peripheral nerve endings, or the entire TRPV1-expressing neuron itself, can be used to control chronic pain. Administration of the potent TRPV1 agonist resiniferatoxin (RTX) to neuronal perikarya or nerve terminals induces calcium cytotoxicity and selective lesioning of the TRPV1-expressing nociceptive primary afferent population. This selective neuroablation has been coined "molecular neurosurgery" and has the advantage of sparing motor, proprioceptive, and other somatosensory functions that are so important for coordinated movement, performing activities of daily living, and maintaining quality of life. This review examines the mechanisms and preclinical data underlying the therapeutic use of RTX and examples of such use for the management of chronic pain in clinical veterinary and human pain states.

Keywords: TRPV1; resiniferatoxin; chronic pain; analgesia

1. Introduction

Nearly two decades of preclinical research supports the involvement of thermoTRP channels in nociceptive transmission and sensitization. The identification of potent, subtype selective agonists and antagonists that demonstrate attractive preclinical pharmacological activity have generated extensive pharmaceutical interest for effective management of chronic pain patients without the need for long-term use of opioid or non-steroidal anti-inflammatory drugs. transient receptor potential cation channel subfamily V member 1 (TRPV1) is the most extensively studied mammalian transient receptor potential channel (TRP) channel with the potential for life changing pain control, particularly in patients with intractable chronic pain states [1–5].

TRPV1 is a calcium permeable non-selective cation channel with expression restricted to small and medium sized sensory neurons in the dorsal root, trigeminal, and vagal ganglia [6–8]. These neurons form the unmyelinated or thinly myelinated C and Aδ sensory nerve fibers that project to most organs and tissues. Functionally, TRPV1 acts as a sensor for noxious heat (>~42 °C) and can also be activated by acidic solutions (pH < 6.5), as well as some endogenous lipid-derived molecules. However, it is the discovery of the agonist actions of some plant derived compounds such as capsaicin and resiniferatoxin (RTX) that are the focus of pharmaceutical development for long-term chronic pain relief. The understanding of the mode of action of the known TRPV1 ligands including RTX is a continually evolving area of research and is pivotal to a successful drug design approach to the management of chronic pain [9–12].

Resiniferatoxin, derived from the *Euphorbia resinifera* plant, is the most potent amongst all known endogenous and synthetic agonists for TRPV1. RTX causes extremely prolonged channel opening and calcium influx, which results in cytotoxicity to the TRPV1-positive pain fibers or cell bodies [13]. When applied to the sensory neuron perikarya, the prolonged calcium influx induced by RTX specifically deletes only the sensory neurons that express the TRPV1 ion channel. Thus, intrathecal and intraganglionic RTX administration leads to selective targeting and permanent deletion of the TRPV1-expressing Aδ and C-fiber neuronal cell bodies in the dorsal root ganglia (DRG) [14,15]. Loss of these sensory neurons interrupts the transmission of pain information from the body to second-order spinal cord neurons, which in turn convey the information to the brain. At the same time, noxious and nonnoxious mechanosensation, proprioception, and locomotor capability are retained [14]. This highly selective chemoablation of specific neurons has been coined "molecular neurosurgery" and RTX coined a "molecular scalpel" in this novel approach that is under study for the permanent control of chronic pain [16].

This review examines the development of RTX to control intractable pain conditions through the permanent deletion of TRPV1 positive sensory nerve fibers. It describes the main studies on RTX mechanism of action and the animal translational research that formed the basis of the human clinical trial currently underway evaluating the use of intrathecal RTX for intractable pain in patients with advanced cancer.

2. Resiniferatoxin Is a Mechanism Based Treatment for Chronic Pain

The vision to develop RTX for control of intractable pain chronic pain states began with studies utilizing live cell microscopic evaluation of stably transfected cell lines expressing a TRPV1eGFP fusion protein [17,18]. Olah et al. used ratiometric imaging of intracellular free calcium and confocal imaging of the TRPV1-green fluorescent fusion protein to demonstrate that the endocannabinoid anandamide, could induce an elevation of intracellular free calcium, resulting in intracellular membrane changes in DRG neurons or transfected cells expressing TRPV1. The subsequent fragmentation of the endoplasmic reticulum and mitochondria could result in intracellular dysfunction and axonal damage of TRPV1-positive DRG neurons. If the cell bodies of nociceptors were exposed to anandamide, cell death could ensue through toxic accumulation of calcium [17].

As an ultrapotent vanilloid, RTX, was shown to bind with nanomolar affinity to TRPV1 or TRPV1eGFP positive cells causing prolonged opening of the TRPV1 ion channel with a rapid and massive increase in intracellular calcium [13]. Confocal imaging revealed that within 1 min, RTX induced vesiculation of the mitochondria and the endoplasmic reticulum of the nociceptive primary sensory neurons endogenously expressing TRPV1 due to a sudden increase in calcium. Within 5–10 min nuclear membrane disruption occurred, and cell lysis was documented within 1–2 h followed by specific deletion of TRPV1-expressing cells [18].

Importantly, the presence of TRPV1 is critical for this RTX action. Without expression of TRPV1, RTX at concentrations 1000 times above the dose used to lesion expressing cells, nerve terminals or axons does not appear to produce any negative effects on non-TRPV1-expressing cells at the cellular level. Non-expressing neurons appear to remain intact even when they are adjacent to TRPV1 expressing neurons that are undergoing damage from RTX activation. These conclusions were reached using the live cell imaging of cultured DRG neurons and the imaging of cells transiently and stably transfected with TRPV1 in the studies described above. In addition, Caudle et al demonstrated that RTX application to DRG cells known to express V1, induced large inward currents that were not induced in DRG cells that do not express the receptor [19].

These data demonstrate that vanilloids can disrupt vital organelles within the cell body of sensory ganglia and RTX, as an ultrapotent vanilloid, might be used to rapidly and selectively delete nociceptive neurons. The next step towards the goal of using RTX in the clinical setting to elicit sustained pain relief was to demonstrate the histopathological and behavioral effects of deletion of subpopulations of primary afferent pain-sensing neurons via central administration of RTX into the cerebrospinal fluid or ganglia in vivo.

3. Preclinical Studies in Laboratory Animals

Sensory neurons in the dorsal root and trigeminal ganglia collect noxious information from well-defined anatomic areas throughout the body. Targeting specific ganglia for treatment with RTX could, therefore, offer relief of well-localized pain. To ablate the sensory neurons, RTX needs to be injected centrally, either directly into the sensory ganglia or administered intrathecally to target the ganglionic nerve roots. Both approaches have been investigated in animal models.

3.1. Corneal Application of Capsaicin

In rats, RTX can be microinjected unilaterally into the trigeminal ganglia using a transcranial stereotaxic approach [14] or a percutaneous approach using an electrical-stimulation needle inserted through the infraorbital foramen [20]. Then, 24 h after injection, an analgesic effect can be documented using the eye-wipe response to corneal application of capsaicin, which is a sensitive test for C-fiber function. Complete suppression of the eye-wiping response evoked by intraocular capsaicin drops was obtained with 200 ng of RTX. The eye-wiping response did not return by the termination of the experiments 350 days after injection suggesting a permanent antinociceptive effect from a single intraganglionic injection. In a similar study, 20 µL RTX solution (0.1 mg/mL concentration) was infused unilaterally in nonhuman primate trigeminal ganglia [21]. Animals were tested for number of eye blinks, eye wipes, and duration of squinting in response to the corneal application of capsaicin for up to 12 weeks after RTX infusion. As it was documented in the rats, the response to capsaicin stimulation in the monkeys was selectively and significantly reduced throughout the duration of the study. The eye-wipe response to corneal application of capsaicin has also been used to document the selective deletion of TRPV1 positive sensory neurons in C57BL/6J mice [22]. The amount of 100 µg RTX or vehicle alone was injected into the cerebrospinal fluid at the cisterna magna. The RTX-treated mice were completely insensitive to the corneal application of capsaicin, while vehicle-treated C57BL/6J mice had a response similar to non-treated animals.

The selectivity of this analgesic approach of sensory neuron ablation was demonstrated with immunohistochemical analysis of the RTX-treated ganglia showing selective elimination of TRPV1-positive neurons. The animals showed no neurological deficits or signs of toxicity. There were no corneal damage or observable alterations in eating or grooming habits that might indicate the presence of a sensory dysesthesia and the loss of capsaicin chemosensitivity did not affect the mechanosensitive response of the corneal reflex. The animals blinked momentarily in response to the liquid droplet itself touching the eye on application.

3.2. Intraplantar Capsaicin and Carrageenan

Following the intrathecal administration of RTX in adult rats, nocifensive behavior was tested with the intraplantar injection of capsaicin [23,24]. A dramatic decrease in pain sensitivity was observed as indicated by reduction in both the duration and number of guarding and licking behaviors exhibited by the rats. The selective alleviation of inflammatory thermal hypersensitivity with intrathecal RTX was also tested [23]. Inflammation was induced by 100 µL of 2% carrageenan in the paw and the intrathecal RTX treated animals showed no change in the paw withdrawal latency due to inflammation.

In these studies, the selectivity of this analgesic approach was demonstrated by further testing, showing that intrathecal RTX did not affect paw withdrawal latency to von Frey filaments after inflammation. This observation is consistent with the notion that RTX treatment does not affect mechanical hypersensitivity due to inflammation because mechanical sensitivity is carried by a distinct set of nociceptors that do not express TRPV1. In addition, immunohistochemistry documented a complete loss of TRPV1 labeling in the dorsal horn of the spinal cord that was localized to the lumbar spinal segments closest to the level of the intrathecal injection [23].

3.3. Noxious Thermal Stimulation

In dogs, behavioral testing was performed to establish baseline paw withdrawal latency to a radiant thermal stimulus. The unrestrained animal was placed on a glass-top table, and a focused radiant halogen heat source was positioned under a paw. When the dog lifted its limb, the time in seconds was recorded, and the heat source was terminated. A maximum exposure time of 20 s was allowed to prevent injury to the animal. Under general anesthesia, RTX was then administered intrathecally into the cisterna magna at 0.1, 1.2, or 3 µg/kg. Two days after treatment, the 1.2 and 3.0 µg/kg doses caused nearly complete loss of sensitivity to noxious thermal stimulation. Compared with pretreatment values, limb withdrawal latency was substantially increased, to the point of cutoff. The effect was maintained when behavior testing was repeated 5, 7, 10, and 12 days after RTX administration [25].

On repeated neurologic examinations following injection, no negative effects from intrathecal RTX were documented. All dogs maintained normal locomotor and proprioceptive activities. At necropsy, all gross and histopathologic findings associated with the spinal cord and spinal canal were consistent with intrathecal catheter placement. In addition, blood and urine collected before one and two weeks after RTX administration revealed no significant increases or decreases of parameters out of the normal range.

3.4. Operant Orofacial Assay

To account for the fact that pain is ultimately experienced as a culmination of complex information from the periphery, Neubert et al. used an operant orofacial assay to evaluate and characterize thermal pain sensitivity in mice [22]. Operant systems utilize a reward-conflict platform, in which animals choose between receiving a reward or escaping an unpleasant stimulus. The animals control the amount of nociceptive stimulation and modify their behavior based on cerebral processing. The mice completed a reward-conflict task whereby they would contact a thermode with their face to access a reward bottle, generating an electrical signal that was acquired for analysis. They documented that TRPV1 knock out mice were insensitive to noxious heat within the activation range of TRPV1 (37–52 °C) and, in addition, mice treated with intracisternal RTX, had significantly higher licks as compared to the vehicle treated animals when tested with the thermode in the noxious heat range.

While operant assays are not new [26,27] the renewed interest in their use stems from the growing frustration over the mounting failures in translating basic scientific data into clinically available analgesics using conventional animal models. The lack of success has been attributed to both unacceptable side effects and lack of efficacy in humans of interventions that appeared to be safe and effective in animal models [28]. The use of operant measures is suggested as one approach to overcome this translational gap based on several examples of discordance between the results obtained using operant versus reflexive measures in the same study, with the operant measure agreeing with the clinical outcome [29].

In addition to designing studies that use operant as opposed to reflexive outcome measures, a variety of other recommendations have been made in the hope of improving the ability of animal studies to predict clinical trial outcomes. These include the utilization of animal models that are more directly applicable to prevalent painful conditions in people, as well as using outcomes that measure spontaneous behaviors and a broader range of "quality of life" [28,30–32]. With these recommendations in mind, the development of intrathecal RTX for intractable chronic pain states moved to studies in companion dogs with the spontaneous development of bone cancer pain.

4. Preclinical Studies in Companion Dogs

4.1. Rationale

Because studies in laboratory animals, mainly rodents, with experimentally induced pain states have only been partially successful in predicting human clinical trial outcomes, supplementing drug development with additional models can provide an informative transitional step for translating novel treatments to human patients. There is growing interest in using the diseases that spontaneously develop in companion (pet) dogs to investigate efficacy of new pharmacological agents and interventional administration approaches. The interest stems from the fact that:

- The spontaneously developed diseases can be pathologically, physiologically and symptomatically analogous to those in people [32–36].
- Medical surveillance of dogs is second only to that of people and illnesses are managed by veterinary specialists using all of the diagnostic approaches of modern medicine [37].
- Dogs share the environment with people and thus the potential environmental risk factors for disease.
- Their large body size simplifies biologic sampling.
- The extended course of disease, compared to rodent models, allows for clinically relevant efficacy data collection, while the shorter overall lifespan of dogs, compared to humans, provides a time course of disease within a time-frame reasonable for efficient data collection.
- Outcome assessment instruments have been specifically developed to capture clinically and translationally relevant pain severity and pain impact data in these models [38].
- Dogs have significant intrabreed homogeneity coupled with marked interbreed heterogeneity, providing unique opportunities to understand the genetic underpinnings of disease [39].
- The spontaneous pain caused by these naturally occurring diseases requires treatment for the animals' sake, and carefully studying novel therapies in these dogs can provide greater insight into the potential efficacy in humans [25,40,41].

Keeping in mind that a goal in using RTX in the clinical setting is to elicit sustained pain relief through deletion of subpopulations of primary afferent pain-sensing neurons, particularly in intractable conditions, an obvious target population is the 75% to 90% of patients with advanced cancer that experience significant, life-altering, cancer-induced pain [42]. The most severe pain is especially associated with tumors involving bone destruction. In the evaluation of RTX efficacy for chronic pain, the naturally occurring companion dog model of bone cancer pain has been instrumental in documenting analgesic efficacy and potential side effects; as well as informing future clinical trial design, justifying the starting dose, and selection of outcome measures and primary endpoints [14,25,40,43].

4.2. Canine Bone Cancer

The spontaneous development of bone cancer is common in companion dogs and bears striking resemblance to bone cancer in humans (Figure 1). In both species, osteosarcoma is histologically indistinguishable and has the same biologic behavior and disease progression [44]. For a variety of reasons, many owners do not choose the standard-of-care management for their dogs with appendicular osteosarcoma, which is amputation followed by chemotherapy. For these animals, the goal is to maintain the dog's comfort and quality of life for as long as possible. The issues associated with managing pain in dogs with bone cancer parallel those that occur in human cancer patients. Over time pain severity becomes refractory to conventional pain management as the disease progresses [44–46]. Dogs often undergo euthanasia within several months of diagnosis due to uncontrolled bone pain and associated loss of function. This evolution of bone pain over weeks to months allows enough time to evaluate the effectiveness of antinociceptive agents through the evolution of the pain process including episodes of break through pain. This time is still short enough, however, to ensure rapid accrual of data through detailed prospective studies.

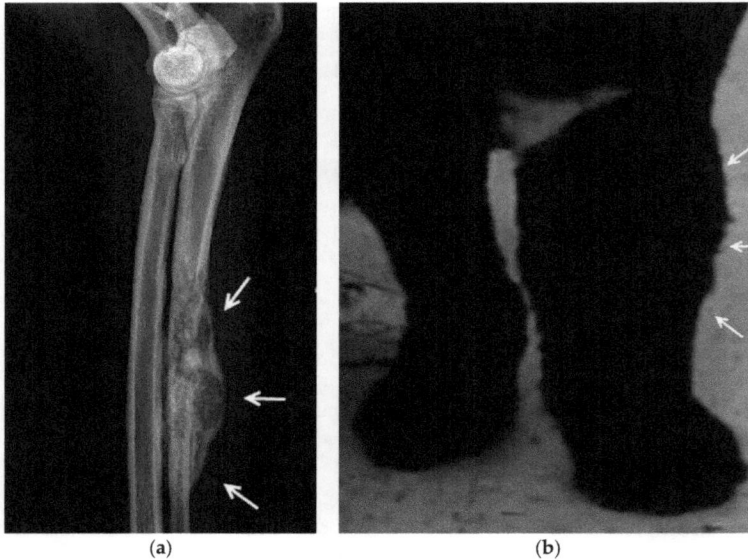

(a)   (b)

Figure 1. An example of canine bone cancer: (**a**) A radiograph of the left radius and ulna reveals a severe moth eaten osteolytic lesion of the ulna (white arrows); (**b**) Compared to the right forelimb there is marked swelling of the left forelimb (white arrows) due to edema associated with the underlying bone tumor.

4.2.1. Outcomes

In addition to identifying animal models that more closely represent the prevalent human disease conditions, much attention has been paid to the choice of outcomes in animal studies with a call to use outcomes that measure spontaneous behaviors and a broader range of 'quality of life' measures as opposed to evoked responses [28,31,32]. In addition to laboratory based measures, such as gait analysis to quantify lameness [47], a variety of clinically relevant outcomes measures have been validated in dogs to capture changes in spontaneous pain-related behaviors and overall quality of life, over extended periods of time, in the animal's home environment. Watch-sized, accelerometer based activity monitors can be unobtrusively worn on the dogs' collar to collect activity data for weeks or months at a time, while the dog performs its routine activities of daily living in its home environment. Increased activity levels can be documented in dogs with chronic painful conditions when appropriate anti-inflammatories and analgesics are administered [41,48]. In addition, much like the proxy assessment of pain behaviors in young children or cognitively impaired populations, owner assessments of chronic pain behaviors in their dogs have been validated [49–51]. These assessments allow the measurement of pain severity and its impact on the dogs function as well as overall quality of life. In some cases, these measures were developed to specifically to not only reliably quantify chronic pain behaviors in dogs, but also to have translational relevance to human studies [38]. Several of these measures were used to quantify the severity of chronic pain and its impact on the function of dogs treated with intrathecal RTX.

4.2.2. Analgesic Efficacy of RTX

To generate preclinical data supporting the fact that intrathecal RTX could provide effective pain relief and improve function in bone cancer pain, a single-blind, controlled study in 72 companion dogs with bone cancer was implemented [40]. Dogs were randomized to standard of care analgesic therapy alone or 1.2 mg/kg intrathecal RTX in addition to standard of care analgesic therapy. To maintain owner blinding, all dogs were admitted to the hospital for randomization and the fur was clipped over the intravenous catheter and intrathecal injection sites. While only the dogs randomized to the RTX group were anesthetized and underwent intrathecal injection, all dogs were hospitalized overnight to allow treated dogs to fully recover and were discharged the next day from the hospital to owners who were unaware as to which group their dog was randomized. Dogs were evaluated two weeks after the randomization visit and then at monthly intervals until death. Unblinding occurred when an owner believed that their dog had an unacceptable level of discomfort and required an intervention or at the time of spontaneous death or euthanasia of the dog.

Five efficacy outcomes were evaluated in this study. Although both of the primary outcomes and the lameness secondary outcome revealed a positive effect of RTX, the owner pain scores did not. This could be attributable to the loss of study power due to seven dogs in the treated group undergoing euthanasia prior to the two-week endpoint and the incidence of spinal headache in some of the RTX treated dogs. The negative behaviors associated with a spinal headache—lethargy, lack of interaction with the family, and inappetance—in the first week after randomization could influence the owners' pain assessment. Overall, dogs in the control group required unblinding significantly sooner than dogs that had been treated with RTX. 78% of dogs in the control group required unblinding and adjustment in analgesic protocol or euthanasia within six weeks of randomization, while only 50% of the dogs treated with RTX required unblinding and adjustment in analgesic protocol or euthanasia in that same time frame. Analgesic efficacy was also documented by an orthopedist, blinded to treatment group, who evaluated lameness through video analysis and determined that 7% of dogs in the control group had improved lameness while 33% of dogs in the RTX-treated group had improved lameness two weeks after randomization. While these differences between groups were statistically significant and support the analgesic efficacy of intrathecal RTX in bone cancer pain, it was clear that there was variability in response in the RTX treated dogs.

The variability in the response to RTX may be associated with the varying degree of TRPV1 expression on the small to medium sized DRG neurons that can be documented with immunocytochemical staining [52]. It is possible that high expressing neurons are the most susceptible to RTX cytotoxicity, while lower expressing neurons may be able to sequester a minor influx of calcium and survive transient exposure to RTX, making them less susceptible. Low expressing neurons may remain intact and continue to transmit clinically relevant pain signals and some neurons that are damaged but repair with time may eventually resume transmitting clinically relevant pain signals. In these cases, it is possible that retreatment would lead to a renewed clinical response. Retreatment was offered for dogs that had initially responded to RTX but had recurrence of chronic pain, however the owners opted not to retreat due to the advanced nature of their dogs' disease.

Upon necropsy, the DRG of treated dogs revealed RTX-related effects. Within one month post injection, degenerating neurons are in the process of being replaced by rosettes of proliferating satellite cells. Neurons with larger cell body diameters remain unaffected, even in the immediate vicinity of a degenerating neuron [25]. These histologic findings reflect the observed, analgesic effect that occurs in the dogs with the retention of other sensory and proprioceptive functions. In fact, the analgesic effect was documented in the dogs with bone cancer without any evidence of development of neurologic abnormalities that can be seen with neurolytic therapies.

4.2.3. Adverse Events

Significant increases in blood pressure and heart rate can occur after intrathecal RTX injection in dogs. These cardiovascular effects peak within minutes of injection and return to baseline over the hour that the dog remains anesthetized through the period of TRPV1 activation. Immediately after extubation, many dogs pant for several hours, during which they develop hypothermia that plateaus 3 to 4 h after extubation. Even the most hypothermic animals—those that drop core body temperature more than 4 °C after injection—otherwise make an uneventful recovery and regain normothermia in 12 to 18 h [40].

A serious adverse event that can be seen with neurolytic therapies is deafferentation pain syndromes. Complete or partial interruption of afferent nerve impulses can lead to central sensitization, with patients experiencing abnormal sensory phenomena such as allodynia, hyperalgesia, dysesthesias, and hyperpathia [53,54]. In animals, deafferentation can lead to self-mutilation, biting the region in which they might feel painful, or paresthetic sensations [55–57]. Behaviors consistent with development of deafferentation pain syndromes did not occur in any dogs treated with RTX. The lack of long-term negative effects is important for the clinical translation of RTX. However, there were several acute perinjection effects of RTX noted. Significant increases in blood pressure and heart rate occurred after intrathecal RTX injection in many dogs. These effects typically peak within five min of injection and then gradually return to baseline over the hour that the dog remains anesthetized through the excitation phase of TRPV1 activation. Upon recovery from general anesthesia, many dogs begin panting heavily and can continue to do so for several hours, during which time they tend to become hypothermic. The hypothermia can be significant and persist for many hours, however it does not prohibit the dogs from otherwise making an uneventful recovery [25,40].

While the preclinical laboratory animal studies provided the necessary mechanistic insights into how to use RTX as a therapeutic agent; the canine companion animal bone cancer studies showed that RTX worked well on the complex pain state that develops due to naturally occurring cancer. These studies were the impetus to move intrathecal RTX into human clinical trials.

5. The Clinical Trial

Intrathecal RTX is undergoing a Phase I clinical trial to treat refractory severe pain in patients with advanced cancer. Serial electrocardiogram, brain and spine MRI, eye exam, blood analysis and neurological exam and tools measuring pain, quality of life, active and mental status are used to assess patients pre- and post-injection. An intrathecal catheter is placed and the injection performed under anesthesia to prevent the acute pain that accompanies excitotoxic actions of RTX on TRPV1 neurons. To date, patients have received 3 to 26 µg of RTX into the intrathecal space. While patients receiving the lower doses experienced variable amounts of pain relief, those who received either 13 or 26 µg injections of RTX, showed a clinically meaningful improvement in quality of life following the single injection. These patients consistently reported less pain and improved mobility. No changes in EKG, MRI, or eye examination were noted. Thermal perception reduction was consistent with cell death of the TRPV1 neurons. There were no other sensory or motor changes post-treatment. These initial findings suggest that intrathecal RTX administration can selectively delete neurons that transmit pain. Additional accruals will further detail the safety and efficacy of RTX to reduce refractory pain and improve quality of life in patients with advanced cancer [52,58,59].

6. Conclusions

The vision to develop RTX for control of intractable pain conditions emerged from live cell imaging documenting that, as an ultra-potent TRPV1 agonist, RTX causes extremely prolonged channel opening and calcium influx resulting in cytotoxicity to the TRPV1-positive pain fibers or cell bodies [13,17,18]. The selectivity and behavioral effects of deletion of subpopulations of primary afferent pain-sensing neurons via central administration of RTX into the cerebrospinal fluid or ganglia was then documented in a variety of animal evoked pain models [14,20,22–25]. The final impetus to carry intrathecal RTX into human clinical trials emerged from the preclinical companion animal canine bone cancer studies [14,25,40]. These studies showed that this analgesic approach worked, not just in evoked pain models, but also in the complex pain state that originates from naturally occurring cancer. At the conclusion of these studies, the various elements necessary for a Phase I clinical trial in humans were assembled. Several cohorts of patients with advanced cancer have been recruited to date with promising results [58,59]. Additional accruals will further detail the safety and efficacy of RTX to reduce refractory pain and improve quality of life in patients with advanced cancer.

Acknowledgments: The authors would like to thank collaborators at NIH Michael Iadarola and Andrew Mannes; Molly Love and Michael DiGregorio at the Veterinary Clinical Investigations Center at the University of Pennsylvania for their intensive involvement in the canine RTX work over the years. The canine work was supported by the Division of Intramural Research, NIDCR, and NIDA (5K08DA017720)

Conflicts of Interest: The author declares no conflict of interest.

References

1. Bevan, S.; Quallo, T.; Andersson, D.A. TRPV1. *Handb. Exp. Pharmacol.* **2014**, *222*, 207–245. [PubMed]
2. Brederson, J.D.; Kym, P.R.; Szallasi, A. Targeting TRP channels for pain relief. *Eur. J. Pharmacol.* **2013**, *716*, 61–76. [CrossRef] [PubMed]
3. Iadarola, M.J.; Mannes, A.J. The vanilloid agonist resiniferatoxin for interventional-based pain control. *Curr. Top. Med. Chem.* **2011**, *11*, 2171–2179. [CrossRef] [PubMed]
4. Szallasi, A.; Sheta, M. Targeting TRPV1 for pain relief: Limits, losers and laurels. *Expert Opin. Investig. Drugs* **2012**, *21*, 1351–1369. [CrossRef] [PubMed]
5. Wong, G.Y.; Gavva, N.R. Therapeutic potential of vanilloid receptor TRPV1 agonists and antagonists as analgesics: Recent advances and setbacks. *Brain Res. Rev.* **2009**, *60*, 267–277. [CrossRef] [PubMed]
6. Helliwell, R.J.; McLatchie, L.M.; Clarke, M.; Winter, J.; Bevan, S.; McIntyre, P. Capsaicin sensitivity is associated with the expression of the vanilloid (capsaicin) receptor (VR1) mRNA in adult rat sensory ganglia. *Neurosci. Lett.* **1998**, *250*, 177–180. [CrossRef]
7. Tominaga, M.; Caterina, M.J. Thermosensation and pain. *J. Neurobiol.* **2004**, *61*, 3–12. [CrossRef] [PubMed]
8. Szallasi, A.; Blumberg, P.M. Vanilloid (Capsaicin) receptors and mechanisms. *Pharmacol. Rev.* **1999**, *51*, 159–212. [PubMed]
9. Elokely, K.; Velisetty, P.; Delemotte, L.; Palovcak, E.; Klein, M.L.; Rohacs, T.; Carnevale, V. Understanding TRPV1 activation by ligands: Insights from the binding modes of capsaicin and resiniferatoxin. *Proc. Natl. Acad. Sci. USA* **2016**, *113*, E137–E145. [CrossRef] [PubMed]
10. Gao, Y.; Cao, E.; Julius, D.; Cheng, Y. TRPV1 structures in nanodiscs reveal mechanisms of ligand and lipid action. *Nature* **2016**, *534*, 347–351. [CrossRef] [PubMed]
11. Yang, F.; Xiao, X.; Cheng, W.; Yang, W.; Yu, P.; Song, Z.; Yarov-Yarovoy, V.; Zheng, J. Structural mechanism underlying capsaicin binding and activation of the TRPV1 ion channel. *Nat. Chem. Biol.* **2015**, *11*, 518–524. [CrossRef] [PubMed]
12. Darre, L.; Furini, S.; Domene, C. Permeation and dynamics of an open-activated TRPV1 channel. *J. Mol. Biol.* **2015**, *427*, 537–549. [CrossRef] [PubMed]
13. Karai, L.J.; Russell, J.T.; Iadarola, M.J.; Oláh, Z. Vanilloid receptor 1 regulates multiple calcium compartments and contributes to Ca2+-induced Ca2+ release in sensory neurons. *J. Biol. Chem.* **2004**, *279*, 16377–16387. [CrossRef] [PubMed]
14. Karai, L.; Brown, D.C.; Mannes, A.J.; Connelly, S.T.; Brown, J.; Gandal, M.; Wellisch, O.M.; Neubert, J.K.; Olah, Z.; Iadarola, M.J. Deletion of vanilloid receptor 1-expressing primary afferent neurons for pain control. *J. Clin. Investig.* **2004**, *113*, 1344–1352. [CrossRef] [PubMed]
15. Caterina, M.J.; Rosen, T.A.; Tominaga, M.; Brake, A.J.; Julius, D. A capsaicin-receptor homologue with a high threshold for noxious heat. *Nature* **1999**, *398*, 436–441. [PubMed]
16. Wiley, R.G.; Lappi, D.A. Targeted toxins. *Curr. Protoc. Neurosci.* **2001**. [CrossRef]
17. Olah, Z.; Karai, L.; Iadarola, M.J. Anandamide activates vanilloid receptor 1 (VR1) at acidic pH in dorsal root ganglia neurons and cells ectopically expressing VR1. *J. Biol. Chem.* **2001**, *276*, 31163–31170. [CrossRef] [PubMed]
18. Olah, Z.; Szabo, T.; Karai, L.; Hough, C.; Fields, R.D.; Caudle, R.M.; Blumberg, P.M.; Iadarola, M.J. Ligand-induced dynamic membrane changes and cell deletion conferred by vanilloid receptor 1. *J. Biol. Chem.* **2001**, *276*, 11021–11030. [CrossRef] [PubMed]
19. Caudle, R.M.; Karai, L.; Mena, N.; Cooper, B.Y.; Mannes, A.J.; Perez, F.M.; Iadarola, M.J.; Olah, Z. Resiniferatoxin-induced loss of plasma membrane in vanilloid receptor expressing cells. *Neurotoxicology* **2003**, *24*, 895–908. [CrossRef]

20. Neubert, J.K.; Mannes, A.J.; Keller, J.; Wexel, M.; Iadarola, M.J.; Caudle, R.M. Peripheral targeting of the trigeminal ganglion via the infraorbital foramen as a therapeutic strategy. *Brain Res. Protoc.* **2005**, *15*, 119–126. [CrossRef] [PubMed]

21. Tender, G.C.; Walbridge, S.; Olah, Z.; Karai, L.; Iadarola, M.; Oldfield, E.H.; Lonser, R.R. Selective ablation of nociceptive neurons for elimination of hyperalgesia and neurogenic inflammation. *J. Neurosurg.* **2005**, *102*, 522–525. [CrossRef] [PubMed]

22. Neubert, J.K.; King, C.; Malphurs, W.; Wong, F.; Weaver, J.P.; Jenkins, A.C.; Rossi, H.L.; Caudle, R.M. Characterization of mouse orofacial pain and the effects of lesioning TRPV1-expressing neurons on operant behavior. *Mol. Pain* **2008**, *4*, 43. [CrossRef] [PubMed]

23. Jeffry, J.A.; Yu, S.Q.; Sikand, P.; Parihar, A.; Evans, M.S.; Premkumar, L.S. Selective targeting of TRPV1 expressing sensory nerve terminals in the spinal cord for long lasting analgesia. *PLoS ONE* **2009**, *4*, e7021. [CrossRef] [PubMed]

24. Bishnoi, M.; Bosgraaf, C.A.; Premkumar, L.S. Preservation of acute pain and efferent functions following intrathecal resiniferatoxin-induced analgesia in rats. *J. Pain* **2011**, *12*, 991–1003. [CrossRef] [PubMed]

25. Brown, D.C.; Iadarola, M.J.; Perkowski, S.Z.; Erin, H.; Shofer, F.; Laszlo, K.J.; Olah, Z.; Mannes, A.J. Physiologic and antinociceptive effects of intrathecal resiniferatoxin in a canine bone cancer model. *Anesthesiology* **2005**, *103*, 1052–1059. [CrossRef] [PubMed]

26. Vierck, C.J., Jr.; Hamilton, D.M.; Thornby, J.I. Pain reactivity of monkeys after lesions to the dorsal and lateral columns of the spinal cord. *Exp. Brain Res.* **1971**, *13*, 140–158. [CrossRef] [PubMed]

27. Dubner, R.; Beitel, R.E.; Brown, F.J. A Behavioral Animal Model for the Study of Pain Mechanisms in Primates. In *Pain: New Perspectives in Therapy and Research*; Weisenberg, M., Tursky, B., Eds.; Springer US: Boston, MA, USA, 1976; pp. 155–170.

28. Mogil, J.S. Animal models of pain: Progress and challenges. *Nat. Rev. Neurosci.* **2009**, *10*, 283–294. [CrossRef] [PubMed]

29. Vierck, C.J.; Hansson, P.T.; Yezierski, R.P. Clinical and pre-clinical pain assessment: Are we measuring the same thing? *Pain* **2008**, *135*, 7–10. [CrossRef] [PubMed]

30. Mogil, J.S.; Crager, S.E. What should we be measuring in behavioral studies of chronic pain in animals? *Pain* **2004**, *112*, 12–15. [CrossRef] [PubMed]

31. Blackburn-Munro, G. Pain-like behaviours in animals—How human are they? *Trends Pharmacol. Sci.* **2004**, *25*, 299–305. [CrossRef] [PubMed]

32. Rice, A.S.; Cimino-Brown, D.; Eisenach, J.C.; Kontinen, V.K.; Lacroix-Fralish, M.L.; Machin, I.; Mogil, J.S.; Stöhr, T. Animal models and the prediction of efficacy in clinical trials of analgesic drugs: A critical appraisal and call for uniform reporting standards. *Pain* **2008**, *139*, 243–247. [CrossRef] [PubMed]

33. Khanna, C.; Lindblad-Toh, K.; Vail, D.; London, C.; Bergman, P.; Barber, L.; Breen, M.; Kitchell, B.; McNeil, E.; Modiano, J.F.; Niemi, S. The dog as a cancer model. *Nat. Biotechnol.* **2006**, *24*, 1065–1066. [CrossRef] [PubMed]

34. Loscher, W. Animal models of intractable epilepsy. *Prog. Neurobiol.* **1997**, *53*, 239–258. [CrossRef]

35. Nowend, K.L.; Starr-Moss, A.N.; Murphy, K.E. The function of dog models in developing gene therapy strategies for human health. *Mamm. Genome* **2011**, *22*, 476–485. [CrossRef] [PubMed]

36. Vainio, O. Translational animal models using veterinary patients—An example of canine osteoarthritis (OA). *Scand. J. Pain* **2012**, *3*, 84–89. [CrossRef]

37. Ostrander, E.A.; Galibert, F.; Patterson, D.F. Canine genetics comes of age. *Trends Genet.* **2000**, *16*, 117–124. [CrossRef]

38. Brown, D.C.; Boston, R.; Coyne, J.C.; Farrar, J.T. A novel approach to the use of animals in studies of pain: Validation of the canine brief pain inventory in canine bone cancer. *Pain Med.* **2009**, *10*, 133–142. [CrossRef] [PubMed]

39. Shearin, A.L.; Ostrander, E.A. Leading the way: Canine models of genomics and disease. *Dis. Model. Mech.* **2010**, *3*, 27–34. [CrossRef] [PubMed]

40. Brown, D.C.; Agnello, K.; Iadarola, M.J. Intrathecal resiniferatoxin in a dog model: Efficacy in bone cancer pain. *Pain* **2015**, *156*, 1018–1024. [CrossRef] [PubMed]

41. Brown, D.C.; Agnello, K. Intrathecal substance P-saporin in the dog: Efficacy in bone cancer pain. *Anesthesiology* **2013**, *119*, 1178–1185. [CrossRef] [PubMed]

42. Luger, N.M.; Mach, D.B.; Sevcik, M.A.; Mantyh, P.W. Bone cancer pain: From model to mechanism to therapy. *J. Pain Symptom Manag.* **2005**, *29*, S32–S46. [CrossRef] [PubMed]

43. Mannes, A.J.; Brown, D.C.; Keller, J.; Cordes, L.; Eckenhoff, R.G.; Caudle, R.M.; Iadarola, M.J.; Meng, Q.C. Measurement of resiniferatoxin in serum samples by high-performance liquid chromatography. *J. Chromatogr. B* **2005**, *823*, 184–188. [CrossRef] [PubMed]

44. Withrow, S.J.; Powers, B.E.; Straw, R.C.; Wilkins, R.M. Comparative aspects of osteosarcoma: Dog versus man. *Clin. Orthop. Relat. Res.* **1991**, *270*, 159–168. [CrossRef] [PubMed]

45. MacEwen, E.G. Spontaneous tumors in dogs and cats: Models for the study of cancer biology and treatment. *Cancer Metast. Rev.* **1990**, *9*, 125–136. [CrossRef]

46. Mueller, F.; Fuchs, B.; Kaser-Hotz, B. Comparative biology of human and canine osteosarcoma. *Anticancer Res.* **2007**, *27*, 155–164. [PubMed]

47. Fan, T.M.; Charney, S.C.; De Lorimier, L.P.; Garrett, L.D.; Griffon, D.J.; Gordon-Evans, W.J.; Wypij, J.M. Double-blind placebo-controlled trial of adjuvant pamidronate with palliative radiotherapy and intravenous doxorubicin for canine appendicular osteosarcoma bone pain. *J. Vet. Intern. Med.* **2009**, *23*, 152–160. [CrossRef] [PubMed]

48. Brown, D.C.; Boston, R.C.; Farrar, J.T. Use of an activity monitor to detect response to treatment in dogs with osteoarthritis. *J. Am. Vet. Med. Assoc.* **2010**, *237*, 66–70. [CrossRef] [PubMed]

49. Brown, D.C.; Boston, R.C.; Coyne, J.C.; Farrar, J.T. Development and psychometric testing of an instrument designed to measure chronic pain in dogs with osteoarthritis. *Am. J. Vet. Res.* **2007**, *68*, 631–637. [CrossRef] [PubMed]

50. Brown, D.C.; Boston, R.C.; Coyne, J.C.; Farrar, J.T. Ability of the canine brief pain inventory to detect response to treatment in dogs with osteoarthritis. *J. Am. Vet. Med. Assoc.* **2008**, *233*, 1278–1283. [CrossRef] [PubMed]

51. Wiseman-Orr, M.L.; Scott, E.M.; Reid, J.; Nolan, A.M. Validation of a structured questionnaire as an instrument to measure chronic pain in dogs on the basis of effects on health-related quality of life. *Am. J. Vet. Res.* **2006**, *67*, 1826–1836. [CrossRef] [PubMed]

52. Brown, D.C.; Iadarola, M.J. TRPV1 Agonist Cytotoxicity for Chronic Pain Relief: From Mechanistic Understanding to Clinical Application A2—Szallasi, Arpad. In *TRP Channels as Therapeutic Targets*; Academic Press: Boston, MA, USA, 2015; pp. 99–118.

53. Davar, G.; Maciewicz, R.J. Deafferentation pain syndromes. *Neurol. Clin.* **1989**, *7*, 289–304. [PubMed]

54. Whitworth, L.A.; Feler, C.A. Application of spinal ablative techniques for the treatment of benign chronic painful conditions: history, methods, and outcomes. *Spine* **2002**, *27*, 2607–2612. [CrossRef] [PubMed]

55. Albe-Fessard, D. Neurophysical studies in rats deafferented by dorsal root sections. In *Deafferentation Pain Syndromes: Pathophysiology and Treatments*; Nashold, B., Ovelmen-Levitt, J., Eds.; Raven Press: New York, NY, USA, 1991; pp. 125–139.

56. Forterre, F.; Jaggy, A.; Malik, Y.; Howard, J.; Rüfenacht, S.; Spreng, D. Non-selective cutaneous sensory neurectomy as an alternative treatment for auto-mutilation lesion following arthrodesis in three dogs. *Vet. Comp. Orthop. Traumatol.* **2009**, *22*, 233–237. [CrossRef] [PubMed]

57. Kriz, N.; Yamamotova, A.; Tobias, J.; Rokyta, R. Tail-flick latency and self-mutilation following unilateral deafferentation in rats. *Physiol. Res.* **2006**, *55*, 213–220. [PubMed]

58. Heiss, J.; Iadarola, M.; Cantor, F.; Oughourli, A.; Smith, R.; Mannes, A. A Phase I study of the intrathecal administration of resiniferatoxin for treating severe refractory pain associated with advanced cancer. *J. Pain* **2014**, *15*, S67. [CrossRef]

59. Mannes, A.; Hughes, M.; Quezado, Z.; Berger, A.; Fojo, T.; Smith, R.; Butman, J.; Lonser, R.; Iadarola, M. Resiniferatoxin, a potent TRPV1 agonist: Intrathecal administration to treat severe pain associated with advanced cancer—Case report. *J. Pain* **2010**, *11*, S43. [CrossRef]

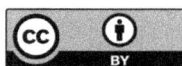

pharmaceuticals

MDPI

Review

TRPV1: A Target for Rational Drug Design

Vincenzo Carnevale [1,*] and Tibor Rohacs [2,*]

1   Institute for Computational Molecular Science, Temple University, Philadelphia, PA 19122, USA
2   New Jersey Medical School, Rutgers University, Newark, NJ 07103, USA
*   Correspondence: vincenzo.carnevale@temple.edu (V.C.); tibor.rohacs@rutgers.edu (T.R.);
    Tel.: +1-215-204-4214 (V.C.); +1-973-972-4464 (T.R.)

Academic Editors: Arpad Szallasi and Susan M. Huang
Received: 13 July 2016; Accepted: 18 August 2016; Published: 23 August 2016

Abstract: Transient Receptor Potential Vanilloid 1 (TRPV1) is a non-selective, Ca^{2+} permeable cation channel activated by noxious heat, and chemical ligands, such as capsaicin and resiniferatoxin (RTX). Many compounds have been developed that either activate or inhibit TRPV1, but none of them are in routine clinical practice. This review will discuss the rationale for antagonists and agonists of TRPV1 for pain relief and other conditions, and strategies to develop new, better drugs to target this ion channel, using the newly available high-resolution structures.

Keywords: TRPV1; capsaicin; vanilloid; pain; nociception

1. Introduction—TRP Channels

Transient Receptor Potential (TRP) channels were discovered while analyzing a visual mutant of drosophila that showed transient response to light, as opposed to the sustained receptor potential in wild type flies [1]. Unlike in mammals, invertebrate vision is initiated by the activation of a Phospholipase C (PLC) enzyme, which hydrolyzes the membrane phospholipid phosphatidylinositol 4,5-bisphosphate (PIP_2) to form the two classical second messengers inositol 1,4,5 trisphosphate (IP_3) and Diacylglycerol (DAG). Despite decades of research, it is still unclear how this enzymatic cascade activates the channel responsible for generating the receptor potential in insects. This channel complex includes dTRP protein, mutation of which was responsible for the transient light response [2]. Based on sequence homology, mammalian orthologues of the dTRP channel were soon cloned; the seven mammalian TRPs with the closest homology to dTRP were designated as Classical, or Canonical TRPs, or TRPCs [3]. Two additional major subfamilies (TRPV and TRPM) and three smaller subfamilies (TRPA, TRPN, and TRPML) were identified; together with TRPCs they comprise the mammalian TRP (super) family. TRP channels are highly diverse; it is impossible to succinctly summarize their functions. Two major general themes however stand out: regulation by the PLC pathway, and involvement in sensory transduction. The closest mammalian homologs of the dTRP channel, TRPCs are all stimulated downstream of PLC coupled receptor activation, and several other TRP channels are modulated by this pathway [4]. TRP channels are involved in a variety of sensory functions; their roles are best established in thermosensation [5]. Mutations in TRP channels cause human diseases as diverse as kidney disease (TRPC6), spontaneous pain syndrome (TRPA1), hypomagnesemia (TRPM6), night blindness (TRPM1) and complex musculoskeletal and neurological disorders (TRPV4) [6]. Given their widespread physiological roles and relatively recent discovery, many of them are promising drug targets [7].

2. Sensory TRP Channels

TRP channels play various roles in all primary senses [8]. They initiate the visual signal in invertebrates, and TRPM1 in retinal on-bipolar cells plays an important role in visual transmission in mammals; its loss of function mutation causes stationary night blindness in humans [9]. TRPM5 knockout mice have altered sweet, bitter and umami taste sensation [10]. TRP channels play important roles in mechanosensation in invertebrates, but their role in mammals is controversial [11]. TRPC2 is important in pheromone sensation in rodents, but in humans it is a pseudogene [8]. As discussed below, the roles of TRP channels are best established in thermosensation, and chemical nociception [5,12]. To place TRPV1 channels in context, we first briefly discuss thermo- and somatosensory TRP channels other than TRPV1.

2.1. Heat Sensitive TRP Channels other than TRPV1

TRPV2 [13] is a capsaicin insensitive homolog of TRPV1, initially identified as a noxious heat sensor. It is activated with a heat threshold higher than that for TRPV1, and it is well expressed in peripheral sensory dorsal root ganglion (DRG) neurons [14]. Behavioral studies however found no difference in temperature sensation between TRPV2$^{-/-}$ and wild type mice, showing that this channel is unlikely to be a physiological heat sensor [15]. TRPV2 knockout mice show various abnormalities, such as macrophage phagocytosis [16], and maintenance of cardiac structure and function [17], highlighting the importance of these channels in functions other than thermosensation.

TRPV3 [18] is expressed in keratinocytes of the skin and it is activated by moderate heat [19]. These channels are sensitized and activated by various oregano, thyme and clove derived skin sensitizers, such as carvacrol, thymol and eugenol. While some studies reported defects in temperature sensation in TRPV3$^{-/-}$ mice, the effect depended on the genetic background [5]. In humans, gain of function mutations of TRPV3 lead to Olmsted syndrome, which is characterized by palmoplantar and periorificial keratoderma, alopecia and severe itching [20].

TRPV4 [21] is an osmosensor, but it is also activated by moderate heat. Similar to TRPV3, it is essentially undetectable in DRG neurons, but well expressed in keratinocytes [5]. TRPV4 knockout mice showed a mild defect in thermal preference [22].

TRPM3 is the most recent addition to the thermo-TRP family. These channels are expressed in small nociceptive DRG neurons; they are activated by heat, and chemical agonists such as pregnenolone sulfate [23]. Genetic deletion of these channels in mice leads to defects in noxious heat sensitivity [24].

2.2. Cold Sensitive TRP Channels

TRPM8 [25] is a well-established sensor of mild environmental cold temperatures. This channel is activated by cold, menthol, and other cooling agents, such as icilin [19,26,27]. Genetic deletion of these channels in mice leads to decreased sensitivity to moderate cold [28–30]. TRPM8 is also the main mediator of menthol-induced analgesia [31].

TRPA1 [32] was originally proposed to function as a noxious cold sensor [33]. This channel is also activated by a variety of noxious and pungent chemical compounds such as mustard oil and acrolein [34]. While it is very well established by now that this channel serves as a noxious chemical sensor, its cold activation is still controversial, detailed discussion of this controversy is beyond the scope of this chapter, and it was reviewed in detail recently [5,32].

TRPC5 channels [35], but not TRPC1/TRPC5 heteromers, were shown to be activated by cold temperatures, but genetic deletion of TRPC5 did not result in a change in cold sensitivity [36].

3. Physiological and Pathophysiological Roles of TRPV1

Similarly to most TRP channels, TRPV1 is an outwardly rectifying Ca^{2+} permeable non-selective cation channel. Its activators most often used in experiments are temperatures over 42 °C, capsaicin, and low extracellular pH. Resiniferatoxin (RTX) is an ultrapotent agonist of TRPV1 [37], it activates the channel at lower concentrations than capsaicin, but its effect also develops much slower [38]. Most likely due to its slowly developing effect [39], RTX is less pungent than capsaicin [40].

TRPV1 is one of the most promiscuous ion channels; it is activated by many endogenous [41] and exogenous compounds, including various painful arthropod toxins [42,43]. Endogenous regulators of TRPV1 include endovanilloids, such as anandamide and 2-Arachidonoylglycerol [44] and lysophosphatidic acid [45]. Most of these endogenous compounds, even at maximally effective concentrations, induce TRPV1 currents smaller than those evoked by saturating capsaicin concentrations. Interestingly, ethanol at high concentrations also activates TRPV1, an effect probably responsible for the pungency of concentrated spirits [46].

TRPV1 has been implicated in a plethora of physiological and pathophysiological functions, which have been extensively reviewed [47,48]. Below we will summarize the functions most relevant to its role as a drug target.

3.1. Functions Related to Expression in Peripheral Sensory Neurons

TRPV1 was first described in small nociceptive DRG and trigeminal ganglion (TG) neurons. Most sensory neurons innervating the urinary bladder also express TRPV1. This channel is also present in a large portion of neurons of the nodose and jugular sensory vagal ganglia [49] innervating the airways (see Section 3.1.3). The following three sections will briefly discuss the roles of TRPV1 in nociception, micturition, and airway hypersensitivity.

3.1.1. Nociceptive Heat Sensation and Thermal Hyperalgesia

Capsaicin, the chemical activator of TRPV1 evokes intense burning pain, and temperatures over ~42 °C induce a steep increase in channel activity with a ~20 fold change upon a 10 °C increase in temperature (Q_{10} ~20) [50]. These properties intuitively suggest that this channel functions as a noxious heat sensor. Surprisingly, initial studies in mice somewhat differed on the effect of genetic deletion of this channel on acute nociceptive heat sensation [51]. One knockout study found that TRPV1$^{-/-}$ mice showed altered responses to heat in the tail flick, radiant heat, and hot plate assays [52]. An independent study however found no difference in acute heat sensitivity between wild type and TRPV1$^{-/-}$ mice [53]. The same study, on the other hand, found that thermal hyperalgesia induced by inflammation was severely altered in the TRPV1 knockout mice [53]. Subsequent research with TRPV1$^{-/-}$ mice supported the role of TRPV1 as a noxious heat sensor having more pronounced defects at higher temperatures [15,54,55]. Also consistent with the role of TRPV1 as a noxious heat sensor is the finding that one of the key side effects of TRPV1 blockers in humans is the increase of the threshold for painful heat, and consequential accidental burns (see Section 4.1) [7].

When TRPV1 expressing sensory neurons were ablated using diphtheria toxin in mice, heat sensitivity was essentially eliminated [56]. The more robust phenotype of this mouse model compared to TRPV1$^{-/-}$ mice suggests the presence of other heat sensing ion channels in TRPV1 expressing neurons.

Thermal hyperalgesia, increased sensitivity to heat, is a hallmark of inflammatory pain. In mouse models, genetic deletion of TRPV1 essentially eliminated thermal hyperalgesia induced by inflammation in two independent TRPV1$^{-/-}$ lines [52,53], demonstrating the importance of these channels in this phenomenon. In principle, there are two mechanisms by which TRPV1 activity can increase and thus induce thermal hypersensitivity: higher expression levels, and increased sensitivity/activity. Increased expression of TRPV1 at the RNA and protein levels has been reported both in inflammatory models [57], and in response to application of inflammatory mediators such as Nerve Growth Factor (NGF) [58]. In addition, NGF was shown to increase the number of functional TRPV1 channels in the plasma membrane by PI3K mediated increase in trafficking [59,60]. In contrast to NGF, stimulation of pro-inflammatory G-protein coupled receptors (GPCRs) increase the sensitivity of TRPV1 to heat, low pH and capsaicin, without increasing the number of functional channels [61]. Direct phosphorylation by Protein Kinase C (PKC) has been shown to play an important role in sensitization of TRPV1 by pro-inflammatory mediators such as bradykinin, prostaglandins and extracellular ATP, all of which act via Gq-coupled receptors [62–64]. Some pro-inflammatory mediators, such as prostaglandin E2 also activate Gs-coupled receptors, and the ensuing cAMP formation and activation of Protein Kinase A (PKA) contributes to sensitization [64–66]. The A kinase anchoring protein 79/150 (AKAP79/150) was shown to be important not only to PKA-, but also for PKC-mediated potentiation of TRPV1 activity [64], highlighting the importance of localized signaling complexes in the regulation of these channels.

In contrast to the very well established role of TRPV1 in inflammatory thermal hyperalgesia, the role of TRPV1 in rodent models of neuropathic pain is less clear. Caterina et al. reported no difference between wild type and TRPV1$^{-/-}$ mice in thermal hyperalgesia induced by partial sciatic nerve ligation [52]. This is consistent with the finding that in rodent models of neuropathic pain TRPV1 expression is often decreased rather than increased [67], even though in some nerve injury models increased TRPV1 expression was also reported [68].

3.1.2. Urinary Bladder

The majority of sensory nerves innervating the urinary bladder express TRPV1, but the expression of this channel in urothelial cells is controversial; if present, it is expressed at much lower levels than in sensory neurons [7]. The role of TRPV1 in normal micturition is not very clear; TRPV1$^{-/-}$ mice display a only mild spotty incontinence [69], and TRPV1 antagonists do not alter micturition in naïve mice [7]. The role of TRPV1 on the other hand is very well established in dysfunctional micturition reflex. Desensitizing TRPV1 expressing nerves using intravesical capsaicin, or RTX have been used to treat incontinence [7]. RTX is better tolerated, because it causes less pain than capsaicin.

3.1.3. Airways

TRPV1 is expressed in neurons of the vagal nerve innervating the airways that give rise to C-fibers. The cell bodies of these neurons are found in the nodose and jugular ganglia. Inhaled capsaicin evokes an urge to cough in humans and guinea pigs, but not in rats [7]. Sensitivity to inhaled capsaicin aerosols is increased in some respiratory disorders, and chronic allergic airway inflammation leads to increased TRPV1 expression [49]. TRPV1 antagonists were reported to inhibit cough evoked by inhaled aerosoled citric acid, but not spontaneous cough [7]. Desensitizing TRPV1 by intranasal application of capsaicin provided symptomatic relief in vasomotor rhinitis, but the procedure was painful and not very well tolerated [70]. Sensory neurons innervating the airways also express TRPA1, consistent with the role of that channel as a major sensor of environmental irritants [71].

3.2. Functions Based on Expression in Other Tissues

There is a relatively large literature on the involvement of TRPV1 in many different functions in a variety of tissues, especially in the central nervous system. Some effects are well established, some of the data are disputed, mainly due to findings obtained from a reporter mouse, where the authors show very restricted expression pattern of TRPV1 in small peptidergic neurons of primary sensory ganglia such as DRG and TG, the caudal hypothalamus, and in a subset of arteriolar smooth muscle cells within thermoregulatory tissues [72]. Below we briefly discuss three topics: 1. body temperature regulation, which is important for understanding the side effects of TRPV1 antagonists, 2. increased metabolism, which is a potential positive effect of TRPV1 agonists 3. the potential role of TRPV1 in ocular injury, which may also be a potential therapeutic application for TRPV1 antagonists.

3.2.1. Body Temperature Regulation

Given that TRPV1 does not normally show significant activity below ~42 °C, it is counterintuitive that this channel plays a major role in regulation of body temperature. Furthermore, TRPV1$^{-/-}$ mice have basal body temperatures indistinguishable from wild-type mice, even though they do not show the characteristic drop in body temperature after capsaicin injection [52]. Mice, in which TRPV1 expressing cells are depleted, also show no difference from wild-type animals in basal body temperature, but they show somewhat altered ability to maintain their body temperatures in response to various challenges [56]. Some investigators concluded that TRPV1 is not a major regulator of body temperature [73].

A major side effect of TRPV1 antagonist of TRPV1, however, is hyperthermia, which in some cases may reach dangerous levels [7]. How is this possible? As not all antagonists have this effect, it is unclear at this point whether this is an on target side effect [7]. It also has to be kept in mind that the temperature threshold of TRPV1 is dynamic; inflammatory mediators for example shift the temperature threshold in a PKC dependent manner. It is quite possible, that TRPV1 channels expressed in cells responsible for body temperature regulation, are in a sensitized state. The role of TRPV1 in thermoregulation has been recently reviewed in detail [74].

3.2.2. Metabolism

There is extensive literature on the effects of capsaicin and TRPV1 on metabolism, diabetes and obesity, as reviewed in [7,75]. A relatively recent meta-analysis of clinical trials concluded that daily consumption of capsaicin or capsiate, a non-pungent vanilloid, modestly increase thermogenesis and decrease appetite, thus can be useful in weight management [76]. Animal studies however show a somewhat more confusing picture. TRPV1$^{-/-}$ mice were shown to be protected from diet-induced obesity [77], but a more recent study found no difference in weight gain on high fat diet between wild type and TRPV1 knockout mice [78]. Neonatal ablation of TRPV1 expressing neurons using capsaicin in rats also resulted in conflicting data: some authors found lower weight, while others found no change in food consumption (reviewed in [79]). Consistent with the human data on the other hand, capsaicin consumption was shown to induce browning of white adipose tissue and reduce obesity in mice in a TRPV1 dependent fashion [80].

3.2.3. Ocular Injury and Eye Disease

Besides their potential use as analgesics, TRPV1 antagonists may also be useful in other pathological conditions [7], one example; eye injury is briefly discussed here. Okada et al. showed that in an alkali burn model of cornea in mice, both genetic deletion of TRPV1, and TRPV1 antagonists inhibited inflammatory cell invasion, myofibroblast generation, and scarring [81]. It was also shown that TRPV1 activation induces EGFR-transactivation in human corneal epithelial cells, which increases cell proliferation [82]. It was also demonstrated that TRPV1 activation in corneal epithelial cells by hypertonic media, similar to those observed in tears of dry eye patients, induces increased pro-inflammatory and chemoattractant release, which may contribute to the development of inflammation in dry eye patients [83]. The role of TRP channels in ocular function and eye disease has been recently reviewed [84].

4. TRPV1 as a Drug Target

There are many different TRPV1 antagonists developed by the pharmaceutical industry, several of them are, or were, in clinical trials, but to our knowledge, none of them are in routine clinical use yet. The topic has been extensively reviewed recently [7,85], here we will only discuss two aspects briefly: the limitations of currently available TRPV1 antagonists, and the rationale for using TRPV1 agonists for pain relief.

4.1. Limitations of TRPV1 Antagonists

Given the importance of TRPV1 in nociception, the rationale for using its antagonists as pain medications is straightforward. TRPV1 antagonists have been shown to provide pain relief in some pain modalities in animal models, but they are not universally effective in all studies. This topic has been extensively reviewed [86–88], here we only mention a small number of examples. In a rat model of osteoarthritis the intraarticular injection of the TRPV1 antagonist JNJ17203212 almost completely eliminated the weight bearing asymmetry in mice [89]. A different TRPV1 antagonist ABT-116, however induced only moderate pain relief in dogs in an experimental model of synovitis [90], and a third TRPV1 antagonist AZD1386 was withdrawn from clinical trials because of the absence of significant clinical benefit in osteoarthritis patients [91]. TRPV1 antagonists inhibited acute pancreatitis-induced pain in rats, but they were ineffective once chronic pancreatitis was established [92]. In mice the TRPV1 antagonist JNJ17203212 was shown to inhibit bone cancer pain [93].

Besides their variable and modality dependent effectiveness, the major limitation of TRPV1 antagonists is the two key side effects: accidental burns and hyperthermia. While accidental burns are usually mild and can be largely avoided by warning the patients to be careful, hyperthermia in some cases can be severe [7]. Is it possible to develop antagonists that are devoid of these side effects? Different antagonists show these side effects to different extents, suggesting that the answer is yes. Accumulating knowledge about the regulation of the channel also raises the possibility of developing better antagonist.

TRPV1 is a multimodal ion channel, the regulation of which is complex. Heat, low pH and capsaicin activate the channel with different mechanisms, thus theoretically it is possible to develop modality dependent inhibitors. For example, an antagonist that does not block heat activation of the channel, is expected not to block nociceptive heat sensation, thus should not cause accidental burns. Such an inhibitor may still have beneficial effects by inhibiting other modalities, such as activation by low pH and by endovanilloids. An inhibitor that selectively blocks the sensitized state of the channel, but not the basal activity, could potentially be also devoid of this side effect. What makes this rationale a little more complex is that it is not very well known what activates these channels in various pain conditions. In addition, it is not currently clear whether the most important side effect, hyperthermia, is an on-target, or off-target effect [7]. One could argue that inhibiting a heat-sensing channel is expected to induce an increase in body temperature, by "tricking" the body into feeling colder, thus increasing temperature to compensate. There are two problems with this thought: first, as mentioned earlier, the temperature threshold of TRPV1 is ~42 °C, well over normal body temperature. Second, it was proposed that antagonists that do not block activation of the channel by low pH are less likely to induce hyperthermia [94]. This, however, seems to be true for some antagonists, but not for others [7].

4.2. Desensitization of TRPV1–Rationale for Using TRPV1 Agonists

Capsaicin containing creams and other topical preparations have long been used as local analgesics. Topical capsaicin, after an initial burning sensation, desensitizes the sensory nerves not only to heat and capsaicin, but other modalities as well [79]. Capsaicin-induced desensitization is a poorly defined and highly complex phenomenon.

Native TRPV1 in DRG neurons and heterologously expressed TRPV1 undergo desensitization when exposed to maximally effective concentrations of capsaicin [50,95], which is defined as decreased current amplitude in the continuous presence of the agonist. Some articles differentiate between acute desensitization, and tachyphylaxis, which is reduced responsiveness to short applications of capsaicin. The best-established mechanism behind desensitization is depletion of PIP_2 by Ca^{2+}-induced activation of PLC. Even though PIP_2 was originally proposed to inhibit TRPV1 [96], it is clear by now that the channel is potentiated by this lipid applied to excised inside-out patches [59,97–100], and the channel requires endogenous phosphoinositides for activity in a cellular context. Capsaicin was shown to activate a PLCδ isoform leading to a robust decrease in the levels of PIP_2 and its precursor PI(4)P in TRPV1 positive DRG neurons [101]. Various inducible phosphoinositide phosphatases that decrease PIP_2 and PI(4)P levels were shown to inhibit TRPV1 activity [97,101–103], and the decrease in PIP_2 levels displayed very good correlation with decreasing current levels [102]. When the whole cell patch pipette is supplemented with PIP_2, or PI(4)P, desensitization of both recombinant TRPV1 [99,104,105] and native TRPV1 in DRG neurons [98] is reduced, but not eliminated, pointing to the contribution of other signaling processes. Paradoxically, the decrease in PIP_2 levels upon PLC activation by GPCRs may also play an auxiliary role in sensitization of TRPV1 by potentiating the effect of PKC [101]. Phosphoinositide regulation of TRPV1 is complex, its detailed discussion is beyond the scope of this article, and was extensively reviewed recently [106].

Other Ca^{2+} dependent processes such as calmodulin (CaM) [107], calcineurin [108,109], and endocytosis [110] may also contribute to desensitization. The distal C-terminus of TRPV1 was shown to bind CaM, and removal of this segment reduced tachyphylaxis, and to a lesser also inhibited acute desensitization [107]. The same study however found that neither the CaM inhibitor W7, nor a dominant negative mutant of CaM inhibited desensitization [107]. An independent study found that CaM applied to excised patches inhibited TRPV1 activity, this inhibition, however was slow, developing over several minutes, and partial [111]. An anti-CaM antibody was also shown to inhibit desensitization [104], and the crystal structure of CaM binding to the distal C-terminus of TRPV1 has been determined [112]. Inhibition of the Ca^{2+}-CaM dependent protein phosphatase calcineurin with cyclosporine and intracellular dialysis of cyclophilin was shown to reduce desensitization of TRPV1 [108,109], but a pseudosubstrate inhibitor of calcineurin failed to inhibit desensitization [113]. Even though current activity was shown to recover from desensitization within ~10 min, if ATP is provided in the patch pipette [114], TRPV1 was also shown to undergo internalization after exposure to capsaicin [110].

TRPV1 activation in DRG neurons does not only lead to desensitization of the TRPV1 channel itself, but the massive Ca^{2+} influx also leads to inhibition of other ion channels via various downstream signaling pathways. There are numerous reports showing that capsaicin application inhibits voltage gated Ca^{2+} channels [115–120]. Voltage gated Na^+ channels were also shown to be partially inhibited upon TRPV1 activation [121]. KCNQ voltage gated K^+ channels were shown to be inhibited upon TRPV1 activation via PIP_2 depletion [122]. Hyperpolarization activated HCN channels [123], P2X ATP activated ion channels [124,125] and TRPA1 [126] were also shown to be inhibited by capsaicin via TRPV1 activation. Mechanosensitive Piezo 1 and Piezo2 channels are also inhibited by TRPV1 activation in a Ca^{2+} dependent manner and supplementing the whole cell patch pipette with PIP_2 alleviated this inhibition [127].

The acute effects of TRPV1 activation on the channel itself and inhibition of other channels may, in principle, contribute to the analgesic effect of topical capsaicin. It has to be noted, however, that the pain relieving effects of high concentrations of topical capsaicin last for several weeks, and local, reversible nerve degeneration has been demonstrated after those treatments [7]. On the other hand, the effects of intravesical RTX treatment for incontinence (see later) are more reversible, and occur without detectable nerve degeneration [7], thus acute inhibition of ion channels is a more feasible explanation for this effect. Note that RTX may cause nerve degeneration when administered via a different route [128].

Even though capsaicin is highly lipophilic, the non-damaged human skin poses a significant barrier to this compound, which is why handling hot chili peppers does not usually cause significant pain in the hands, while capsaicin evokes very intense pain in the mouth, or the eye, when accidentally touched with capsaicin-contaminated hands. The over the counter creams available in US pharmacies usually contain 0.1% capsaicin, which corresponds to ~3.3 mM, which is several orders of magnitude higher concentration than the EC_{50} (~100 nM) when activating the channel in electrophysiological experiments [61]. When placed on human skin, however, these formulations usually evoke only a slowly developing moderate burning sensation, and they require multiple daily applications over several weeks to have an effect [129]. When injected intradermally in a small volume (20 µL), the same, or even lower concentrations of capsaicin (0.01% and 0.1%) were shown to induce a dose-dependent nerve degeneration after a single injection [130]. Overall, capsaicin from sporadic application of low concentration creams may not reach the nerve terminals at high enough concentrations to induce clinically relevant desensitization. It was proposed that these creams are more likely to exert some pain relief via counter irritation [79], which may involve the release of somatostatin, which exerts antinociceptive and anti-inflammatory effects [131,132]. Developing TRPV1 agonists with better penetration through the skin is one area where rational drug design may play a role. It has to be noted however, that when applied in a large quantity and for a long time (48 h), a low concentration (0.1%) capsaicin preparation was also shown to induce long lasting, slowly reversible nerve degeneration [133].

There are several high concentration patches and injectable capsaicin formulations either in clinical trial or approved; these are discussed in detail elsewhere [7]. The high concentration capsaicin patch Qutenza (8%) which requires a single one hour application and its effect lasts for several weeks, for example is approved for post-herpetic neuralgia [129], but did not receive FDA approval for HIV-related pain [7]. Unlike the topical capsaicin creams containing low concentrations of the drug mentioned above, the Qutenza having 8% capsaicin causes degeneration of TRPV1-expressing nociceptive nerve endings even after a 1 h application, which is only slowly reversible, explaining the long duration of action of the drug [134].

The effects of TRPV1 agonists also depend on the application site and age of experimental animals. In newborn rats, systemic injection of RTX, or capsaicin, destroys TRPV1 positive cells, and has been used as a model to study nociception [79,135]. Intrathecal application of RTX or capsaicin induces degeneration of the central terminals of TRPV1 positive DRG neurons, and thus eliminates transmission of signals from these cells [136]. CT-guided local administration of RTX to DRGs in pigs was shown to reduce withdrawal from noxious heat in corresponding dermatomes [137].

4.3. Structure Based Rational Design of TRPV1 Modulators

Despite the advances in membrane protein crystallography, and the enormous interest in TRP channels, no full-length TRP channel has been crystallized, until very recently [138]. Advances in cryo-electron microscopy (cryoEM) however made it possible to obtain structures sufficiently accurate to resolve side chain conformations. TRPV1 was the first ion channel for which such structure was available [139,140], followed by TRPA1 [141] and TRPV2 [142,143]. The most recent cryoEM structure of TRPV1 was determined in lipid nanodiscs, a native-like lipid environment [144].

The advances in structural biology of TRP channels opens up the possibility to rationally design both agonists and antagonist for TRPV1 and other TRP channels.

4.3.1. CryoEM Structure of TRPV1: First Insights on the Gating Mechanism

Facilitated by recent technical developments in single-particle cryoEM, the structure of the mammalian TRPV1 cation channel has been recently solved in three distinct conformational states: closed state without any agonist, capsaicin-bound partially open state, and fully open state with two agonists RTX and double-knot-toxin bound to the channel [139,140]. These structures have provided an unprecedented atomistic view of both the initial and terminal states of channel gating. TRPV1 is a member of the evolutionary superfamily of 6TM channels, i.e., it is distantly related to the family of voltage gated ion channels [145]. The functional assembly of the channel is a tetramer of subunits containing each six transmembrane helices, termed S1 through S6. As a clade of 6TM channels, TRP channels (and thus TRPV1) inherited the overall architecture from voltage sensitive ancestral genes (Figure 1). Thus, besides the pore domain, constituted by the tetrameric assembly of the S5 and S6 helices, TRPV1 shows four identical peripheral domains that are structurally homologous to voltage sensor domains. These are formed by helices S1 through S4 and are connected to the pore domain through an amphiphilic helix parallel to the membrane called S4–S4 linked domain [139].

In contrast to voltage gated ion channels, the S1–S4 domain does not undergo significant conformational changes upon activation. However, in the agonist-activated states of the channel, pore-forming helices move apart from each other, breaking a seal of hydrophobic residues and opening the so-called gate [139]. The molecular mechanism responsible for channel opening upon ligand binding is thus seemingly different from that underlying voltage sensitive activation. In spite of the abundant structural information so far collected, the nature of the close-to-open structural transition and, most importantly, the role played in this transition by the channel-ligand interactions is still the object of intense investigation.

A)

B)

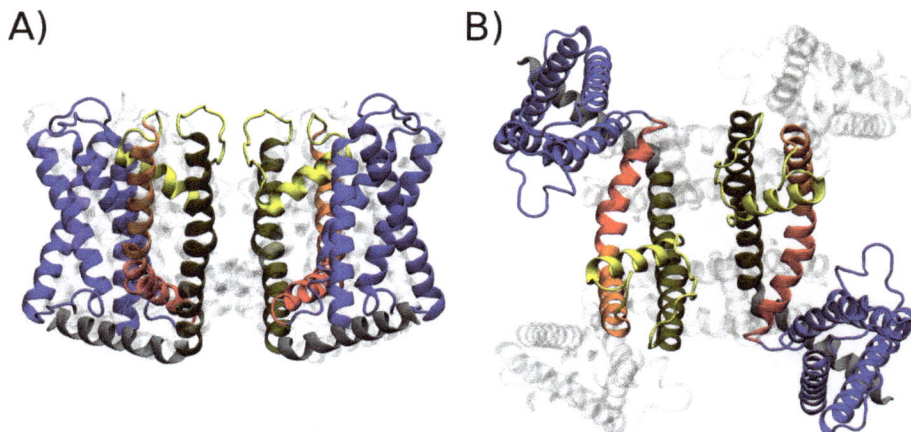

Figure 1. Molecular architecture of the Transient Receptor Potential Vanilloid 1 channel (TRPV1). Cartoon representation of the structure of the transmembrane region of TRPV1 as determined via cryoEM in lipid nanodiscs: (**A**) side view; and (**B**) top view. For clarity, only two subunits are highlighted in solid color while the other two are rendered as grey shading. Different colors highlight the major structural elements described in the text: S1–S4 domain (blue), linker domain (red), S5 (orange), pore helix and selectivity filter (yellow), S6 (brown) and TRP domain (grey).

Before the structure of TRPV1 became available, biochemical studies had already localized the interaction sites of various TRPV1 small molecule agonists: capsaicin, RTX, and *N*-arachidonoyl dopamine activate the channel from the intracellular face in a pocket usually referred to as vanilloid binding site [139]. The best-characterized TRPV1 ligand is arguably the agonist capsaicin [79]. Intriguingly, the molecule capsazepine, which is structurally very similar to capsaicin, while showing a reasonably large affinity, does not cause channel opening. Therefore, by competing for binding to the vanilloid site with TRPV1 activators, it exerts a modulatory effect opposite to that of capsaicin (i.e., inhibits the channel, it is a vanilloid antagonist) [146]. In other words, while retaining a relatively large affinity for TRPV1, capsazepine does not elicit the structural response leading to channel opening. While this lack of activity as activator is of clear pharmacological relevance—antagonizing the effect of endogenous vanilloids is one of the putative strategies to achieve analgesia—its molecular determinants remain to be understood and thus we are still far from a rational design of antagonists.

Indeed, despite the fact that single particle cryo electron microscopy has unveiled the three-dimensional structures of the channel in the apo form and in complex with capsaicin, RTX and capsazepine, the electron density maps for these structures did not have initially enough information to unambiguously determine the position of structural waters and to unambiguously determine the conformation of all the side chains of the residues lining the vanilloid pocket. Nevertheless, this structural information paved the way for subsequent computational docking and molecular dynamics studies in which the comparison between different agonists and between agonists and antagonists has been used to rationalize the different behavior of the ligands. These structural studies are opening up a new era for pain killer design in which the accurate knowledge of the specific binding modes gives insights into the design principles of agonists and antagonists [147].

4.3.2. Binding Mode of Capsaicin and RTX

The initial electron density determined by Cao et al. [139] did not possess a resolution large enough to unambiguously determine the spatial location and orientation of capsaicin and RTX. This lack of information motivated a series of computational and joint computational/experimental studies that not only resulted in a more detailed structural picture of vanilloid binding to TRPV1, but also allowed to formulate informed hypotheses about their mode of action. In this regard, one of the most important milestones has been the work of Yang et al. [148], which has shown that capsaicin binds "head down" (with the vanillyl group pointing toward the intracellular milieu) and that the most relevant interactions between the ligand and the channel involve the amide group of capsaicin and the side chain of Thr550 and the hydroxyl from the vanilloid group and the side chain of Glu570. The relevance of these ligand channel interactions was quantitatively assessed via double mutant cycle analysis [149].

A subsequent molecular dynamics investigation by Darre and Domene [150] provided additional elements of support to the notion that that the amide group of capsaicin plays a crucial role in ligand binding: molecular dynamics trajectories and free energy calculations showed that Thr550 and Tyr511 engage in hydrogen bonding interactions, respectively, with the amine and carbonyl groups of capsaicin through bridging water molecules. These water-mediated interactions were confirmed by an independent study by Elokely et al. [38] in which a statistical physics based model was used to find binding regions for tightly bound water molecules. In addition to these polar interactions, this study investigated the role of hydrophobic interactions involving residues from S4 and the linker domain. In particular five residues were predicted and shown experimentally to affect significantly binding upon mutation (Leu515, Leu553, Tyr554, Ile573 and Phe587), thereby providing a stringent test for the structural model. The emerging picture is a tight fit of the vanilloid group in a hydrophobic pocket formed mainly by residues from the C-term region of S4 and the linker. This set of interactions was shown to be crucial for both capsaicin and RTX. Importantly, the largest effect was observed for Leu553 and Tyr554 from S4 and Ile573 from the linker domain.

4.3.3. Mechanism of Activation by Vanilloids

The computational studies based on docking and molecular dynamics highlighted a small set of persistent ligand-channel interactions, which were subsequently experimentally tested. This information enabled to formulate hypotheses on the molecular mechanism of vanilloids and provided a rationale for the novel structural information that became recently available. Indeed, Gao et al. [144] determined the structure of TRPV1 in the apo form and in complex with RTX and capsazepine in a lipid nanodisc environment (Figure 2). The use of this supermolecular assembly, which faithfully reproduces the native lipid bilayer environment of the channel, enabled the authors to obtain extremely well defined electron densities and thus to identify the location and orientation of the ligands with remarkable accuracy. This study confirmed the theoretical prediction that RTX interacts one side with the S1–S4 domain (with residues Ser512, Arg557, Leu515, Val518, and Met547 as well as Leu669, and Thr550) and on the other side with linker residue Ile573 (Figure 2A). Importantly, this observation brings support to the hypothesis raised in the previous computational studies [38,148,150] that the role of agonists is to act as "molecular glue" between the linker and the S1–S4 domain. Importantly, the cryoEM structures provided evidence of a feature deemed crucial for the agonist effect in Yang et al. 2015 [148], i.e., the fact that the vanilloid head group catalyzes the formation of a salt bridge between Glu570 and Arg577, an interaction that contributes to make the S1–S4 and the linker domains a single rigid unit. Importantly, the structure of TRPV1 in complex with capsazepine revealed no salt bridge between these two side chains and, in general, less extensive interactions with the linker domain (Figure 2B).

The overall emerging picture confirms the "pull-and-contact" model proposed initially by Yang et al. [148] in which the binding of vanilloids, by acting as "molecular glue", promotes the lateral movement of the linker toward the S1–S4 domain. As shown previously for voltage gated ion channels, this conformational transition of the linker domain is able to release the steric hindrance that prevents the splay of the S6 bundle. In other words, in the resting state the four linker domains surround the S6 four-helix bundle lining the pore and act as a "cuff". Once the linker domains are displaced, the constriction is removed and the S6 helix bundle is free to expand [151]. Strikingly, two independent studies have provided compelling confirmation of this model by engineering RTX sensitivity into TRPV2—a channel that is natively insensitive to this vanilloid. In the first study, Yang et al. [152] introduced the residues Ser512, Phe543, Thr550 and Glu570 (TRPV1 numbering) in the corresponding positions of TRPV2. The resulting construct was shown to be activated by RTX (although the ligand-induced open state was relatively unstable). In the second work, Zhang et al. [153] reported completely consistent observations by engineering a quadruple mutant that introduces Ser512, Met547, Thr550 and Glu570 in the background of TRPV2.

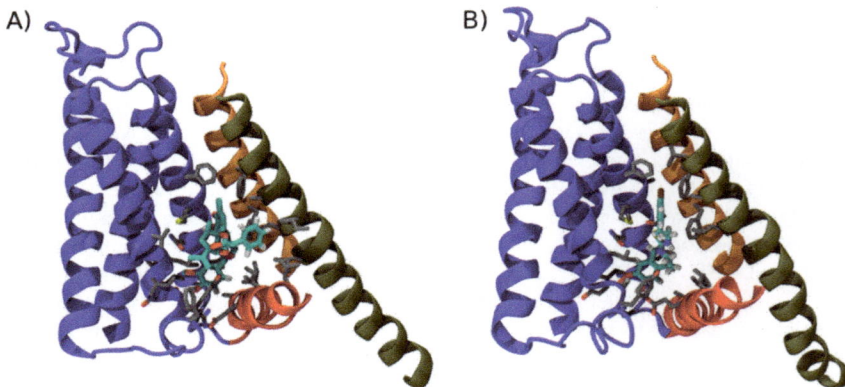

Figure 2. Binding mode of TRPV1 modulators. Structure of TRPV1 in complex with: RTX (**A**); and capsazepine (**B**). For clarity only the structural element surrounding the vanilloid binding site are shown in cartoon representation using the same color code used in Figure 1. Amino acid side chains contacting the ligands are shown as sticks; to highlight the location of ligand in the two structures, the carbon atoms of RTX and capsezepine are highlighted by the cyan color. Note how the conformations of RTX and capsazepine are very similar, except for a phenyl group, which, in RTX, contacts the side chains of S6.

4.3.4. Structure Driven Design of Novel Modulators

The accurate structural information available at this point for TRPV1 in complex with agonists and antagonists, together with an experimentally testable—and to some extent verified—microscopic model of the vanilloid action has already prompted several structure-based studies in the last two years and will, no doubt, catalyze an explosion of rational drug design campaigns in the foreseeable future.

The first study entirely based on this newly available information was that of Feng et al. [154]. The authors of this study used docking and molecular dynamics simulations to extract detailed information about the interactions of two groups of ligands known to have agonist or antagonist action. The accurate three-dimensional structures obtained from these calculations were then used to generate a so-called pharmacophore, an abstract representation of the molecular features most relevant for binding and activity. Thanks to this pharmacophore, the authors were able to screen a virtual library of compounds and extract promising hits. In particular two compounds were found experimentally to be relatively potent (two halogenated diaryl-nitro compounds), that were also investigated through docking and molecular dynamics simulations. The two compounds resulted in $98.2\% \pm 2.7\%$ and $79.9\% \pm 4.9\%$ inhibition at a concentration of 30 μM, i.e., they antagonized capsaicin (30 nM) in a calcium uptake assay. These compounds also proved to have relatively high affinity with K_i values for capsaicin antagonism of 2.60 ± 0.62 μM and 4.50 ± 0.88 μM. Simulations showed that the compounds interacted stably with Tyr511 and Thr550 via hydrogen bonds. Moreover, the ligands established strong hydrophobic interactions with Met514 and Leu547, i.e., some of the side chains previously shown to affect capsaicin affinity upon mutation. Importantly, these relatively potent antagonists, formed strong hydrogen bonds with Arg557, thereby inhibiting the salt bridge with Glu570 found to be crucial for activation by Cao et al. 2016. Consistently, inactive compounds were not observed to form this hydrogen bond with Arg557.

Building on their initial screen Feng et al. [155] further investigated diaryl molecules and screened a library of diarylurea compounds. The rationale for the choice of this class of molecules is the observation, coming from the previous computational studies, of the crucial energetic role played by the interaction between the capsaicin amide group and the side chain of Thr550. The hypothesis was that, given the relevance of this polar interaction, replacing the amide group with urea should increase affinity and thus potency. Using the hydroxyl of Thr550 as anchoring point for the urea, the library developed chemical diversity by changing the substituents of the two aryl-groups. In addition, in this case, docking and molecular dynamics showed that Tyr511, Leu518, Leu547, Thr550, Asn551, Arg557, and Leu670 were the most important side chains for recognition of the ligand by TRPV1.

A second group identified *N*-(3-fluoro-4-methylsulfonamidomethylphenyl)urea as a novel template for TRPV1 antagonists and developed chemical diversity in various regions of this molecule to generate a library to be screened [156,157]. Importantly, when the binding of this compound was analyzed with computational docking, the urea group forms hydrogen bonds with Tyr511, thereby properly orienting the molecule and favoring the interaction between the two flanking phenyl groups and the hydrophobic regions of the binding site. Importantly, all the residues shown to be crucial for capsaicin binding turned out to form stabilizing interactions with the novel molecules. The *N*-benzylmethanesulfonamide group was found to occupy the crevice lined by the side chains of Tyr511, Tyr554, Ile564, and Ile569. Moreover, the oxygen of the sulfonamide group was shown to be engaged in a hydrogen bond with Ser512, the 3-trifluoromethyl group was found to interact with Leu547 and the methyl group of Thr550 and the 4-methylpiperidine ring in was observed to be in contact with Tyr511, Met514, and Leu515.

Overall, these recent studies have provided proof of concept that the detailed structural information that became available greatly simplifies the search for TRPV1 modulators and molecules with potency comparable to capsaicin can be now easily identified. Despite these success stories, predicting the activity of the ligand, i.e., the agonist vs. antagonist action, remains challenging on purely structural basis. To make progress in this issue additional studies will be needed to develop a quantitative microscopic model that explains activation of TRPV1 by vanilloids.

Acknowledgments: Research in the authors' laboratories were funded by National Science Foundation Grants ACI-1440059 (to V.C.) and NIH Grants R01NS055159 and R01GM093290 (to T.R.).

Conflicts of Interest: The authors declare no conflict of interest.

References

1. Montell, C.; Rubin, G.M. Molecular characterization of the Drosophila TRP locus: A putative integral membrane protein required for phototransduction. *Neuron* **1989**, *2*, 1313–1323. [CrossRef]
2. Montell, C. Drosophila visual transduction. *Trends Neurosci.* **2012**, *35*, 356–363. [CrossRef] [PubMed]
3. Clapham, D.E.; Runnels, L.W.; Strubing, C. The TRP ion channel family. *Nat. Rev. Neurosci.* **2001**, *2*, 387–396. [CrossRef] [PubMed]
4. Rohacs, T. Regulation of transient receptor potential channels by the phospholipase C pathway. *Adv. Biol. Regul.* **2013**, *53*, 341–355. [CrossRef] [PubMed]
5. Vriens, J.; Nilius, B.; Voets, T. Peripheral thermosensation in mammals. *Nat. Rev. Neurosci.* **2014**, *15*, 573–589. [CrossRef] [PubMed]
6. Nilius, B.; Owsianik, G.; Voets, T.; Peters, J.A. Transient receptor potential cation channels in disease. *Physiol. Rev.* **2007**, *87*, 165–217. [CrossRef] [PubMed]
7. Nilius, B.; Szallasi, A. Transient receptor potential channels as drug targets: From the science of basic research to the art of medicine. *Pharmacol. Rev.* **2014**, *66*, 676–814. [CrossRef] [PubMed]
8. Clapham, D.E. TRP channels as cellular sensors. *Nature* **2003**, *426*, 517–524. [CrossRef] [PubMed]

9. Koike, C.; Obara, T.; Uriu, Y.; Numata, T.; Sanuki, R.; Miyata, K.; Koyasu, T.; Ueno, S.; Funabiki, K.; Tani, A.; et al. TRPM1 is a component of the retinal ON bipolar cell transduction channel in the mGluR6 cascade. *Proc. Natl. Acad. Sci. USA* **2010**, *107*, 332–337. [CrossRef] [PubMed]

10. Zhang, Y.; Hoon, M.A.; Chandrashekar, J.; Mueller, K.L.; Cook, B.; Wu, D.; Zuker, C.S.; Ryba, N.J. Coding of sweet, bitter, and umami tastes: Different receptor cells sharing similar signaling pathways. *Cell* **2003**, *112*, 293–301. [CrossRef]

11. Sachs, F. Stretch-activated ion channels: What are they? *Physiology* **2010**, *25*, 50–56. [CrossRef] [PubMed]

12. Julius, D. TRP channels and pain. *Annu. Rev. Cell Dev. Biol.* **2013**, *29*, 355–384. [CrossRef] [PubMed]

13. Kojima, I.; Nagasawa, M. TRPV2. *Handb. Exp. Pharmacol.* **2014**, *222*, 247–272. [PubMed]

14. Caterina, M.J.; Rosen, T.A.; Tominaga, M.; Brake, A.J.; Julius, D. A capsaicin-receptor homologue with a high threshold for noxious heat. *Nature* **1999**, *398*, 436–441. [PubMed]

15. Park, U.; Vastani, N.; Guan, Y.; Raja, S.N.; Koltzenburg, M.; Caterina, M.J. TRP vanilloid 2 knock-out mice are susceptible to perinatal lethality but display normal thermal and mechanical nociception. *J. Neurosci.* **2011**, *31*, 11425–11436. [CrossRef] [PubMed]

16. Link, T.M.; Park, U.; Vonakis, B.M.; Raben, D.M.; Soloski, M.J.; Caterina, M.J. TRPV2 has a pivotal role in macrophage particle binding and phagocytosis. *Nat. Immunol.* **2010**, *11*, 232–239. [CrossRef] [PubMed]

17. Katanosaka, Y.; Iwasaki, K.; Ujihara, Y.; Takatsu, S.; Nishitsuji, K.; Kanagawa, M.; Sudo, A.; Toda, T.; Katanosaka, K.; Mohri, S.; et al. TRPV2 is critical for the maintenance of cardiac structure and function in mice. *Nat. Commun.* **2014**, *5*, 3932. [CrossRef] [PubMed]

18. Yang, P.; Zhu, M.X. TRPV3. *Handb. Exp. Pharmacol.* **2014**, *222*, 273–291. [PubMed]

19. Xu, H.; Ramsey, I.S.; Kotecha, S.A.; Moran, M.M.; Chong, J.A.; Lawson, D.; Ge, P.; Lilly, J.; Silos-Santiago, I.; Xie, Y.; et al. TRPV3 is a calcium-permeable temperature-sensitive cation channel. *Nature* **2002**, *418*, 181–186. [CrossRef] [PubMed]

20. Lin, Z.; Chen, Q.; Lee, M.; Cao, X.; Zhang, J.; Ma, D.; Chen, L.; Hu, X.; Wang, H.; Wang, X.; et al. Exome sequencing reveals mutations in TRPV3 as a cause of Olmsted syndrome. *Am. J. Hum. Genet.* **2012**, *90*, 558–564. [CrossRef] [PubMed]

21. Garcia-Elias, A.; Mrkonjic, S.; Jung, C.; Pardo-Pastor, C.; Vicente, R.; Valverde, M.A. The TRPV4 channel. *Handb. Exp. Pharmacol.* **2014**, *222*, 293–319. [PubMed]

22. Lee, H.; Iida, T.; Mizuno, A.; Suzuki, M.; Caterina, M.J. Altered thermal selection behavior in mice lacking transient receptor potential vanilloid 4. *J. Neurosci.* **2005**, *25*, 1304–1310. [CrossRef] [PubMed]

23. Oberwinkler, J.; Philipp, S.E. TRPM3. *Handb. Exp. Pharmacol.* **2014**, *222*, 427–459. [PubMed]

24. Vriens, J.; Owsianik, G.; Hofmann, T.; Philipp, S.E.; Stab, J.; Chen, X.; Benoit, M.; Xue, F.; Janssens, A.; Kerselaers, S.; et al. TRPM3 is a nociceptor channel involved in the detection of noxious heat. *Neuron* **2011**, *70*, 482–494. [CrossRef] [PubMed]

25. Almaraz, L.; Manenschijn, J.A.; de la Pena, E.; Viana, F. TRPM8. *Handb. Exp. Pharmacol.* **2014**, *222*, 547–579. [PubMed]

26. McKemy, D.D.; Neuhausser, W.M.; Julius, D. Identification of a cold receptor reveals a general role for TRP channels in thermosensation. *Nature* **2002**, *416*, 52–58. [CrossRef] [PubMed]

27. Peier, A.M.; Moqrich, A.; Hergarden, A.C.; Reeve, A.J.; Andersson, D.A.; Story, G.M.; Earley, T.J.; Dragoni, I.; McIntyre, P.; Bevan, S.; et al. A TRP channel that senses cold stimuli and menthol. *Cell* **2002**, *108*, 705–715. [CrossRef]

28. Bautista, D.M.; Siemens, J.; Glazer, J.M.; Tsuruda, P.R.; Basbaum, A.I.; Stucky, C.L.; Jordt, S.E.; Julius, D. The menthol receptor TRPM8 is the principal detector of environmental cold. *Nature* **2007**, *448*, 204–208. [CrossRef]

29. Colburn, R.W.; Lubin, M.L.; Stone, D.J., Jr.; Wang, Y.; Lawrence, D.; D'Andrea, M.R.; Brandt, M.R.; Liu, Y.; Flores, C.M.; Qin, N. Attenuated cold sensitivity in TRPM8 null mice. *Neuron* **2007**, *54*, 379–386. [CrossRef] [PubMed]

30. Dhaka, A.; Murray, A.N.; Mathur, J.; Earley, T.J.; Petrus, M.J.; Patapoutian, A. TRPM8 is required for cold sensation in mice. *Neuron* **2007**, *54*, 371–378. [CrossRef] [PubMed]

31. Liu, B.; Fan, L.; Balakrishna, S.; Sui, A.; Morris, J.B.; Jordt, S.E. TRPM8 is the principal mediator of menthol-induced analgesia of acute and inflammatory pain. *Pain* **2013**, *154*, 2169–2177. [CrossRef]

32. Zygmunt, P.M.; Hogestatt, E.D. TRPA1. *Handb. Exp. Pharmacol.* **2014**, *222*, 583–630. [PubMed]
33. Story, G.M.; Peier, A.M.; Reeve, A.J.; Eid, S.R.; Mosbacher, J.; Hricik, T.R.; Earley, T.J.; Hergarden, A.C.; Andersson, D.A.; Hwang, S.W.; et al. ANKTM1, a TRP-like channel expressed in nociceptive neurons, is activated by cold temperatures. *Cell* **2003**, *112*, 819–829. [CrossRef]
34. Jordt, S.E.; Bautista, D.M.; Chuang, H.H.; McKemy, D.D.; Zygmunt, P.M.; Hogestatt, E.D.; Meng, I.D.; Julius, D. Mustard oils and cannabinoids excite sensory nerve fibres through the TRP channel ANKTM1. *Nature* **2004**, *427*, 260–265. [CrossRef] [PubMed]
35. Zholos, A.V. TRPC5. *Handb. Exp. Pharmacol.* **2014**, *222*, 129–156. [PubMed]
36. Zimmermann, K.; Lennerz, J.K.; Hein, A.; Link, A.S.; Kaczmarek, J.S.; Delling, M.; Uysal, S.; Pfeifer, J.D.; Riccio, A.; Clapham, D.E. Transient receptor potential cation channel, subfamily C, member 5 (TRPC5) is a cold-transducer in the peripheral nervous system. *Proc. Natl. Acad. Sci. USA* **2011**, *108*, 18114–18119. [CrossRef] [PubMed]
37. Szallasi, A.; Blumberg, P.M. Resiniferatoxin, a phorbol-related diterpene, acts as an ultrapotent analog of capsaicin, the irritant constituent in red pepper. *Neuroscience* **1989**, *30*, 515–520. [CrossRef]
38. Elokely, K.; Velisetty, P.; Delemotte, L.; Palovcak, E.; Klein, M.L.; Rohacs, T.; Carnevale, V. Understanding TRPV1 activation by ligands: Insights from the binding modes of capsaicin and resiniferatoxin. *Proc. Natl. Acad. Sci. USA* **2016**, *113*, E137–E145. [CrossRef] [PubMed]
39. Ursu, D.; Knopp, K.; Beattie, R.E.; Liu, B.; Sher, E. Pungency of TRPV1 agonists is directly correlated with kinetics of receptor activation and lipophilicity. *Eur. J. Pharmacol.* **2010**, *641*, 114–122. [CrossRef] [PubMed]
40. Szallasi, A.; Blumberg, P.M. Resiniferatoxin and its analogs provide novel insights into the pharmacology of the vanilloid (capsaicin) receptor. *Life Sci.* **1990**, *47*, 1399–1408. [CrossRef]
41. Morales-Lazaro, S.L.; Simon, S.A.; Rosenbaum, T. The role of endogenous molecules in modulating pain through transient receptor potential vanilloid 1 (TRPV1). *J. Physiol.* **2013**, *591*, 3109–3121. [CrossRef] [PubMed]
42. Siemens, J.; Zhou, S.; Piskorowski, R.; Nikai, T.; Lumpkin, E.A.; Basbaum, A.I.; King, D.; Julius, D. Spider toxins activate the capsaicin receptor to produce inflammatory pain. *Nature* **2006**, *444*, 208–212. [CrossRef] [PubMed]
43. Yang, S.; Yang, F.; Wei, N.; Hong, J.; Li, B.; Luo, L.; Rong, M.; Yarov-Yarovoy, V.; Zheng, J.; Wang, K.; et al. A pain-inducing centipede toxin targets the heat activation machinery of nociceptor TRPV1. *Nat. Commun.* **2015**, *6*, 8297. [CrossRef] [PubMed]
44. Starowicz, K.; Nigam, S.; Di Marzo, V. Biochemistry and pharmacology of endovanilloids. *Pharmacol. Ther.* **2007**, *114*, 13–33. [CrossRef] [PubMed]
45. Nieto-Posadas, A.; Picazo-Juarez, G.; Llorente, I.; Jara-Oseguera, A.; Morales-Lazaro, S.; Escalante-Alcalde, D.; Islas, L.D.; Rosenbaum, T. Lysophosphatidic acid directly activates TRPV1 through a C-terminal binding site. *Nat. Chem. Biol.* **2012**, *8*, 78–85. [CrossRef] [PubMed]
46. Trevisani, M.; Smart, D.; Gunthorpe, M.J.; Tognetto, M.; Barbieri, M.; Campi, B.; Amadesi, S.; Gray, J.; Jerman, J.C.; Brough, S.J.; et al. Ethanol elicits and potentiates nociceptor responses via the vanilloid receptor-1. *Nat. Neurosci.* **2002**, *5*, 546–551. [CrossRef] [PubMed]
47. Caterina, M.J.; Julius, D. The vanilloid receptor: a molecular gateway to the pain pathway. *Annu. Rev. Neurosci.* **2001**, *24*, 487–517. [CrossRef] [PubMed]
48. Bevan, S.; Quallo, T.; Andersson, D.A. TRPV1. *Handb. Exp. Pharmacol.* **2014**, *222*, 207–245. [PubMed]
49. Lee, L.Y.; Gu, Q. Role of TRPV1 in inflammation-induced airway hypersensitivity. *Curr. Opin. Pharmacol.* **2009**, *9*, 243–249. [CrossRef] [PubMed]
50. Caterina, M.J.; Schumacher, M.A.; Tominaga, M.; Rosen, T.A.; Levine, J.D.; Julius, D. The capsaicin receptor: A heat-activated ion channel in the pain pathway. *Nature* **1997**, *389*, 816–824. [PubMed]
51. Dhaka, A.; Viswanath, V.; Patapoutian, A. TRP ion channels and temperature sensation. *Annu. Rev. Neurosci.* **2006**, *29*, 135–161. [CrossRef] [PubMed]
52. Caterina, M.J.; Leffler, A.; Malmberg, A.B.; Martin, W.J.; Trafton, J.; Petersen-Zeitz, K.R.; Koltzenburg, M.; Basbaum, A.I.; Julius, D. Impaired nociception and pain sensation in mice lacking the capsaicin receptor. *Science* **2000**, *288*, 306–313. [CrossRef] [PubMed]
53. Davis, J.B.; Gray, J.; Gunthorpe, M.J.; Hatcher, J.P.; Davey, P.T.; Overend, P.; Harries, M.H.; Latcham, J.; Clapham, C.; Atkinson, K.; et al. Vanilloid receptor-1 is essential for inflammatory. *Nature* **2000**, *405*, 183–187. [CrossRef] [PubMed]

54. Hoffmann, T.; Kistner, K.; Miermeister, F.; Winkelmann, R.; Wittmann, J.; Fischer, M.J.; Weidner, C.; Reeh, P.W. TRPA1 and TRPV1 are differentially involved in heat nociception of mice. *Eur. J. Pain* **2013**, *17*, 1472–1482. [CrossRef] [PubMed]

55. Marics, I.; Malapert, P.; Reynders, A.; Gaillard, S.; Moqrich, A. Acute heat-evoked temperature sensation is impaired but not abolished in mice lacking TRPV1 and TRPV3 channels. *PLoS ONE* **2014**, *9*, e99828.

56. Mishra, S.K.; Tisel, S.M.; Orestes, P.; Bhangoo, S.K.; Hoon, M.A. TRPV1-lineage neurons are required for thermal sensation. *EMBO J.* **2011**, *30*, 582–593. [CrossRef] [PubMed]

57. Yu, L.; Yang, F.; Luo, H.; Liu, F.Y.; Han, J.S.; Xing, G.G.; Wan, Y. The role of TRPV1 in different subtypes of dorsal root ganglion neurons in rat chronic inflammatory nociception induced by complete Freund's adjuvant. *Mol. Pain* **2008**, *4*, 61. [CrossRef] [PubMed]

58. Amaya, F.; Shimosato, G.; Nagano, M.; Ueda, M.; Hashimoto, S.; Tanaka, Y.; Suzuki, H.; Tanaka, M. NGF and GDNF differentially regulate TRPV1 expression that contributes to development of inflammatory thermal hyperalgesia. *Eur. J. Neurosci.* **2004**, *20*, 2303–2310. [CrossRef] [PubMed]

59. Stein, A.T.; Ufret-Vincenty, C.A.; Hua, L.; Santana, L.F.; Gordon, S.E. Phosphoinositide 3-kinase binds to TRPV1 and mediates NGF-stimulated TRPV1 trafficking to the plasma membrane. *J. Gen. Physiol.* **2006**, *128*, 509–522. [CrossRef] [PubMed]

60. Zhang, X.; Huang, J.; McNaughton, P.A. NGF rapidly increases membrane expression of TRPV1 heat-gated ion channels. *EMBO J.* **2005**, *24*, 4211–4223. [CrossRef] [PubMed]

61. Tominaga, M.; Wada, M.; Masu, M. Potentiation of capsaicin receptor activity by metabotropic ATP receptors as a possible mechanism for ATP-evoked pain and hyperalgesia. *Proc. Natl. Acad. Sci. USA* **2001**, *98*, 6951–6956. [CrossRef] [PubMed]

62. Cesare, P.; Dekker, L.V.; Sardini, A.; Parker, P.J.; McNaughton, P.A. Specific involvement of PKC-ε in sensitization of the neuronal response to painful heat. *Neuron* **1999**, *23*, 617–624. [CrossRef]

63. Numazaki, M.; Tominaga, T.; Toyooka, H.; Tominaga, M. Direct phosphorylation of capsaicin receptor VR1 by protein kinase Cε and identification of two target serine residues. *J. Biol. Chem.* **2002**, *277*, 13375–13378. [CrossRef]

64. Zhang, X.; Li, L.; McNaughton, P.A. Proinflammatory mediators modulate the heat-activated ion channel TRPV1 via the scaffolding protein AKAP79/150. *Neuron* **2008**, *59*, 450–461. [CrossRef] [PubMed]

65. Rathee, P.K.; Distler, C.; Obreja, O.; Neuhuber, W.; Wang, G.K.; Wang, S.Y.; Nau, C.; Kress, M. PKA/AKAP/VR-1 module: A common link of Gs-mediated signaling to thermal hyperalgesia. *J. Neurosci.* **2002**, *22*, 4740–4745. [PubMed]

66. Varga, A.; Bolcskei, K.; Szoke, E.; Almasi, R.; Czeh, G.; Szolcsanyi, J.; Petho, G. Relative roles of protein kinase A and protein kinase C in modulation of transient receptor potential vanilloid type 1 receptor responsiveness in rat sensory neurons in vitro and peripheral nociceptors in vivo. *Neuroscience* **2006**, *140*, 645–657. [CrossRef] [PubMed]

67. Costigan, M.; Befort, K.; Karchewski, L.; Griffin, R.S.; D'Urso, D.; Allchorne, A.; Sitarski, J.; Mannion, J.W.; Pratt, R.E.; Woolf, C.J. Replicate high-density rat genome oligonucleotide microarrays reveal hundreds of regulated genes in the dorsal root ganglion after peripheral nerve injury. *BMC Neurosci.* **2002**, *3*, 16. [CrossRef] [PubMed]

68. Kim, H.Y.; Park, C.K.; Cho, I.H.; Jung, S.J.; Kim, J.S.; Oh, S.B. Differential Changes in TRPV1 expression after trigeminal sensory nerve injury. *J. Pain* **2008**, *9*, 280–288. [CrossRef] [PubMed]

69. Birder, L.A.; Nakamura, Y.; Kiss, S.; Nealen, M.L.; Barrick, S.; Kanai, A.J.; Wang, E.; Ruiz, G.; De Groat, W.C.; Apodaca, G.; et al. Altered urinary bladder function in mice lacking the vanilloid receptor TRPV1. *Nat. Neurosci.* **2002**, *5*, 856–860. [CrossRef] [PubMed]

70. Marabini, S.; Ciabatti, P.G.; Polli, G.; Fusco, B.M.; Geppetti, P. Beneficial effects of intranasal applications of capsaicin in patients with vasomotor rhinitis. *Eur. Arch. Otorhinolaryngol.* **1991**, *248*, 191–194. [PubMed]

71. Bessac, B.F.; Jordt, S.E. Breathtaking TRP channels: TRPA1 and TRPV1 in airway chemosensation and reflex control. *Physiology* **2008**, *23*, 360–370. [CrossRef] [PubMed]

72. Cavanaugh, D.J.; Chesler, A.T.; Braz, J.M.; Shah, N.M.; Julius, D.; Basbaum, A.I. Restriction of transient receptor potential vanilloid-1 to the peptidergic subset of primary afferent neurons follows its developmental downregulation in nonpeptidergic neurons. *J. Neurosci.* **2011**, *31*, 10119–10127. [CrossRef] [PubMed]

73. Romanovsky, A.A.; Almeida, M.C.; Garami, A.; Steiner, A.A.; Norman, M.H.; Morrison, S.F.; Nakamura, K.; Burmeister, J.J.; Nucci, T.B. The transient receptor potential vanilloid-1 channel in thermoregulation: A thermosensor it is not. *Pharmacol. Rev.* **2009**, *61*, 228–261. [CrossRef] [PubMed]
74. Szolcsanyi, J. Effect of capsaicin on thermoregulation: an update with new aspects. *Temperature* **2015**, *2*, 277–296. [CrossRef] [PubMed]
75. Suri, A.; Szallasi, A. The emerging role of TRPV1 in diabetes and obesity. *Trends Pharmacol. Sci.* **2008**, *29*, 29–36. [CrossRef] [PubMed]
76. Ludy, M.J.; Moore, G.E.; Mattes, R.D. The effects of capsaicin and capsiate on energy balance: Critical review and meta-analyses of studies in humans. *Chem. Senses* **2012**, *37*, 103–121. [CrossRef] [PubMed]
77. Motter, A.L.; Ahern, G.P. TRPV1-null mice are protected from diet-induced obesity. *FEBS Lett.* **2008**, *582*, 2257–2262. [CrossRef] [PubMed]
78. Marshall, N.J.; Liang, L.; Bodkin, J.; Dessapt-Baradez, C.; Nandi, M.; Collot-Teixeira, S.; Smillie, S.J.; Lalgi, K.; Fernandes, E.S.; Gnudi, L.; et al. A role for TRPV1 in influencing the onset of cardiovascular disease in obesity. *Hypertension* **2013**, *61*, 246–252. [CrossRef] [PubMed]
79. Szallasi, A.; Blumberg, P.M. Vanilloid (Capsaicin) receptors and mechanisms. *Pharmacol. Rev.* **1999**, *51*, 159–212. [PubMed]
80. Baskaran, P.; Krishnan, V.; Ren, J.; Thyagarajan, B. Capsaicin Induces Browning of White Adipose Tissue and Counters Obesity by activating TRPV1 dependent mechanism. *Br. J. Pharmacol.* **2016**. [CrossRef] [PubMed]
81. Okada, Y.; Reinach, P.S.; Shirai, K.; Kitano, A.; Kao, W.W.; Flanders, K.C.; Miyajima, M.; Liu, H.; Zhang, J.; Saika, S. TRPV1 involvement in inflammatory tissue fibrosis in mice. *Am. J. Pathol.* **2011**, *178*, 2654–2664. [CrossRef] [PubMed]
82. Yang, H.; Wang, Z.; Capo-Aponte, J.E.; Zhang, F.; Pan, Z.; Reinach, P.S. Epidermal growth factor receptor transactivation by the cannabinoid receptor (CB1) and transient receptor potential vanilloid 1 (TRPV1) induces differential responses in corneal epithelial cells. *Exp. Eye Res.* **2010**, *91*, 462–471. [CrossRef] [PubMed]
83. Pan, Z.; Wang, Z.; Yang, H.; Zhang, F.; Reinach, P.S. TRPV1 activation is required for hypertonicity-stimulated inflammatory cytokine release in human corneal epithelial cells. *Investig. Ophthalmol. Vis. Sci.* **2011**, *52*, 485–493. [CrossRef] [PubMed]
84. Reinach, P.S.; Mergler, S.; Okada, Y.; Saika, S. Ocular transient receptor potential channel function in health and disease. *BMC Ophthalmol.* **2015**, *15* (Suppl. 1), 153. [CrossRef] [PubMed]
85. Moran, M.M.; McAlexander, M.A.; Biro, T.; Szallasi, A. Transient receptor potential channels as therapeutic targets. *Nat. Rev. Drug Discov.* **2011**, *10*, 601–620. [CrossRef] [PubMed]
86. Szallasi, A.; Sheta, M. Targeting TRPV1 for pain relief: limits, losers and laurels. *Expert Opin. Investig. Drugs* **2012**, *21*, 1351–1369. [CrossRef] [PubMed]
87. Szolcsanyi, J.; Pinter, E. Transient receptor potential vanilloid 1 as a therapeutic target in analgesia. *Expert Opin. Ther. Targets* **2013**, *17*, 641–657. [CrossRef] [PubMed]
88. Kort, M.E.; Kym, P.R. TRPV1 antagonists: clinical setbacks and prospects for future development. *Prog. Med. Chem.* **2012**, *51*, 57–70. [PubMed]
89. Kelly, S.; Chapman, R.J.; Woodhams, S.; Sagar, D.R.; Turner, J.; Burston, J.J.; Bullock, C.; Paton, K.; Huang, J.; Wong, A.; et al. Increased function of pronociceptive TRPV1 at the level of the joint in a rat model of osteoarthritis pain. *Ann. Rheum. Dis.* **2015**, *74*, 252–259. [PubMed]
90. Cathcart, C.J.; Johnston, S.A.; Reynolds, L.R.; Al-Nadaf, S.; Budsberg, S.C. Efficacy of ABT-116, an antagonist of transient receptor potential vanilloid type 1, in providing analgesia for dogs with chemically induced synovitis. *Am. J. Vet. Res.* **2012**, *73*, 19–26. [CrossRef] [PubMed]
91. Miller, F.; Bjornsson, M.; Svensson, O.; Karlsten, R. Experiences with an adaptive design for a dose-finding study in patients with osteoarthritis. *Contemp. Clin. Trials* **2014**, *37*, 189–199. [CrossRef] [PubMed]
92. Schwartz, E.S.; La, J.H.; Scheff, N.N.; Davis, B.M.; Albers, K.M.; Gebhart, G.F. TRPV1 and TRPA1 antagonists prevent the transition of acute to chronic inflammation and pain in chronic pancreatitis. *J. Neurosci.* **2013**, *33*, 5603–5611. [CrossRef] [PubMed]
93. Ghilardi, J.R.; Rohrich, H.; Lindsay, T.H.; Sevcik, M.A.; Schwei, M.J.; Kubota, K.; Halvorson, K.G.; Poblete, J.; Chaplan, S.R.; Dubin, A.E.; et al. Selective blockade of the capsaicin receptor TRPV1 attenuates bone cancer pain. *J. Neurosci.* **2005**, *25*, 3126–3131. [CrossRef] [PubMed]

94. Lehto, S.G.; Tamir, R.; Deng, H.; Klionsky, L.; Kuang, R.; Le, A.; Lee, D.; Louis, J.C.; Magal, E.; Manning, B.H.; et al. Antihyperalgesic effects of (*R*,*E*)-*N*-(2-hydroxy-2,3-dihydro-1*H*-inden-4-yl)-3-(2-(piperidin-1-yl)-4-(trifluorom ethyl)phenyl)-acrylamide (AMG8562), a novel transient receptor potential vanilloid type 1 modulator that does not cause hyperthermia in rats. *J. Pharmacol. Exp. Ther.* **2008**, *326*, 218–229. [CrossRef] [PubMed]

95. Koplas, P.A.; Rosenberg, R.L.; Oxford, G.S. The role of calcium in the desensitization of capsaicin responses in rat dorsal root ganglion neurons. *J. Neurosci.* **1997**, *17*, 3525–3537. [PubMed]

96. Chuang, H.H.; Prescott, E.D.; Kong, H.; Shields, S.; Jordt, S.E.; Basbaum, A.I.; Chao, M.V.; Julius, D. Bradykinin and nerve growth factor release the capsaicin receptor from PtdIns(4,5)P2-mediated inhibition. *Nature* **2001**, *411*, 957–962. [CrossRef] [PubMed]

97. Klein, R.M.; Ufret-Vincenty, C.A.; Hua, L.; Gordon, S.E. Determinants of molecular specificity in phosphoinositide regulation. Phosphatidylinositol (4,5)-bisphosphate (PI(4,5)P2) is the endogenous lipid regulating TRPV1. *J. Biol. Chem.* **2008**, *283*, 26208–26216. [CrossRef] [PubMed]

98. Lukacs, V.; Rives, J.M.; Sun, X.; Zakharian, E.; Rohacs, T. Promiscuous activation of transient receptor potential vanilloid 1 channels by negatively charged intracellular lipids, the key role of endogenous phosphoinositides in maintaining channel activity. *J. Biol. Chem.* **2013**, *288*, 35003–35013. [CrossRef] [PubMed]

99. Lukacs, V.; Thyagarajan, B.; Varnai, P.; Balla, A.; Balla, T.; Rohacs, T. Dual regulation of TRPV1 by phosphoinositides. *J. Neurosci.* **2007**, *27*, 7070–7080. [CrossRef] [PubMed]

100. Poblete, H.; Oyarzun, I.; Olivero, P.; Comer, J.; Zuniga, M.; Sepulveda, R.V.; Baez-Nieto, D.; Gonzalez Leon, C.; Gonzalez-Nilo, F.; Latorre, R. Molecular determinants of phosphatidylinositol 4,5-bisphosphate (PI(4,5)P2) binding to transient receptor potential V1 (TRPV1) channels. *J. Biol. Chem.* **2014**, *290*, 2086–2098. [CrossRef] [PubMed]

101. Lukacs, V.; Yudin, Y.; Hammond, G.R.; Sharma, E.; Fukami, K.; Rohacs, T. Distinctive changes in plasma membrane phosphoinositides underlie differential regulation of TRPV1 in nociceptive neurons. *J. Neurosci.* **2013**, *33*, 11451–11463. [CrossRef] [PubMed]

102. Yao, J.; Qin, F. Interaction with phosphoinositides confers adaptation onto the TRPV1 pain receptor. *PLoS Biol.* **2009**, *7*, e1000046. [CrossRef] [PubMed]

103. Hammond, G.R.; Fischer, M.J.; Anderson, K.E.; Holdich, J.; Koteci, A.; Balla, T.; Irvine, R.F. PI4P and PI(4,5)P2 are essential but independent lipid determinants of membrane identity. *Science* **2012**, *337*, 727–730. [CrossRef] [PubMed]

104. Lishko, P.V.; Procko, E.; Jin, X.; Phelps, C.B.; Gaudet, R. The ankyrin repeats of TRPV1 bind multiple ligands and modulate channel sensitivity. *Neuron* **2007**, *54*, 905–918. [CrossRef] [PubMed]

105. Yu, Y.; Carter, C.R.; Youssef, N.; Dyck, J.R.; Light, P.E. Intracellular long-chain acyl CoAs activate TRPV1 channels. *PLoS ONE* **2014**, *9*, e96597. [CrossRef] [PubMed]

106. Rohacs, T. Phosphoinositide regulation of TRPV1 revisited. *Pflugers. Arch.* **2015**, *467*, 1851–1869. [CrossRef] [PubMed]

107. Numazaki, M.; Tominaga, T.; Takeuchi, K.; Murayama, N.; Toyooka, H.; Tominaga, M. Structural determinant of TRPV1 desensitization interacts with calmodulin. *Proc. Natl. Acad. Sci. USA* **2003**, *100*, 8002–8006. [CrossRef] [PubMed]

108. Docherty, R.J.; Yeats, J.C.; Bevan, S.; Boddeke, H.W. Inhibition of calcineurin inhibits the desensitization of capsaicin-evoked currents in cultured dorsal root ganglion neurones from adult rats. *Pflugers. Arch.* **1996**, *431*, 828–837. [CrossRef] [PubMed]

109. Mohapatra, D.P.; Nau, C. Desensitization of capsaicin-activated currents in the vanilloid receptor TRPV1 is decreased by the cyclic AMP-dependent protein kinase pathway. *J. Biol. Chem.* **2003**, *278*, 50080–50090. [CrossRef] [PubMed]

110. Sanz-Salvador, L.; Andres-Borderia, A.; Ferrer-Montiel, A.; Planells-Cases, R. Agonist-and Ca^{2+}-dependent desensitization of TRPV1 channel targets the receptor to lysosomes for degradation. *J. Biol. Chem.* **2012**, *287*, 19462–19471. [CrossRef] [PubMed]

111. Rosenbaum, T.; Gordon-Shaag, A.; Munari, M.; Gordon, S.E. Ca^{2+}/calmodulin modulates TRPV1 activation by capsaicin. *J. Gen. Physiol.* **2004**, *123*, 53–62. [CrossRef] [PubMed]

112. Lau, S.Y.; Procko, E.; Gaudet, R. Distinct properties of Ca^{2+}-calmodulin binding to N- and C-terminal regulatory regions of the TRPV1 channel. *J. Gen. Physiol.* **2012**, *140*, 541–555. [CrossRef] [PubMed]

113. Piper, A.S.; Yeats, J.C.; Bevan, S.; Docherty, R.J. A study of the voltage dependence of capsaicin-activated membrane currents in rat sensory neurones before and after acute desensitization. *J. Physiol.* **1999**, *518 Pt 3*, 721–733. [CrossRef] [PubMed]

114. Liu, B.; Zhang, C.; Qin, F. Functional recovery from desensitization of vanilloid receptor TRPV1 requires resynthesis of phosphatidylinositol 4,5-bisphosphate. *J. Neurosci.* **2005**, *25*, 4835–4843. [CrossRef] [PubMed]

115. Bleakman, D.; Brorson, J.R.; Miller, R.J. The effect of capsaicin on voltage-gated calcium currents and calcium signals in cultured dorsal root ganglion cells. *Br. J. Pharmacol.* **1990**, *101*, 423–431. [CrossRef] [PubMed]

116. Comunanza, V.; Carbone, E.; Marcantoni, A.; Sher, E.; Ursu, D. Calcium-dependent inhibition of T-type calcium channels by TRPV1 activation in rat sensory neurons. *Pflugers. Arch.* **2011**, *462*, 709–722. [CrossRef] [PubMed]

117. Docherty, R.J.; Robertson, B.; Bevan, S. Capsaicin causes prolonged inhibition of voltage-activated calcium currents in adult rat dorsal root ganglion neurons in culture. *Neuroscience* **1991**, *40*, 513–521. [CrossRef]

118. Hagenacker, T.; Splettstoesser, F.; Greffrath, W.; Treede, R.D.; Busselberg, D. Capsaicin differentially modulates voltage-activated calcium channel currents in dorsal root ganglion neurones of rats. *Brain Res.* **2005**, *1062*, 74–85. [CrossRef] [PubMed]

119. Wu, Z.Z.; Chen, S.R.; Pan, H.L. Transient receptor potential vanilloid type 1 activation down-regulates voltage-gated calcium channels through calcium-dependent calcineurin in sensory neurons. *J. Biol. Chem.* **2005**, *280*, 18142–18151. [CrossRef] [PubMed]

120. Wu, Z.Z.; Chen, S.R.; Pan, H.L. Signaling mechanisms of down-regulation of voltage-activated Ca^{2+} channels by transient receptor potential vanilloid type 1 stimulation with olvanil in primary sensory neurons. *Neuroscience* **2006**, *141*, 407–419. [CrossRef] [PubMed]

121. Liu, L.; Oortgiesen, M.; Li, L.; Simon, S.A. Capsaicin inhibits activation of voltage-gated sodium currents in capsaicin-sensitive trigeminal ganglion neurons. *J. Neurophysiol.* **2001**, *85*, 745–758. [PubMed]

122. Zhang, X.F.; Han, P.; Neelands, T.R.; McGaraughty, S.; Honore, P.; Surowy, C.S.; Zhang, D. Coexpression and activation of TRPV1 suppress the activity of the KCNQ2/3 channel. *J. Gen. Physiol.* **2011**, *138*, 341–352. [CrossRef] [PubMed]

123. Kwak, J. Capsaicin blocks the hyperpolarization-activated inward currents via TRPV1 in the rat dorsal root ganglion neurons. *Exp. Neurobiol.* **2012**, *21*, 75–82. [CrossRef] [PubMed]

124. Piper, A.S.; Docherty, R.J. One-way cross-desensitization between P2X purinoceptors and vanilloid receptors in adult rat dorsal root ganglion neurones. *J. Physiol.* **2000**, *523 Pt 3*, 685–696. [CrossRef] [PubMed]

125. Stanchev, D.; Blosa, M.; Milius, D.; Gerevich, Z.; Rubini, P.; Schmalzing, G.; Eschrich, K.; Schaefer, M.; Wirkner, K.; Illes, P. Cross-inhibition between native and recombinant TRPV1 and P2X(3) receptors. *Pain* **2009**, *143*, 26–36. [CrossRef] [PubMed]

126. Akopian, A.N.; Ruparel, N.B.; Jeske, N.A.; Hargreaves, K.M. Transient receptor potential TRPA1 channel desensitization in sensory neurons is agonist dependent and regulated by TRPV1-directed internalization. *J. Physiol.* **2007**, *583*, 175–193. [CrossRef] [PubMed]

127. Borbiro, I.; Badheka, D.; Rohacs, T. Activation of TRPV1 channels inhibit mechanosensitive Piezo channel activity by depleting membrane phosphoinositides. *Sci. Signal.* **2015**, *8*, ra15. [CrossRef]

128. Pecze, L.; Pelsoczi, P.; Kecskes, M.; Winter, Z.; Papp, A.; Kaszas, K.; Letoha, T.; Vizler, C.; Olah, Z. Resiniferatoxin mediated ablation of TRPV1+ neurons removes TRPA1 as well. *Can. J. Neurol. Sci.* **2009**, *36*, 234–241. [CrossRef] [PubMed]

129. Anand, P.; Bley, K. Topical capsaicin for pain management: therapeutic potential and mechanisms of action of the new high-concentration capsaicin 8% patch. *Br. J. Anaesth.* **2011**, *107*, 490–502. [CrossRef] [PubMed]

130. Simone, D.A.; Nolano, M.; Johnson, T.; Wendelschafer-Crabb, G.; Kennedy, W.R. Intradermal injection of capsaicin in humans produces degeneration and subsequent reinnervation of epidermal nerve fibers: Correlation with sensory function. *J. Neurosci.* **1998**, *18*, 8947–8959. [PubMed]

131. Pinter, E.; Helyes, Z.; Szolcsanyi, J. Inhibitory effect of somatostatin on inflammation and nociception. *Pharmacol. Ther.* **2006**, *112*, 440–456. [CrossRef] [PubMed]

132. Szolcsanyi, J.; Pinter, E.; Helyes, Z.; Petho, G. Inhibition of the function of TRPV1-expressing nociceptive sensory neurons by somatostatin 4 receptor agonism: Mechanism and therapeutical implications. *Curr. Top. Med. Chem.* **2011**, *11*, 2253–2263. [CrossRef] [PubMed]

133. Gibbons, C.H.; Wang, N.; Freeman, R. Capsaicin induces degeneration of cutaneous autonomic nerve fibers. *Ann. Neurol.* **2010**, *68*, 888–898. [CrossRef] [PubMed]
134. Uceyler, N.; Sommer, C. High-dose capsaicin for the treatment of neuropathic pain: What we know and what we need to know. *Pain Ther.* **2014**, *3*, 73–84. [CrossRef] [PubMed]
135. Jancso, G.; Kiraly, E.; Jancso-Gabor, A. Pharmacologically induced selective degeneration of chemosensitive primary sensory neurones. *Nature* **1977**, *270*, 741–743. [CrossRef] [PubMed]
136. Cavanaugh, D.J.; Lee, H.; Lo, L.; Shields, S.D.; Zylka, M.J.; Basbaum, A.I.; Anderson, D.J. Distinct subsets of unmyelinated primary sensory fibers mediate behavioral responses to noxious thermal and mechanical stimuli. *Proc. Natl. Acad. Sci. USA* **2009**, *106*, 9075–9080. [CrossRef] [PubMed]
137. Brown, J.D.; Saeed, M.; Do, L.; Braz, J.; Basbaum, A.I.; Iadarola, M.J.; Wilson, D.M.; Dillon, W.P. CT-guided injection of a TRPV1 agonist around dorsal root ganglia decreases pain transmission in swine. *Sci. Transl. Med.* **2015**, *7*, 305ra145. [CrossRef] [PubMed]
138. Saotome, K.; Singh, A.K.; Yelshanskaya, M.V.; Sobolevsky, A.I. Crystal structure of the epithelial calcium channel TRPV6. *Nature* **2016**, *534*, 506–511. [CrossRef] [PubMed]
139. Cao, E.; Liao, M.; Cheng, Y.; Julius, D. TRPV1 structures in distinct conformations reveal activation mechanisms. *Nature* **2013**, *504*, 113–118. [CrossRef] [PubMed]
140. Liao, M.; Cao, E.; Julius, D.; Cheng, Y. Structure of the TRPV1 ion channel determined by electron cryo-microscopy. *Nature* **2013**, *504*, 107–112. [CrossRef] [PubMed]
141. Paulsen, C.E.; Armache, J.P.; Gao, Y.; Cheng, Y.; Julius, D. Structure of the TRPA1 ion channel suggests regulatory mechanisms. *Nature* **2015**, *520*, 511–517. [CrossRef] [PubMed]
142. Zubcevic, L.; Herzik, M.A., Jr.; Chung, B.C.; Liu, Z.; Lander, G.C.; Lee, S.Y. Cryo-electron microscopy structure of the TRPV2 ion channel. *Nat. Struct. Mol. Biol.* **2016**, *23*, 180–186. [CrossRef] [PubMed]
143. Huynh, K.W.; Cohen, M.R.; Jiang, J.; Samanta, A.; Lodowski, D.T.; Zhou, Z.H.; Moiseenkova-Bell, V.Y. Structure of the full-length TRPV2 channel by cryo-EM. *Nat. Commun.* **2016**, *7*, 11130. [CrossRef] [PubMed]
144. Gao, Y.; Cao, E.; Julius, D.; Cheng, Y. TRPV1 structures in nanodiscs reveal mechanisms of ligand and lipid action. *Nature* **2016**, *534*, 347–351. [CrossRef] [PubMed]
145. Kasimova, M.A.; Granata, D.; Carnevale, V. Voltage-gated sodium channels: Evolutionary history and distinctive sequence features. *Curr. Top. Membr.* **2016**, http://dx.doi.org/10.1016/bs.ctm.2016.05.002.
146. Bevan, S.; Hothi, S.; Hughes, G.; James, I.F.; Rang, H.P.; Shah, K.; Walpole, C.S.; Yeats, J.C. Capsazepine: A competitive antagonist of the sensory neurone excitant capsaicin. *Br. J. Pharmacol.* **1992**, *107*, 544–552. [CrossRef] [PubMed]
147. Diaz-Franulic, I.; Caceres-Molina, J.; Sepulveda, R.V.; Gonzalez-Nilo, F.; Latorre, R. Structure driven pharmacology of transient receptor potential channel vanilloid 1 (TRPV1). *Mol. Pharmacol.* **2016**. [CrossRef] [PubMed]
148. Yang, F.; Xiao, X.; Chen, W.; Yang, W.; Yu, P.; Song, Z.; Yarov-Yarovoy, V.; Zheng, J. Structural mechanism underlying capsaicin binding and activation of the TRPV1 ion channel. *Nat. Chem. Biol.* **2015**, *11*, 518–524. [CrossRef] [PubMed]
149. Ranganathan, R.; Lewis, J.H.; MacKinnon, R. Spatial localization of the K$^+$ channel selectivity filter by mutant cycle-based structure analysis. *Neuron* **1996**, *16*, 131–139. [CrossRef]
150. Darre, L.; Domene, C. Binding of capsaicin to the TRPV1 ion channel. *Mol. Pharm.* **2015**, *12*, 4454–4465. [CrossRef] [PubMed]
151. Fowler, P.W.; Sansom, M.S. The pore of voltage-gated potassium ion channels is strained when closed. *Nat. Commun.* **2013**, *4*, 1872. [CrossRef] [PubMed]
152. Yang, F.; Vu, S.; Yarov-Yarovoy, V.; Zheng, J. Rational design and validation of a vanilloid-sensitive TRPV2 ion channel. *Proc. Natl. Acad. Sci. USA* **2016**, *113*, E3657–E3666. [CrossRef] [PubMed]
153. Zhang, F.; Hanson, S.M.; Jara-Oseguera, A.; Krepkiy, D.; Bae, C.; Pearce, L.V.; Blumberg, P.M.; Newstead, S.; Swartz, K.J. Engineering vanilloid-sensitivity into the rat TRPV2 channel. *eLife* **2016**, *5*, e16409. [CrossRef] [PubMed]
154. Feng, Z.; Pearce, L.V.; Xu, X.; Yang, X.; Yang, P.; Blumberg, P.M.; Xie, X.Q. Structural insight into tetrameric hTRPV1 from homology modeling, molecular docking, molecular dynamics simulation, virtual screening, and bioassay validations. *J. Chem. Inf. Model.* **2015**, *55*, 572–588. [CrossRef] [PubMed]

Pharmaceuticals **2016**, *9*, 52

155. Feng, Z.; Pearce, L.V.; Zhang, Y.; Xing, C.; Herold, B.K.; Ma, S.; Hu, Z.; Turcios, N.A.; Yang, P.; Tong, Q.; et al. Multi-functional diarylurea small molecule inhibitors of TRPV1 with therapeutic potential for neuroinflammation. *AAPS J.* **2016**, *18*, 898–913. [CrossRef] [PubMed]
156. Ann, J.; Ki, Y.; Yoon, S.; Kim, M.S.; Lee, J.U.; Kim, C.; Lee, S.; Jung, A.; Baek, J.; Hong, S.; et al. 2-Sulfonamidopyridine C-region analogs of 2-(3-fluoro-4-methylsulfonamidophenyl)propanamides as potent TRPV1 antagonists. *Bioorg. Med. Chem.* **2016**, *24*, 1231–1240. [CrossRef] [PubMed]
157. Ann, J.; Sun, W.; Zhou, X.; Jung, A.; Baek, J.; Lee, S.; Kim, C.; Yoon, S.; Hong, S.; Choi, S.; et al. Discovery of *N*-(3-fluoro-4-methylsulfonamidomethylphenyl)urea as a potent TRPV1 antagonistic template. *Bioorg. Med. Chem. Lett.* **2016**, *26*, 3603–3607. [CrossRef] [PubMed]

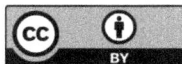

pharmaceuticals

MDPI

Review

Nociceptive TRP Channels: Sensory Detectors and Transducers in Multiple Pain Pathologies

Aaron D. Mickle [1,2], Andrew J. Shepherd [1,2] and Durga P. Mohapatra [1,2,3,4,*]

1 Department of Anesthesiology, Washington University School of Medicine, 660 S. Euclid Avenue, St. Louis, MO 63110, USA; amickle@wustl.edu (A.D.M.); a.shepherd@wustl.edu (A.J.S.)
2 Washington University Pain Center, Department of Anesthesiology, Washington University School of Medicine, 660 S. Euclid Avenue, St. Louis, MO 63110, USA
3 Center for Investigation of Membrane Excitability Diseases, Washington University School of Medicine, 660 S. Euclid Avenue, St. Louis, MO 63110, USA
4 Siteman Cancer Center, Washington University School of Medicine, 660 S. Euclid Avenue, St. Louis, MO 63110, USA
* Correspondence: d.p.mohapatra@wustl.edu; Tel.: +1-314-362-8229; Fax: +1-314-362-8334

Academic Editors: Arpad Szallasi and Susan M. Huang
Received: 24 August 2016; Accepted: 9 November 2016; Published: 14 November 2016

Abstract: Specialized receptors belonging to the transient receptor potential (TRP) family of ligand-gated ion channels constitute the critical detectors and transducers of pain-causing stimuli. Nociceptive TRP channels are predominantly expressed by distinct subsets of sensory neurons of the peripheral nervous system. Several of these TRP channels are also expressed in neurons of the central nervous system, and in non-neuronal cells that communicate with sensory nerves. Nociceptive TRPs are activated by specific physico-chemical stimuli to provide the excitatory trigger in neurons. In addition, decades of research has identified a large number of immune and neuromodulators as mediators of nociceptive TRP channel activation during injury, inflammatory and other pathological conditions. These findings have led to aggressive targeting of TRP channels for the development of new-generation analgesics. This review summarizes the complex activation and/or modulation of nociceptive TRP channels under pathophysiological conditions, and how these changes underlie acute and chronic pain conditions. Furthermore, development of small-molecule antagonists for several TRP channels as analgesics, and the positive and negative outcomes of these drugs in clinical trials are discussed. Understanding the diverse functional and modulatory properties of nociceptive TRP channels is critical to function-based drug targeting for the development of evidence-based and efficacious new generation analgesics.

Keywords: TRP channel; pain; nociception; inflammatory pain; neuropathic pain; visceral pain; cancer pain; migraine; dental pain; peripheral sensitization

1. Introduction

Pain constitutes an "unpleasant sensory and emotional experience associated with actual or potential tissue damage", as defined by The International Association for the Study of Pain [1]. As a sensory modality, pain represents an integral part of life. It serves as a protective mechanism and an associative condition, as well as an alarm system for a wide range of pathological conditions. In addition, pathologies and/or disease conditions that exclusively lead to pain also exist. The first and foremost process is the peripheral detection and transduction of noxious stimuli that are determined as painful by the higher-order structures in the central nervous system (CNS). The terminology that has been widely used to define this process is "nociception", which accounts for the neural mechanisms and pathways for the encoding and processing of noxious stimuli [1]. Nociception constitutes the primary physiological and/or pathophysiological process for the somatic, visceral and trigeminal sensory systems. The specialized receptive fields as well as the molecular entities therein are widely regarded as nociceptors. Sensory neurons of the peripheral nervous system (PNS) that transmit nociceptive signals lie in distinct populations of sensory ganglia. These neurons send peripheral afferents to the somatic, visceral, and craniofacial regions, and also connect to the spinal cord and brain stem. These neurons are the critical anatomical/structural mediators of sensory signal transmission between the PNS and CNS.

Nociceptive neurons are functionally characterized by the type of sensory receptors and ion channels expressed on the plasma membrane throughout the cell body (somata) and nerve fibers. These receptors/channels are vital for the detection of various noxious stimuli. These neurons also possess the molecular machinery to convert the noxious signals into electrical signals and transmit this information to the CNS. Nociceptive receptors/channels, membrane proteins belonging to the Transient Receptor Potential (TRP) family, constitute the major group of molecular detectors/ transducers. The first TRP channel discovered was a defective phototransduction channel from a mutant form of *Drosophila* that exhibited an abnormally transient membrane potential change in response to bright light, and was subsequently found preserved/conserved in many animal species [2,3]. TRPs are non-selective cation channels with relatively high Ca^{2+}-permeability, and are expressed in a wide variety of cell/tissue types, both on the plasma membrane and intracellular organelle membranes [4,5]. They also share identical overall membrane topology, consisting of tetramers of 6-transmembrane (6-TM) segment polypeptide subunits with a central ion conduction pore, which is similar to voltage-gated K^+ channels. Since their discovery, the TRP family of proteins have now grown significantly, and to date consist of six sub-families with 28 mammalian members; categorized as canonical (TRPC), vanilloid (TRPV), ankyrin (TRPA), melastatin (TRPM), polycystin (TRPP), and mucolipin (TRPML) [4,5]. In general, TRP channels are primary transducers of most known sensory modalities such as vision, hearing, olfaction, taste and touch, to a wide range of innocuous-to-noxious stimuli, and are therefore one of the most extensively studied receptor families in sensory biology [5–7]. The diversity in TRP channels is mainly linked to the greatest level of amino acid sequence differences in their cytoplasmic N- and C-termini. Based on their ability to detect and transduce specific nociceptive modalities, members of only three TRP sub-families, TRPV, TRPA and TRPM, have been grouped into the category of "nociceptive TRP channels". Activation of nociceptive TRP channels by specific noxious and/or pain-producing stimuli serves as the principal mode of detection/transduction of pain under physiological and pathophysiological conditions. In addition, modifications in channel function and trafficking properties, as well as changes in gene expression of nociceptive TRP channels are considered to be highly critical for peripheral nociceptive and pain processing under a wide variety of pathological conditions. Since in-depth studies have already been conducted to characterize the role of nociceptive TRP channels in multiple pain and migraine pathologies, they constitute attractive targets for new-generation analgesics and anti-migraine drug developments [8–13]. This review summarizes a comprehensive knowledge on the molecular characterization of nociceptive TRP channels, their constitutive and modulatory functions, expression and tissue distribution, as well as how these channels and their specific properties are critically involved in various pain conditions. Recent developments in analgesic targeting of nociceptive TRP channels are also outlined here.

2. Nociceptive TRP Channels

2.1. History, Identification and Cloning

Excitation of sensory nerves by multiple chemical and physical stimuli was first described over 100 years ago [14]. In addition to heat and cold stimuli, one of the first chemical compounds described to activate sensory neurons was capsaicin. Extensive research studies conducted between 1960 and the mid-1990s showed specific actions of capsaicin on sensory neurons, and thereby proposed the existence of a specialized receptor—"the capsaicin receptor" [15]. Even before molecular cloning, studies suggested that the capsaicin receptor was a TRP-like receptor channel, since capsaicin's actions on sensory nerves were effectively blocked by the non-selective TRP channel blocker ruthenium red [16]. Ultimately, in 1997 the molecular identity of the capsaicin receptor was revealed by expression cloning using a cDNA library generated from rodent sensory neurons [17], and named as "vanilloid receptor subtype-1" (VR1). Subsequently VR1 was assigned as the first member of the new TRP channel family TRPV, and referred to as TRPV1. Along with gene discovery, further characterization of TRPV1 revealed the ability of this channel to be activated by multimodal pain-producing stimuli, as well as integration of such stimuli at the channel protein level [17,18]. This discovery provided the much-awaited catalyst for the subsequent discovery of a series of nociceptive TRP channels for several noxious and painful stimuli. The next TRP channel cloned was TRPV2 and characterized as the high noxious temperature transducer on rodent sensory neurons [19]. Utilizing TRPV1 and TRPV2 cDNA sequences, the TRPV4 expressed-sequence tag (EST) from GenBank, and subsequently the cDNA for TRPV4 from rat kidney cDNA library were identified as osmotically-activated TRP channels (VR-OAC and OTRPC4) [20,21]. Similar approaches also led to the identification and cloning of TRPV5 and TRPV6 [22–24]. It was also proposed that cold temperatures and menthol, the cooling compound in mint leaves, activate another receptor on sensory neurons [25]. It was subsequently confirmed with the cloning and characterization of the "cold-menthol receptor-1", later designated as TRPM8 [26,27]. With both heat- and cold-activation receptors identified, the obvious next question centered on the identity of receptor(s) that could be activated by temperatures in the neutral range. This led to the identification/cloning of TRPV3 from human sensory neurons and rodent keratinocytes, based on a sequence homology cloning strategy utilizing TRPV1–6 sequences [28,29]. Although originally cloned from human lung fibroblasts as a cell growth-controlling protein [30], identification and cloning of ankyrin-containing transmembrane protein-1 (ANKTM1), later designated as TRPA1, from rodent sensory neurons led to the discovery of a noxious cold- and mechano-sensitive channel [31]. Similarly, the EST of TRPM3 channel was initially cloned and characterized from a human kidney cDNA library, as a Ca^{2+} permeable channel, and subsequently as the receptor for several steroids, including pregnenolone sulfate [32–34]. Much later, the thermo-sensing and nociceptive properties of TRPM3 were identified and characterized [35]. Overall, the nociceptive TRP channel group represents a critical mass of receptors sensing diverse painful and non-painful modalities, and are thus extensively studied, as well as explored as therapeutic targets.

2.2. Characterization of Channel Function: Activation by Diverse Physico-Chemical Stimuli

Distinct physico-chemical activation represents the crucial functional property of nociceptive TRP channels, a property that was exploited to the fullest to aid in their identification and cloning. In addition, algogenic chemicals found in natural sources, such as plants and spices, greatly influenced the functional characterization and provided identification of these channels. The majority of these channels turn out to be polymodal, in terms of their activation. The exhaustive list of exogenous and endogenous activators of nociceptive TRP channels and their underlying structure-functional mechanisms have recently been detailed [11]. Here we summarize only the endogenous or pathophysiological activators of nociceptive TRP channels (Figure 1). Starting with the major polymodal nociceptive TRP channel, TRPV1, which is directly activated by noxious temperatures ($\geq$43 °C) and an acidic extracellular environment (~pH 6.0 or less) [9,17,18,36], as well as by a basic intracellular environment (~pH 7.8 or more) [37]. A number of endovanilloids and endocannabinoids generated by lipid metabolism pathways and/or under inflammatory conditions also directly activate TRPV1 [9,38–40]. In heterologous expression systems, TRPV1 can also be activated by reactive oxygen and nitrogen species (ROS/RNS), although whether such activation operates in sensory neurons still remains a matter of debate [41]. Activation of TRPV1 leads to the influx of Ca^{2+} and Na^+ (with relatively high permeability for Ca^{2+}) through the channel pore [17,42,43], which then results in neuronal plasma membrane depolarization and subsequent opening of Na_v/Ca_v channels to initiate AP firing. Following activation, the TRPV1 channel undergoes rapid Ca^{2+}-dependent desensitization, resulting in diminished AP firing [17,18,43–45]. In contrast, the TRPV2 channel can only be activated by higher noxious temperatures (>52 °C), with no endogenous ligands identified so far [19,34]. Activation of TRPV2 also leads to cellular influx of Ca^{2+} and Na^+ with relatively high Ca^{2+} permeability [19]. Similarly, warm temperatures account for the activation of TRPV3 (32 °C to 40 °C) and TRPV4 (≥33 °C), which then lead to cellular influx of Ca^{2+} and Na^+ with high relative Ca^{2+} permeability [5,46,47], resulting in membrane depolarization and subsequent AP firing. In addition, TRPV4 can be activated by osmotic changes and mechanical forces such as pressure and shear stress [47–50].

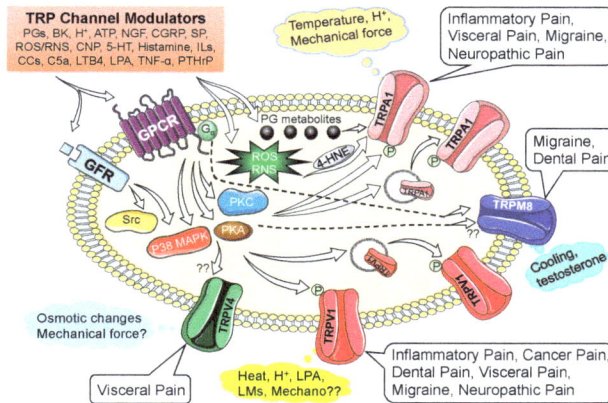

Figure 1. Scheme depicting specific activators and modulators of various nociceptive transient receptor potential (TRP) channels on mammalian sensory neurons. Involvement of individual TRP channels in specific pain-related pathologies are indicated/listed within call-out boxes. Abbreviations: 5-HT, serotonin; ATP, adenosine triphosphate; BK, bradykinin; CCs, chemokines; CGRP, calcitonin gene-related peptide; CNP, C-type natriuretic peptide; GFR, growth factor receptor; GPCR, G protein-coupled receptor; H^+, protons; ILs, interleukins; LMs, lipid mediators; LPA, lysophosphatidic acid; LTB4, leukotriene B4; NGF, nerve growth factor; p38 MAPK, p38 mitogen-activated protein kinase; PGs, prostaglandins; PKA, cAMP-dependent protein kinase; PKC, protein kinase C; PTHrP, parathyroid hormone-related peptide; ROS, reactive oxygen species; RNS, reactive nitrogen species; SP, substance P or neurokinin; Src; *src*-type protein kinase; TRPA1, transient receptor potential sub-family ankyrin, member-1; TRPM8, transient receptor potential sub-family melastatin, member-8; TRPV1, transient receptor potential sub-family vanilloid, member-1; TRPV4, transient receptor potential sub-family vanilloid, member-4.

Although preliminary studies suggested pregnenolone sulfate was the endogenous activator of TRPM3, warm/noxious temperature (>30 °C) activation of the channel has also been shown subsequently [33–35]. Activation of TRPM3, like TRPVs, lead to cellular influx of Ca^{2+} and Na^+ with relatively high Ca^{2+} permeability [33,35]. In contrast, TRPM8 can be activated by innocuous cooling (26 °C–15 °C) to noxious cold temperatures (15 °C–8 °C), leading to cellular influx of Ca^{2+} and Na^+ with high relative Ca^{2+} permeability [26,27,51]. In addition, TRPM8 can be directly activated by testosterone in human prostate cell lines and rat DRG neurons [52,53].

TRPA1 was originally described as a cold-sensing ion channel [31,54,55], although others have debated this conclusion [56]. Comparative analysis of TRPA1 from different species showed that rodent, but not primate TRPA1 could be activated at noxious cold temperatures, which was directly linked to regions within the 5th transmembrane domain and pore region of the channel protein [57]. In contrast, a recent report suggests that human TRPA1 exhibits a U-shaped temperature-activation curve [58]. It shows robust channel activation at noxious cold temperatures (≤15 °C), relative inactivity at mild cooling temperatures (20 °C–25 °C), then increased channel opening at neutral-to-warm temperatures (25 °C–35 °C), and finally a decrease in channel open probability at noxious warm temperatures [58]. Earlier, mouse TRPA1 was shown to be insensitive to warm temperatures [59]. Similarly, acidic pH has also been shown to activate TRPA1 in a species-dependent manner; human, but not rodent TRPA1 is sensitive to acidic pH [60], and a dose-dependent increase in channel gating was found for increasing proton concentration associated with CO_2 or other weak organic acids [61,62]. ROS, a redox mediator released during injury/inflammation activates TRPA1 via cysteine oxidation or formation of disulphide bonds between cysteine residues in the channel protein [63–65]. Furthermore, it has been suggested that ROS-mediated lipid peroxidation leads to 4-hydroxynonenal (4-HNE) production, which then covalently modifies the cytoplasmic cysteine residues to activate TRPA1 [64,66]. Reactive nitrogen species have also been shown to activate the channel by S-nitrosylation [63–65,67]. In addition to nitric oxide (NO), another "gasotransmitter", hydrogen sulphide (H_2S), has also been suggested to activate TRPA1 channel [68,69]. Also, prostaglandin (PG) metabolic products, such as 15dPGJ2, PGA2 and PGA1 have shown to directly activate TRPA1 [70,71]. Elevated levels of intracellular Ca^{2+} have been suggested to activate TRPA1 directly via interaction with one of the three Ca^{2+}-binding EF-hand domains in the cytoplasmic N-terminus of the channel protein [72]. In addition to temperature and chemical activation, TRPA1 channel has also been shown to be a transducer of mechanical force [73,74], and mechanical activation of the channel has been suggested to be modulated by other algesic stimuli [75]. Like other nociceptive TRP channels, activation of TRPA1 also results in increased cellular influx of Ca^{2+} and Na^+ with relatively high Ca^{2+} permeability, leading to sensory neuron membrane depolarization and subsequent AP firing. It has also been suggested that the Ca^{2+} permeability of TRPA1 increases with repeated agonist stimulation [76].

Taken together, a comprehensive scheme for pathological activation of nociceptive TRP channels in sensory neurons can be proposed. Tissue acidosis, which leads to increased H^+ levels, can directly activate TRPV1 and TRPA1 (but only in humans). Similarly, inflammatory and tissue injury conditions produce elevated levels of H^+, ATP, PG metabolites, ROS/RNS, HNO, H_2S, and several lipid metabolites, which can lead to combined activation of TRPV1 and TRPA1 channels. Increased intracellular Ca^{2+} levels, due to activity of multiple TRP channels during pathological conditions, could further activate/potentiate TRPA1 channels. Furthermore, mechanical activation of one or more nociceptive TRP channels, TRPV4, TRPA1 and TRPV1, could be achieved due to the action of pro-algesic agents. Collectively, it is highly likely that multiple nociceptive TRP channels are activated during pathological conditions, which presumably constitute the mechanism for a stronger and long-lasting nociceptor excitation.

2.3. Similarities and Differences in Channel Expression and Localization

Most nociceptive TRP channels are predominantly expressed in small- and medium-diameter peripheral sensory neurons in the trigeminal ganglia (TG), dorsal root ganglia (DRG), sympathetic ganglia (SG) and nodose ganglia (NG). Significant expression of several nociceptive TRP channels has also been shown in the CNS and other tissue and cell types, such as keratinocytes, vascular endothelial cells, bladder epithelial cells and fibroblasts. Furthermore, TRPV1-3 have also been shown to be expressed in human dental pulp [9,11]. TRPV1 protein expression has been detected in peptidergic sensory afferents innervating bones [77], although expression of other nociceptive TRP channels there remains unexplored. Significant overlap between TRPV1 and TRPA1 expression in small/medium-diameter nociceptive neurons in the DRG and TG has been observed. In contrast, TRPM8 shows minimal overlap with TRPV1 and TRPA1 expression in these ganglia [9,78]. Expression of TRPV4 in DRG neurons has been a matter of debate, with initial reports showing functional TRPV4 expression in DRG neurons [50,79], and a subsequent report suggesting no functional TRPV4 expression in mammalian DRG neurons [80]. Information on expression of TRPV2-6, and TRPM3 channels in specific populations of sensory neurons and CNS neurons is still lacking. A recent surge in the utilization of transcriptome analysis has enabled unbiased, large-scale determination of gene expression signatures in DRG neurons from rodents and humans [81,82]. Furthermore, this approach has recently been expanded to localization of mRNA in the DRG cell body vs peripheral nerve fibers, in order to determine not only the expression, but also the sub-cellular localization of nociceptive TRP channel gene transcripts [83]. In contrast, information on expression and localization of these channels at the protein level is less conclusive. Antibody-based assessment of expression and localization of proteins has been the predominant approach, which is often inconclusive, due to inadequate/improper validation of specificity for these biological reagents. The nociceptive TRP channels are membrane proteins, and are localized to the neuronal/cell plasma membrane [84]. However, a significant fraction of channels, at least for TRPV1 and TRPA1 and TRPA1 have also been reported to be present in intracellular organelle membranes, which upon injury/inflammation undergo translocation to the plasma membrane [85–88]. Similar to the dearth of information on expression of other nociceptive TRP channels in the nervous system, their sub-cellular localization and modes of intracellular trafficking remain poorly understood. With the currently available information on nociceptive TRP channel expression and localization, it can be proposed that multiple pathological activators could activate TRPV1 and TRPA1 channels on the same sub-set of afferents, as well as on distinct TRPV1- or TRPA1-expressing sensory neurons. Overlapping expression of nociceptive TRP channels also provides an opportunity for cross-sensitization of TRPV1 and TRPA1 (example: by Ca^{2+}) to maximize nociceptor excitation. In addition, inflammatory mediator-induced increases in the trafficking of TRPV1 and TRPA1 channels could increase the excitatory strength of nociceptors, referred to as "nociceptive tone".

3. Modulation of Nociceptive TRP Channel Activity and Expression

Nociceptive TRP channel activation on peripheral nerve fiber endings, at least for TRPV1 and TRPA1, has been directly linked to release of neuropeptides, such as calcitonin gene-related peptide (CGRP) and neurokinin or substance P (SP). Local elevation of CGRP and SP levels leads to vasodilatation and activation of a variety of immune cells, which results in the release of several pro-inflammatory mediators, growth factors, and bioactive peptides, as well as oxidative stress conditions. Most of these mediators activate specific G protein-coupled receptors (GPCRs) and growth factor receptors (GFRs) on sensory nerves, leading to downstream activation (or inhibition) of several protein kinases and phosphatases. These cellular signal transduction effectors induce post-translational modifications on multiple nociceptive channel proteins, leading to an increase in the activation of these channels (Figure 1), which results in an increase in nociceptor firing [9,11,13]. Specifically, modification of TRPV1 by protein kinases A and C (PKA & PKC), cyclin-dependent kinase-5 (Cdk5), *Src* kinase, and phosphoinositide kinases (PI3/4/5Ks) have all been shown to enhance activation of the channel by: (a) decreasing the temperature threshold of channel activation to physiological temperatures (~35 °C to 37 °C); (b) activating the channel at mildly/moderately acidic pH; and/or (c) enhancing plasma membrane delivery of the channel protein (Figure 1) [11,45,85,86,89–97]. Ca^{2+} influx through TRPA1 and subsequent activation of PKA has also been shown to modulate TRPV1 channel function [98]. In addition to kinases, lipases such as phospholipase C (PLC) have been shown to both promote and inhibit TRPV1 channel function. Hydrolysis of phosphatidylinositol bis-phosphate (PIP2) to inositol triphosphate (IP3) and diacylglycerol (DAG) by PLC sensitizes TRPV1 channel function via PKC, and by releasing constitutive inhibition of the channel from physical coupling with PIP2 [99]. In contrast, other studies have shown that plasma membrane PIP2 is necessary for TRPV1 channel activation [100]. Ca^{2+} influx through TRPV1 has been shown to activate protein phosphatase 2B (PP2B or calcineurin), which then dephosphorylates the channel protein to induce channel desensitization. Conversely, PKA phosphorylation of calcineurin-sensitive residues on TRPV1 protein has been shown to reverse this desensitization, thereby leading to sustained channel opening following activation [97]. All these changes culminate in constitutive activation of TRPV1 under pathophysiological conditions, thereby resulting in sustained nociceptor firing [9,11,13]. In contrast, GABA release from sensory afferents, downstream of TRPV1-mediated Ca^{2+} influx, has been shown to activate $GABA_B$ receptors, leading to attenuation of NGF/serotonin/bradykinin-PKC-modulation of TRPV1 channel activity [101].

ROS/RNS and mechanical stimuli have been shown to activate TRPA1 [75]. Inflammatory mediators such as bradykinin have been shown to sensitize TRPA1 channel function [54], presumably via phosphorylation of the channel protein by PKC. However, another report suggested the involvement of PLC and PKA, but not PKC, in TRPA1 channel sensitization of TRPA1 [102]. Although the basis for such contrasting observations is not clear, it has been proposed that PLC/PKA-modulation of TRPA1 channel activation is achieved by increased trafficking of the channel protein to the cell plasma membrane (Figure 1) [87]. In addition to the modulatory actions on TRPV1 channel, PIP2 has also been shown to reduce the agonist sensitivity of TRPA1 channel activation [103]. Pro-inflammatory lipid metabolites such as lipoxygenases that are enriched during tissue injury and/or inflammatory conditions, have also been shown to activate TRPA1, in addition to TRPV1 [104]. Intracellular influx of Ca^{2+} itself has also been shown to be an intrinsic modulator of TRPA1 channel function [72].

Modulation of TRPM8 channel function has remained somewhat controversial, due to multiple conflicting observations. PKC has been shown to downregulate TRPM8 activity [105–107]; although one study did not find any effect of pharmacological inhibitors of PKC on TRPM8 channel function [108]. Unlike TRPV1 and TRPA1, TRPM8 function was found to be unaffected by PKA signaling [109–112]. Activation of $G\alpha_{q/11}$-coupled receptors by various inflammatory mediators such as bradykinin, histamine, serotonin, and ATP, has been suggested to inhibit TRPM8 channel activity via direct interaction of the $G\alpha_q$ subunit with the channel protein (Figure 1) [113]. Such a phenomenon is thought to constitute a mechanism underlying reduced cold sensation under injury/inflammatory conditions. Modulation of TRPM8 channel function by endovanilloids and endocannabinoids have also been shown [114]. In addition, phospholipase A2 (PLA_2) activity has been shown to enhance TRPM8 channel activity [115,116]. Furthermore, lipid metabolic products downstream of PLA_2 activity, such as lysophospholipids have been shown to raise the temperature activation threshold of TRPM8 closer to body temperature [115]. An increase in PLC activity has also been linked to a decrease in TRPM8 channel activity [51,117–119].

Modulation of TRPV2 channel function by PKA has been shown in immune cells [120], although any role of such modulation in the context of nociceptor biology remains to be determined. Mediators of inflammatory signaling, lipid metabolites and PKC have also been shown to enhance TRPV3 channel activity [34,46], and similar to TRPV2, the role of such channel modulation in the context of nociceptor biology remains to be determined. Both PKA and *Src* phosphorylation of TRPV4, downstream of PGE_2 and protease-activated receptor 2 (PAR2) signaling, have also been shown to modulate channel function [50,121–123]. In addition, PKC-dependent upregulation of TRPV4 channel activity has also been suggested [47]. All such modulatory actions of TRPV4 have been suggested to increase nociceptor firing in response to mechanical stimuli and/or osmotic changes. However, with a recent report suggesting no activation of TRPV4 in mouse DRG neurons to known chemical agonists and osmotic forces [80], the role of TRPV4 modulation in nociceptor function and AP firing remains to be confirmed.

In addition to direct functional modulation, upregulation of gene and protein expression of nociceptive TRP channels also serves as another mechanism for long-term modulation of nociceptor firing. Sustained intracellular Ca^{2+} influx/elevation due to prolonged/episodic activation of TRPV1 has been suggested to enhance the expression of several nociceptive TRP channel and related genes. TRPV1 expression (both at the mRNA and protein level) is enhanced in sensory neurons following tissue injury and inflammation [9,11,13]. Furthermore, an increase in the proportion of sensory neurons expressing functional TRPV1 channel has also been shown following injury/inflammation, as well as upon exposure to inflammatory mediators [9,11,13]. In addition, recent studies have shown rapid translation of TRPV1 mRNA in peripheral sensory fibers in response to pro-inflammatory mediators such as interleukin-6 (IL-6) and NGF, thereby increasing the magnitude of nociceptor excitation [124,125].

Altogether, modulation of nociceptive TRP channels by a plethora of inflammatory mediators provides diverse mechanisms for robust and sustained activation of these channels during multiple pathological conditions. An unified scheme could be proposed: Pathological conditions lead to:

(1) local activation of TRPV1 and TRPA1 at physiological temperatures, mild-to-moderate acidic and oxidative stress conditions; (2) prolonged channel activation, due to reduced desensitization; (3) enhanced channel activation, due to increases in the expression and surface trafficking of TRPV1 and TRPA1 proteins; (4) cross-sensitization of channel activation (by Ca^{2+} and other intracellular signal transduction molecules), and (5) increased gene expression and local mRNA translation for these channels. Collectively, these processes result in an increase in nociceptive tone/excitation and prolonged nociceptor firing. These complex processes underlie mechanisms for peripheral sensory transduction, and provide both opportunities and challenges for the pharmacotherapeutic targeting of multiple painful pathologies.

4. Involvement of Nociceptive TRP Channels in Painful Pathologies

Nociceptive TRP channels have been shown to be involved in several pain-related pathological conditions/modalities, including inflammatory, neuropathic, visceral and dental pain, as well as pain associated with cancer [9,11,13]. Such information is mainly derived from numerous findings utilizing specific antagonists of individual nociceptive TRP channels in animal models of pain-related pathologies, as well as induction of such pathologies in mice with genetic deletion/alteration of individual nociceptive TRP channels. Both activation and/or modulation of nociceptive TRP channels during pathological conditions has been suggested to underlie the mechanisms associated with specific pain conditions, however, only a handful of direct in vivo evidence in support of these assertions is available.

4.1. Inflammatory Pain

In inflammatory pain conditions, the involvement of TRPV1 is the foremost and most well-established of all the TRP channels. Administration of small-molecule competitive antagonists of TRPV1 has been shown to attenuate thermal hyperalgesia induced by: (a) inflammatory conditions with administration of complete Freund's adjuvant (CFA), formalin, zymosan etc.; and (b) local injection of individual inflammatory mediators in rodents [9,11,13]. Mice lacking the functional TRPV1 gene ($Trpv1^{-/-}$) exhibit dramatic attenuation of thermal hyperalgesia in response to injection of a number of inflammatory mediators, with no alteration in noxious temperature responses observed in un-injected or saline-injected animals [9,11,13,126,127]. Similar results were also observed upon induction of cutaneous inflammation with administration of CFA, formalin, zymosan, etc. in $Trpv1^{-/-}$ mice. In addition to TRPV1, TRPM3 is also involved in the development of inflammatory thermal hyperalgesia, as $Trpm3^{-/-}$ mice demonstrate significant deficits in this pain modality [35]. The involvement of TRPV1 in mechanical hypersensitivity was initially ruled out, taking into consideration the initial findings from the phenotypic characterization of $Trpv1^{-/-}$ mice [126,127]. However, a large number of studies utilizing multiple animal models of inflammatory pain-like conditions have since suggested a critical role for TRPV1 in inflammatory mechanical hypersensitivity. These studies show attenuation of mechanical hypersensitivity by: (a) specific small molecule antagonists of TRPV1; and/or (b) administration of inflammatory mediators (or induction of inflammatory/disease conditions) in $Trpv1^{-/-}$ mice [85,128–134]. In addition to TRPV1, TRPA1 has also been proposed to be involved in inflammatory mechanical hyperalgesia. Pharmacological inhibitors of TRPA1 have been shown to attenuate CFA-induced mechanical hypersensitivity in rodents [135,136]. Furthermore, TRPA1 has also been suggested to mediate cold hyperalgesia under persistent inflammatory conditions in rodents [137,138]. Another aspect of the crucial role of TRPA1 in inflammatory pain states is the resultant inflammatory pain in chronic itch. It has been demonstrated that TRPA1 is critical to the development of neuropathic inflammation associated with allergic contact dermatitis [139]. TRPA1 has also been shown to be integral to the development of chloroquine-induced itch; in both transduction of itch and changes that occur in the skin associated with chronic itch [140,141]. In addition to TRPV1 and TRPA1 channels, the involvement of TRPV4 in inflammatory pain has also been proposed. In $Trpv4^{-/-}$ mice, increased latency to escape from hot plate following tissue injury and inflammation has been observed, which suggests a role for TRPV4 in the development of thermal hyperalgesia [142]. The role of TRPV4 in mechanical hyperalgesia, in responses to osmotic stimuli, both hypotonic and hypertonic, under injury/inflammatory conditions has also been proposed [49,50]. In osteoarthritis models, both TRPV1 and TRPA1 have been shown to play an important role. Genetic and pharmacological inhibition of TRPV1 can reduce arthritis-like symptoms [143–145]. In animal models both TRPV1 and TRPA1 activation results in increased release of TNF-α, a pro-inflammatory cytokine important for the development of osteoarthritis [145]. Further, there is evidence of TRPV1 involvement in osteoarthritis patient populations, including a TRPV1 variant associated with increased knee osteoarthritis, and increased expression of TRPV1 in the knee synovium of patients with osteoarthritis [144,146]. Additionally, topical capsaicin creams have long been used to relieve joint pain by desensitizing TRPV1-expressing nociceptors. Moreover, no edema or hypersensitivity were observed in $Trpv1^{-/-}$ mice following joint inflammation, strengthening the assertion that TRPV1 is critically involved in the pathogenesis of arthritis-like inflammatory conditions [144].

Table 1. Small molecule modulators of TRP channels as drugs in clinical development.

Agonist/Antagonist (Producer/Company)	Channel (Mode of Action)	Current Clinical Use/Trial Status	Specific Painful Pathology	References
AMG517 (Amgen)	TRPV1 (channel blocker)	Phase Ib/Phase II-terminated	Dental pain	[147–150]
ABT102 (Abbott)	TRPV1 (channel blocker)	Phase I—completed; Phase II—unknown	Healthy volunteers	[148–152]
GRC 6211 (Lilly/Glenmark)	TRPV1 (channel blocker)	Phase I-Phase II	Dental pain	[148–150]
SB-705498 (GlaxoSmithKline)	TRPV1 (channel blocker)	Phase II—completed	Dental pain/Toothache	[149,150,153]
		Phase II—terminated	Rectal pain	[154]
MK-2295 (Merck-Neurogen)	TRPV1 (channel blocker)	Phase II—completed	Postoperative dental pain	[149,150,155]
AZD1386 (Astra-Zeneca)	TRPV1 (channel blocker)	Phase I—completed	Esophageal pain	[149,150,156,157]
		Phase II—completed	Dental pain	[149,158,159]
		Phase II—terminated	Osteoarthritis, knee pain	[149,150,160]
		Phase II—terminated	Neuropathic pain	[161]
NEO06860 (Neomed Institute)	TRPV1 (blockade of channel activation by capsaicin, but not by heat and protons)	Phase I—completed Phase II—ongoing	Osteoarthritis, knee pain	[162,163]
NGX 4010 (NeurogesX; Acorda Therapeutics/ Astellas Pharma)	TRPV1 (agonist; capsaicin transdermal patch)	Phase III—completed (launched for clinical use in PHN)	PHN-associated neuropathic pain	[164,165]
		Phase III—completed	HIV-associated neuropathic pain	[165–167]
Resiniferatoxin (NIDCR-NIH)	TRPV1 (potent agonist)	Phase I—ongoing	Advanced cancer pain	[168–170]
Zucapsaicin (Sanofi-Aventis; Winston Pharmaceuticals)	TRPV1 (agonist; nasal and topical capsaicin patch & cream)	Phase III—completed (launched for clinical use in osteoarthritis)	Osteoarthritis, knee pain	[171]
		Phase III—completed	Episodic cluster headache	[172]
		Phase II—completed	PHN-associated neuropathic pain	[173]
GRC-17536 (Glenmark)	TRPA1 (channel locker)	Phase II—completed	Diabetic peripheral neuropathic pain	[174]
SAR292833 (Sanofi)	TRPV3 (channel blocker)	Phase II—completed	Neuropathic pain	[175]
PF-05PR105679 (Pfizer)	TRPM8 (channel blocker)	Phase I—completed	Healthy volunteers	[176,177]

For an extended list of drugs targeting TRP channels and their development status, refer to earlier reports [150,178].

Based on these pre-clinical findings, several small molecule antagonists of nociceptive TRP channels, mainly targeting TRPV1, have been tested in clinical trials for multiple inflammatory pain conditions, such as dental pain and osteoarthritis (Table 1). Most first-generation TRPV1 antagonists showed alteration in body temperatures, more specifically hyperthermia, and ultimately resulted in poor outcomes and/or termination of clinical trials [148–150,178]. In a phase II clinical trial, the TRPV1 antagonist AZD1386 failed to cause significant pain relief in patients with osteoarthritis [149,160], suggesting a more complex role for TRPV1, as well as involvement of other nociceptive channels/receptors in osteoarthritis. One positive scientific outcome from these failures in clinical trials can be attributed to the discovery and expansion of knowledge on the thermo-regulatory role of TRPV1. Furthermore, a clear and cautious warning has been relayed by these clinical findings—an in-depth basic scientific knowledge on these nociceptive ion channels/receptors is absolutely required before exploring these channels as clinical therapeutic targets. Therefore, a rational, specific, pathological function-based approach is required for targeting the modality-specific activation and/or modulatory properties of TRPV1 channel, in order to circumvent the thermoregulatory side effects. Recent development of drugs such as NEO06860 [162,163] and A1165442 [179], which are more potent antagonists of TRPV1 activation by capsaicin and protons, but not by heat, support these assertions. Contrarily, clinical development of a TRPV1 agonist, zucapsaicin, has been successful, and is currently in clinical use for osteoarthritis [171]. This drug is applied topically, which leads to excessive transient activation of TRPV1 on peripheral nerve fibers, followed by channel desensitization and/or nerve fiber degeneration. Whether the same outcome could be achieved by targeted attenuation of TRPV1 function on peripheral sensory nerves by a systemically administered small molecule antagonist in multiple inflammatory conditions remains to be elucidated. Other than TRPV1, modulators of other TRP channel have so far not been tested in clinical trials.

4.2. Neuropathic Pain

Neuropathic pain conditions result primarily from nerve injury due to structural damage and/or constriction, either related to neurological, viral and metabolic disease states or with the use of chemotherapeutic drugs. A number of different nociceptive TRP channels have been implicated in neuropathic pain states. Multiple studies utilizing TRPV1 antagonists in rodents and induction of neuropathy in $Trpv1^{-/-}$ mice have demonstrated a significant role for TRPV1 in neuropathic pain, mainly associated with diabetes and chemotherapeutic drug use (reviewed in [9,47]).

Pharmacological inhibitors of TRPA1 have also been shown to be effective in attenuating mechanical hyperalgesia associated with neuropathic pain conditions [139,140]. TRPA1 can be activated by ROS/RNS, which is associated with several disease pathologies, one of which is diabetes [180]. Chemotherapeutic drugs such as oxaliplatin, vincristine and paclitaxel can also increase ROS/RNS production. Studies have shown that TRPA1 is critically involved in mechanical allodynia associated with such chemotherapeutic drug-induced neuropathic pain [181–183]. Cold hyperalgesia associated with nerve injury- and nerve ligation-induced neuropathic conditions in rodents have also been shown to require TRPA1, but not TRPM8, with pharmacological and antisense knock-down approaches [138,184]. Both TRPM8 and TRPA1 have been implicated in the cold allodynia associated with chemotherapeutic drug-induced neuropathic pain, although recent evidence suggests that it may primarily be confined to TRPA1 [185]. However, some studies have shown attenuated cold hypersensitivity responses in $Trpm8^{-/-}$ mice in chronic constriction injury (CCI), and during the second phase of CFA injection [186]. Involvement of other nociceptive TRP channels in nerve injury/neuropathic conditions has not yet been established.

Based on various pre-clinical findings, small molecule blockers of TRPV1, TRPA1 and TRPV3 have been tested in clinical trials for various neuropathic pain conditions (Table 1). The only TRPV1 antagonist to enter phase II clinical trials was AZD1386, which was subsequently terminated [161], and the underlying results/reasons were not published. More recently, phase II clinical trials on the TRPA1 antagonist GRC-17536 [174], and the TRPV3 antagonist SAR292833 [175] for neuropathic pain conditions have been completed. The results/outcome from these trials still remain unpublished. On the other hand, topical TRPV1 agonists, such as zucapsaicin and NGX 4010, have been quite successful in clinical trials for neuropathic pain conditions. NGX 4010 has already been launched for clinical use in human PHN-neuropathic pain conditions [164,165], and zucapsaicin has successfully completed phase II trials [173]. Therefore, it remains to be determined if antagonists of these specific nociceptive TRP channels could provide effective relief from neuropathic pain conditions. Furthermore, the site of action of drugs targeting nociceptive TRP channels, i.e., peripheral nerve fibers vs spinal cord, remains an area of concern, since central sensitization mechanisms operating at the level of spinal cord dorsal horn are highly critical in the maintenance of neuropathic pain conditions [9].

4.3. Visceral Pain

TRPV1 is the most well studied nociceptive TRP channel in multiple visceral pain-like conditions. Studies utilizing pharmacological inhibition and genetic deletion of TRPV1 have been shown to decrease responses to colorectal distension in naïve and inflamed mice [187]. Further, studies have shown that inhibition of TRPV1 can decrease severity of disease in a variety of animal models for the initiation and maintenance of visceral hypersensitivity after injury [188]. TRPV1 has even been linked to severity of colorectal disease in human patients, where enhanced TRPV1 expression was positively correlated with disease severity [189]. To further link TRPV1 to visceral pain, multiple studies have shown that $Trpv1^{-/-}$ mice show reduced pain-like behaviors in animal models of cystitis and inflammatory bowel disease [190–192]. While $Trpv1^{-/-}$ mice demonstrate reduced pain-like behaviors during visceral inflammation, they show unexpectedly elevated levels of inflammatory markers compared to wild-type mice, which indicates that TRPV1 plays a more complex role in visceral sensitivity [193,194]. TRPV1 also plays a critical role in pain and alterations in bladder activity after inflammation [195–197]. Resiniferatoxin, a potent TRPV1 agonist that causes long lasting desensitization and/or degeneration of TRPV1-expressing nerve fibers, has been shown to decrease pain-like behaviors, as well as the number of bladder contractions in animals with bladder cystitis [196,198]. This evidence indicates that TRPV1 channel and TRPV1-expressing nerve fibers are vital to the development and maintenance of visceral pain. In addition to TRPV1, TRPV4 has been suggested to be involved in visceral pain hypersensitivity. Induction of pancreatitis and irritable bowel syndrome in $Trpv4^{-/-}$ mice lead to attenuated nociceptive responses when compared to wild-type mice, suggesting the involvement of TRPV4 in these visceral pain pathologies [199,200].

Several studies have also implicated TRPA1 and TRPM8 channels in visceral pain conditions. TRPA1 is expressed in a population of visceral nociceptors and it has been shown that pathological activation of TRPA1 induces neurogenic inflammation associated with irritable bowel syndrome and colitis, and the resultant inflammatory pain [201,202]. In combination with TRPV1, TRPA1 has been suggested to contribute to pain hypersensitivity downstream of PAR-2-stimulated pancreatitis [203]. The bacterial cell wall carbohydrate lipopolysaccharide (LPS) was found to activate TRPA1 directly, and was thus proposed as a mechanism for irritation/pain-like condition associated with bacterial infections [204]. In addition, TRPA1 has also been shown to be a critical component of chemosensory airway reflexes in response to irritants. TRPA1 on TG neurons has been shown to mediate sneezing and coughing reflexes [205]. Interestingly, $TRPA1^{-/-}$ mice do not exhibit the antinociceptive effects of acetaminophen and tetrahydrocannabinol (THC), suggesting a possible mechanism underlying analgesic properties of these drugs [206]. Peppermint oil, an agonist of TRPM8, can decrease pain in irritable bowel syndrome; however, these effects could be mediated by other channels, such as GABA$_A$ receptors [207]. Additionally, there is some evidence that TRPM8 antagonists can reduce visceral pain-like behaviors in rats, such as overactive bladder and painful bladder syndrome [208]. So far, two TRPV1 antagonists have been tested in clinical trials for visceral pain conditions. The drug AZD1386 was tested in phase I clinical trials for esophageal pain conditions. This trial was completed; however the results/outcome still remain unreported [156,157]. The other TRPV1 antagonist SB-705498 entered into phase II clinical trial for rectal pain conditions; however, this trial was subsequently terminated and results have not yet been published. One of the major reasons for the slow progress of TRP channel antagonists in clinical trials for visceral pain conditions could be the lack of in-depth mechanistic studies on the involvement of nociceptive TRP channels in specific visceral pain conditions.

4.4. Pain Associated with Cancers and Other Pathological Conditions

4.4.1. Cancer Pain

A number of studies have shown that TRPV1 plays an integral role in cancer pain. Specifically, studies have looked at cancer pain using rodent bone cancer models, and found that TRPV1 is critical for the development of cutaneous thermal and mechanical sensitivity, as well as paw guarding behavior [209,210]. There are many chemokines, cytokines and other factors that are released in the bone cancer microenvironment including prostaglandins, bradykinin, NGF, lysophosphatidic acid, and parathyroid hormone-related peptide, which have been shown to (or could presumably) sensitize TRPV1 currents leading to increased nociceptor firing [85,209,211–213]. Additionally, these mediators could potentially induce post-translational changes in TRPV1 and/or increase protein expression, which could lead to nociceptor sensitization. The tumor microenvironment is generally acidic, which could lead to sensitization of proton-activated TRPV1 currents [209]. Additionally, preclinical trials of intrathecal resiniferatoxin, the potent TRPV1 agonist, have shown it to be very effective in a canine model of bone cancer pain [168,214]. Based on these findings, phase I clinical trials have been initiated to determine the efficacy of periganglionic/intrathecal administration of resiniferatoxin in advanced cancer patients with bone pain [169,170]. Involvement of other nociceptive TRP channels in cancer pain has not been shown so far. One of the major challenges in this area has been the lack of pre-clinical models that more closely mimic the pathophysiology of advanced human cancer.

4.4.2. Dental Pain

TRPV1 has also been linked to dental pain. Studies have shown that TRPV1 is expressed in 45%–85% of sensory neurons that innervate the tooth pulp, and increased expression of the channel has been reported in a rat model of pulpitis [215–218]. Although there is already strong evidence for the direct involvement of TRPV1 in dental pain, modulation of channel function by inflammatory/injury mediators could provide additional mechanistic understanding, which altogether makes TRPV1 an attractive target for pharmaceutical interventions. In support of enriched expression of TRPV1 on dental sensory nerves and its possible involvement in dental pain, multiple TRPV1 antagonists have been investigated in clinical trials. The TRPV1 antagonist AZD1386 was effective at providing relief for molar extraction pain compared to placebo, however the analgesia was not long lasting [159]. Other TRPV1 antagonists, GRC 6211, MK-2295 and SB-705498, have been investigated in phase II clinical trials [150,153,155], with two of these trials already completed [153,155]. However, the outcome/results from these studies still remain unpublished/un-reported. In addition to TRPV1, TRPA1 and TRPM8 have also been linked to dental pain, as they are expressed on many of the same fibers as TRPV1 in trigeminal neurons, however the precise mechanistic evidence in support of their direct involvement with dental pain is still lacking [217,219]. With the recent development and testing of TRPA1 and TRPM8 antagonists in pain conditions is likely to promote the testing of these drugs in clinical trials for dental pain conditions.

4.4.3. Migraine

TRPV1, TRPM8 and TRPA1 have all been linked to migraine pathophysiology. Expression of TRPV1 and modulation of its function, trafficking and expression by multiple mediators in trigeminal neurons have been proposed to be involved in the development of migraine pathophysiology [10]. TRPV1 activation in neurons leads to release of CGRP, a critical neuropeptide in the development of trigemino-vascular excitation [10]. Accordingly, TRPV1 antagonists have been shown to be effective in alleviating migraine-like symptoms in rats [220]. Based on these basic and pre-clinical findings, a number of TRPV1 modulators have been investigated in clinical trials for migraine/headache conditions. So far, the only drug showing encouraging results is zucapsaicin, the channel agonist, for episodic cluster headache conditions [172]. Although a phase III clinical trial has been completed, the detailed outcome/results from this investigation still remain unpublished. Intriguingly, a gene variant of TRPM8 was discovered to have a positive correlation with migraine susceptibility in women [221]. However, it is not known whether this variant leads to any functional and nociceptive changes in TG neurons, and its direct involvement in migraine pathophysiology remains unexplored.

TRPA1 is expressed in trigeminal neurons and localized on dural afferents, where its activation has been shown to result in headache-like behaviors in mice [219,222]. Experimental drugs that serve as NO donors, such as nitroglycerine, have been extensively studied for their migraine-inducing properties. Both in humans and animals, NO directly activates TRPA1 via S-nitrosylation, and therefore, could serve as a mechanism for trigeminal excitation and migraine [8]. Interestingly, another recent study demonstrated the critical role of TRPA1 activation via monocyte/macrophage-induced oxidative stress conditions under trigeminal nerve constriction injury model in rodents [223]. Again, recent development of TRPA1 and TRPM8 antagonists for pain conditions is likely to promote testing of these drugs in clinical trials for specific migraine and headache conditions. Involvement of other nociceptive TRP channels in development of migraine and headache pathophysiology still remains unknown.

5. Nociceptive TRP Channels in Non-Painful Pathologies and Physiological Processes

Although characterized as critical detectors and transducers of nociceptive stimuli, these channels/receptors have also been implicated in several physiological and non-painful pathological conditions. TRPV1 has now been shown to play a role in body temperature regulation. Initial studies utilizing $Trpv1^{-/-}$ mice suggested no involvement of TRPV1 in body temperature regulation [126,127]. During the process of drug development targeting TRP channels, it became clear that TRPV1 is critically involved in the regulation of body temperature, since systemic administration of small molecule antagonists of TRPV1 led to transient hyperthermia [147–150]. This in fact led to the failure of first-generation TRPV1-targeting drugs in clinical trials [147–150]. Subsequent studies have now suggested spinal cord TRPV1 as the critical mediator of noxious temperature detection [224]. In addition, TRPV1 in the brain stem has also been suggested to play an important role in thermoregulation, although expression and function of TRPV1 in the brain still remains a matter of debate [225]. TRPV1 has also been shown to exhibit high expression in sensory neurons innervating the airways, and is therefore involved in the cough reflex. Pharmacological blockade of TRPV1 has been shown to reduce cough in rodent models [226–229], supporting this assertion. Upregulation of TRPV1 protein expression has also been observed in asthma and gastro-esophageal reflux disease [226,228]. TRPV1 involvement in stomach cancers has also been suggested [228]. Interestingly, $Trpv1^{-/-}$ mice exhibit increased sensitivity to insulin [230], raising the possibility of its involvement in diabetes. In fact, evidence suggests that TRPV1 activation could play a protective role in type I diabetes. However, other studies have suggested that activation of TRPV1 could be detrimental in type 2 diabetes conditions [228]. No significant contribution of TRPV2 has been suggested in pathological pain and nociceptive signal processing in vivo, as substantiated by observations utilizing $Trpv2^{-/-}$ mice, which display normal thermal and mechanical nociceptive behaviors [231]. However, TRPV2 has been proposed to influence macrophage function and phagocytosis [232].

In addition to TRPV1, involvement of TRPM8 in thermoregulation has also been suggested, although in the opposite direction. Deficiencies in cold sensation were observed in $Trpm8^{-/-}$ mice, with a decrease in avoidance behavior to moderately cold temperatures was observed in these animals [186,233,234]. Additionally, a selective TRPM8 antagonist showed no significant alteration in body temperature when administered to healthy volunteers, further suggesting it may not be a critical regulator for the maintenance of body temperature [176]. Avoidance of cold temperatures (below 0 °C) could still be observed in $Trpm8^{-/-}$ mice. This could be due to other cold sensitive channels, or any compensatory changes due to specific deletion of the $Trpm8$ gene. In this regard, a role of two other channels has been proposed: (a) leak K^+ channels, such as TRAAK and TREK1, which close at very low temperatures; and (b) TRPA1, which is sensitive to noxious cold temperatures [31,235]. In spite of the important role of TRPM8 in cold hypersensitivity, this channel has also been suggested as the mediator of cold- and menthol-induced analgesia. Cooling, as well as administration of menthol has been shown to reduce acute and inflammatory pain in rodent formalin injection pain models. Interestingly, such analgesic effects of mild cooling are absent for the inflammatory pain phase after formalin injection, but still present for the acute phase in $Trpm8^{-/-}$ mice [233]. Apart from the well-defined role of TRPA1 in pain and cold hypersensitivities, this channel has also been suggested to play a critical role in vertebrate hair cell mechanotransduction and hearing [236,237]. However, subsequent studies utilizing targeted deletion of the *Trpa1* gene in mice showed no involvement of TRPA1 in hair cell mechanotransduction [238]. TRPA1 has been shown to be a sensor of wide range of environmental irritants and proalgesic agents (reviewed in [239,240]).

6. Concluding Remarks

Identification and cloning of nociceptive receptors, mainly belonging to the TRP channel family, in the last decade and-a-half has tremendously advanced our understanding of the biology of nociception and multi-modal pain sensation. In-depth characterization of functional properties of these receptor channels, and describing their expression in various tissue and individual cell types within the nervous system has pushed us closer to connecting all the dots of somatosensory, visceral and trigeminal sensory pathways. In addition, extensive utilization of mouse genetics in sensory biology has been incredibly helpful in this process. Simultaneous development of pharmacological interventions targeting nociceptive TRP channels has not only been closing in on new-generation analgesic drug developments, but also providing vital information on the in vivo mechanisms of sensory signal processing. Although there is still a great deal to uncover in the biology of nociception, the startling and relatively recent progress in expansion in knowledge in this area of research will undoubtedly lead to more efficacious and evidence-based management of multiple pain pathologies.

Acknowledgments: Research on nociceptive TRP channels in our laboratory are/were supported by grant funding from the US National Institutes of Health (NIH/NINDS-NS069869 to DPM; NIH/NCI-CA171927 and NIH/NINDS-NS045549 to ADM), US Department of Defense (DoD/PCRP-PC101096 to DPM), American Pain Society (APS-FLP1483 to DPM), and the International Association for the Study of Pain (IASP-1881650 to DPM). The authors express their apologies to the authors of several research and review papers, and book chapters in the TRP channel field, whose work could not be cited here due to space limitations.

Conflicts of Interest: The authors declare that they have no conflict of interest.

References

1. Loeser, J.D.; Treede, R.D. The kyoto protocol of IASP basic pain terminology. *Pain* **2008**, *137*, 473–477. [CrossRef] [PubMed]
2. Cosens, D.J.; Manning, A. Abnormal electroretinogram from a drosophila mutant. *Nature* **1969**, *224*, 285–287. [CrossRef] [PubMed]
3. Minke, B. The history of the drosophila TRP channel: The birth of a new channel superfamily. *J. Neurogenet.* **2010**, *24*, 216–233. [CrossRef] [PubMed]
4. Venkatachalam, K.; Montell, C. TRP channels. *Annu. Rev. Biochem.* **2007**, *76*, 387–417. [CrossRef] [PubMed]
5. Wu, L.J.; Sweet, T.B.; Clapham, D.E. International union of basic and clinical pharmacology. LXXVI. Current progress in the mammalian TRP ion channel family. *Pharmacol. Rev.* **2010**, *62*, 381–404. [CrossRef] [PubMed]
6. Clapham, D.E. TRP channels as cellular sensors. *Nature* **2003**, *426*, 517–524. [CrossRef] [PubMed]
7. Montell, C. Physiology, phylogeny, and functions of the TRP superfamily of cation channels. *Sci. STKE* **2001**, *90*, re1. [CrossRef] [PubMed]
8. Benemei, S.; De Cesaris, F.; Fusi, C.; Rossi, E.; Lupi, C.; Geppetti, P. TRPA1 and other TRP channels in migraine. *J. Headache Pain* **2013**, *14*, 71. [CrossRef] [PubMed]
9. Julius, D. TRP channels and pain. *Ann. Rev. Cell Dev. Biol.* **2013**, *29*, 355–384. [CrossRef] [PubMed]
10. Meents, J.E.; Neeb, L.; Reuter, U. TRPV1 in migraine pathophysiology. *Trends Mol. Med.* **2010**, *16*, 153–159. [CrossRef] [PubMed]
11. Mickle, A.D.; Shepherd, A.J.; Mohapatra, D.P. Sensory TRP channels: The key transducers of nociception and pain. *Prog. Mol. Biol. Transl. Sci.* **2015**, *131*, 73–118. [PubMed]
12. Moran, M.M.; McAlexander, M.A.; Biro, T.; Szallasi, A. Transient receptor potential channels as therapeutic targets. *Nat. Rev. Drug Discov.* **2011**, *10*, 601–620. [CrossRef] [PubMed]

13. Patapoutian, A.; Tate, S.; Woolf, C.J. Transient receptor potential channels: Targeting pain at the source. *Nat. Rev. Drug Discov.* **2009**, *8*, 55–68. [CrossRef] [PubMed]

14. Sherrington, C. *The Integrative Action of the Nervous System*; Oxford University Press: Oxford, UK, 1906.

15. Dray, A. Mechanism of action of capsaicin-like molecules on sensory neurons. *Life Sci.* **1992**, *51*, 1759–1765. [CrossRef]

16. Amann, R.; Maggi, C.A. Ruthenium red as a capsaicin antagonist. *Life Sci.* **1991**, *49*, 849–856. [CrossRef]

17. Caterina, M.J.; Schumacher, M.A.; Tominaga, M.; Rosen, T.A.; Levine, J.D.; Julius, D. The capsaicin receptor: A heat-activated ion channel in the pain pathway. *Nature* **1997**, *389*, 816–824. [PubMed]

18. Tominaga, M.; Caterina, M.J.; Malmberg, A.B.; Rosen, T.A.; Gilbert, H.; Skinner, K.; Raumann, B.E.; Basbaum, A.I.; Julius, D. The cloned capsaicin receptor integrates multiple pain-producing stimuli. *Neuron* **1998**, *21*, 531–543. [CrossRef]

19. Caterina, M.J.; Rosen, T.A.; Tominaga, M.; Brake, A.J.; Julius, D. A capsaicin-receptor homologue with a high threshold for noxious heat. *Nature* **1999**, *398*, 436–441. [PubMed]

20. Liedtke, W.; Choe, Y.; Marti-Renom, M.A.; Bell, A.M.; Denis, C.S.; Sali, A.; Hudspeth, A.J.; Friedman, J.M.; Heller, S. Vanilloid receptor-related osmotically activated channel (VR-OAC), a candidate vertebrate osmoreceptor. *Cell* **2000**, *103*, 525–535. [CrossRef]

21. Strotmann, R.; Harteneck, C.; Nunnenmacher, K.; Schultz, G.; Plant, T.D. OTRPC4, a nonselective cation channel that confers sensitivity to extracellular osmolarity. *Nat. Cell Biol.* **2000**, *2*, 695–702. [PubMed]

22. Muller, D.; Hoenderop, J.G.; Meij, I.C.; van den Heuvel, L.P.; Knoers, N.V.; den Hollander, A.I.; Eggert, P.; Garcia-Nieto, V.; Claverie-Martin, F.; Bindels, R.J. Molecular cloning, tissue distribution, and chromosomal mapping of the human epithelial Ca^{2+} channel (ECAC1). *Genomics* **2000**, *67*, 48–53. [CrossRef] [PubMed]

23. Peng, J.B.; Chen, X.Z.; Berger, U.V.; Vassilev, P.M.; Tsukaguchi, H.; Brown, E.M.; Hediger, M.A. Molecular cloning and characterization of a channel-like transporter mediating intestinal calcium absorption. *J. Biol. Chem.* **1999**, *274*, 22739–22746. [CrossRef] [PubMed]

24. Weber, K.; Erben, R.G.; Rump, A.; Adamski, J. Gene structure and regulation of the murine epithelial calcium channels ECAC1 and 2. *Biochem. Biophys. Res. Commun.* **2001**, *289*, 1287–1294. [CrossRef] [PubMed]

25. Reid, G.; Flonta, M.L. Physiology. Cold current in thermoreceptive neurons. *Nature* **2001**, *413*, 480. [CrossRef] [PubMed]

26. Peier, A.M.; Moqrich, A.; Hergarden, A.C.; Reeve, A.J.; Andersson, D.A.; Story, G.M.; Earley, T.J.; Dragoni, I.; McIntyre, P.; Bevan, S.; et al. A TRP channel that senses cold stimuli and menthol. *Cell* **2002**, *108*, 705–715. [CrossRef]

27. McKemy, D.D.; Neuhausser, W.M.; Julius, D. Identification of a cold receptor reveals a general role for TRP channels in thermosensation. *Nature* **2002**, *416*, 52–58. [CrossRef] [PubMed]

28. Peier, A.M.; Reeve, A.J.; Andersson, D.A.; Moqrich, A.; Earley, T.J.; Hergarden, A.C.; Story, G.M.; Colley, S.; Hogenesch, J.B.; McIntyre, P.; et al. A heat-sensitive TRP channel expressed in keratinocytes. *Science* **2002**, *296*, 2046–2049. [CrossRef] [PubMed]

29. Xu, H.; Ramsey, I.S.; Kotecha, S.A.; Moran, M.M.; Chong, J.A.; Lawson, D.; Ge, P.; Lilly, J.; Silos-Santiago, I.; Xie, Y.; et al. TRPV3 is a calcium-permeable temperature-sensitive cation channel. *Nature* **2002**, *418*, 181–186. [CrossRef] [PubMed]

30. Jaquemar, D.; Schenker, T.; Trueb, B. An ankyrin-like protein with transmembrane domains is specifically lost after oncogenic transformation of human fibroblasts. *J. Biol. Chem.* **1999**, *274*, 7325–7333. [CrossRef] [PubMed]

31. Story, G.M.; Peier, A.M.; Reeve, A.J.; Eid, S.R.; Mosbacher, J.; Hricik, T.R.; Earley, T.J.; Hergarden, A.C.; Andersson, D.A.; Hwang, S.W.; et al. ANKTM1, a TRP-like channel expressed in nociceptive neurons, is activated by cold temperatures. *Cell* **2003**, *112*, 819–829. [CrossRef]

32. Grimm, C.; Kraft, R.; Sauerbruch, S.; Schultz, G.; Harteneck, C. Molecular and functional characterization of the melastatin-related cation channel TRPM3. *J. Biol. Chem.* **2003**, *278*, 21493–21501. [CrossRef] [PubMed]

33. Wagner, T.F.; Loch, S.; Lambert, S.; Straub, I.; Mannebach, S.; Mathar, I.; Dufer, M.; Lis, A.; Flockerzi, V.; Philipp, S.E.; et al. Transient receptor potential M3 channels are ionotropic steroid receptors in pancreatic beta cells. *Nat. Cell Biol.* **2008**, *10*, 1421–1430. [CrossRef] [PubMed]

34. Vriens, J.; Appendino, G.; Nilius, B. Pharmacology of vanilloid transient receptor potential cation channels. *Mol. Pharmacol.* **2009**, *75*, 1262–1279. [CrossRef] [PubMed]

35. Vriens, J.; Owsianik, G.; Hofmann, T.; Philipp, S.E.; Stab, J.; Chen, X.; Benoit, M.; Xue, F.; Janssens, A.; Kerselaers, S.; et al. TRPM3 is a nociceptor channel involved in the detection of noxious heat. *Neuron* **2011**, *70*, 482–494. [CrossRef] [PubMed]
36. Jordt, S.E.; Tominaga, M.; Julius, D. Acid potentiation of the capsaicin receptor determined by a key extracellular site. *Proc. Natl. Acad. Sci. USA* **2000**, *97*, 8134–8139. [CrossRef] [PubMed]
37. Dhaka, A.; Uzzell, V.; Dubin, A.E.; Mathur, J.; Petrus, M.; Bandell, M.; Patapoutian, A. TRPV1 is activated by both acidic and basic ph. *J. Neurosci.* **2009**, *29*, 153–158. [CrossRef] [PubMed]
38. Huang, S.M.; Bisogno, T.; Trevisani, M.; Al-Hayani, A.; De Petrocellis, L.; Fezza, F.; Tognetto, M.; Petros, T.J.; Krey, J.F.; Chu, C.J.; et al. An endogenous capsaicin-like substance with high potency at recombinant and native vanilloid VR1 receptors. *Proc. Natl. Acad. Sci. USA* **2002**, *99*, 8400–8405. [CrossRef] [PubMed]
39. Hwang, S.W.; Cho, H.; Kwak, J.; Lee, S.Y.; Kang, C.J.; Jung, J.; Cho, S.; Min, K.H.; Suh, Y.G.; Kim, D.; et al. Direct activation of capsaicin receptors by products of lipoxygenases: Endogenous capsaicin-like substances. *Proc. Natl. Acad. Sci. USA* **2000**, *97*, 6155–6160. [CrossRef] [PubMed]
40. Zygmunt, P.M.; Petersson, J.; Andersson, D.A.; Chuang, H.; Sorgard, M.; Di Marzo, V.; Julius, D.; Hogestatt, E.D. Vanilloid receptors on sensory nerves mediate the vasodilator action of anandamide. *Nature* **1999**, *400*, 452–457. [PubMed]
41. Kozai, D.; Ogawa, N.; Mori, Y. Redox regulation of transient receptor potential channels. *Antioxid. Redox Ssignal.* **2014**, *21*, 971–986. [CrossRef] [PubMed]
42. Chung, M.-K.; Guler, A.D.; Caterina, M.J. TRPV1 shows dynamic ionic selectivity during agonist stimulation. *Nat. Neurosci.* **2008**, *11*, 555–564. [CrossRef] [PubMed]
43. Mohapatra, D.P.; Wang, S.Y.; Wang, G.K.; Nau, C. A tyrosine residue in TM6 of the vanilloid receptor TRPV1 involved in desensitization and calcium permeability of capsaicin-activated currents. *Mol. Cell. Neurosci.* **2003**, *23*, 314–324. [CrossRef]
44. Koplas, P.A.; Rosenberg, R.L.; Oxford, G.S. The role of calcium in the desensitization of capsaicin responses in rat dorsal root ganglion neurons. *J. Neurosci.* **1997**, *17*, 3525–3537. [PubMed]
45. Loo, L.; Shepherd, A.J.; Mickle, A.D.; Lorca, R.A.; Shutov, L.P.; Usachev, Y.M.; Mohapatra, D.P. The C-type natriuretic peptide induces thermal hyperalgesia through a noncanonical gbetagamma-dependent modulation of TRPV1 channel. *J. Neurosci.* **2012**, *32*, 11942–11955. [CrossRef] [PubMed]
46. Yang, P.; Zhu, M.X. TRPV3. In *Handbook of Experimental Pharmacology*; Springer: Berlin, Germany, 2014; Volume 222, pp. 273–291.
47. Bourinet, E.; Altier, C.; Hildebrand, M.E.; Trang, T.; Salter, M.W.; Zamponi, G.W. Calcium-permeable ion channels in pain signaling. *Physiol. Rev.* **2014**, *94*, 81–140. [CrossRef] [PubMed]
48. Ho, T.C.; Horn, N.A.; Huynh, T.; Kelava, L.; Lansman, J.B. Evidence TRPV4 contributes to mechanosensitive ion channels in mouse skeletal muscle fibers. *Channels* **2012**, *6*, 246–254. [CrossRef] [PubMed]
49. Alessandri-Haber, N.; Joseph, E.; Dina, O.A.; Liedtke, W.; Levine, J.D. TRPV4 mediates pain-related behavior induced by mild hypertonic stimuli in the presence of inflammatory mediator. *Pain* **2005**, *118*, 70–79. [CrossRef] [PubMed]
50. Alessandri-Haber, N.; Yeh, J.J.; Boyd, A.E.; Parada, C.A.; Chen, X.; Reichling, D.B.; Levine, J.D. Hypotonicity induces TRPV4-mediated nociception in rat. *Neuron* **2003**, *39*, 497–511. [CrossRef]
51. Yudin, Y.; Rohacs, T. Regulation of TRPM8 channel activity. *Mol. Cell. Endocrinol.* **2012**, *353*, 68–74. [CrossRef] [PubMed]
52. Asuthkar, S.; Elustondo, P.A.; Demirkhanyan, L.; Sun, X.; Baskaran, P.; Velpula, K.K.; Thyagarajan, B.; Pavlov, E.V.; Zakharian, E. The TRPM8 protein is a testosterone receptor: I. Biochemical evidence for direct TRPM8-testosterone interactions. *J. Biol. Chem.* **2015**, *290*, 2659–2669. [CrossRef] [PubMed]
53. Asuthkar, S.; Demirkhanyan, L.; Sun, X.; Elustondo, P.A.; Krishnan, V.; Baskaran, P.; Velpula, K.K.; Thyagarajan, B.; Pavlov, E.V.; Zakharian, E. The TRPM8 protein is a testosterone receptor: II. Functional evidence for an ionotropic effect of testosterone on TRPM8. *J. Biol. Chem.* **2015**, *290*, 2670–2688. [CrossRef] [PubMed]
54. Bandell, M.; Story, G.M.; Hwang, S.W.; Viswanath, V.; Eid, S.R.; Petrus, M.J.; Earley, T.J.; Patapoutian, A. Noxious cold ion channel TRPA1 is activated by pungent compounds and bradykinin. *Neuron* **2004**, *41*, 849–857. [CrossRef]
55. Karashima, Y.; Talavera, K.; Everaerts, W.; Janssens, A.; Kwan, K.Y.; Vennekens, R.; Nilius, B.; Voets, T. TRPA1 acts as a cold sensor in vitro and in vivo. *Proc. Natl. Acad. Sci. USA* **2009**, *106*, 1273–1278. [CrossRef] [PubMed]

56. Dunham, J.; Leith, J.; Lumb, B.; Donaldson, L. Transient receptor potential channel A1 and noxious cold responses in rat cutaneous nociceptors. *Neuroscience* **2010**, *165*, 1412–1419. [CrossRef] [PubMed]

57. Chen, J.; Kang, D.; Xu, J.; Lake, M.; Hogan, J.O.; Sun, C.; Walter, K.; Yao, B.; Kim, D. Species differences and molecular determinant of TRPA1 cold sensitivity. *Nat. Commun.* **2013**, *4*, 2501. [CrossRef] [PubMed]

58. Moparthi, L.; Kichko, T.I.; Eberhardt, M.; Hogestatt, E.D.; Kjellbom, P.; Johanson, U.; Reeh, P.W.; Leffler, A.; Filipovic, M.R.; Zygmunt, P.M. Human TRPA1 is a heat sensor displaying intrinsic u-shaped thermosensitivity. *Sci. Rep.* **2016**, *6*, 28763. [CrossRef] [PubMed]

59. Jabba, S.; Goyal, R.; Sosa-Pagan, J.O.; Moldenhauer, H.; Wu, J.; Kalmeta, B.; Bandell, M.; Latorre, R.; Patapoutian, A.; Grandl, J. Directionality of temperature activation in mouse TRPA1 ion channel can be inverted by single-point mutations in ankyrin repeat six. *Neuron* **2014**, *82*, 1017–1031. [CrossRef] [PubMed]

60. De la Roche, J.; Eberhardt, M.J.; Klinger, A.B.; Stanslowsky, N.; Wegner, F.; Koppert, W.; Reeh, P.W.; Lampert, A.; Fischer, M.J.M.; Leffler, A. The molecular basis for species-specific activation of human TRPA1 protein by protons involves poorly conserved residues within transmembrane domains 5 and 6. *J. Biol. Chem.* **2013**, *288*, 20280–20292. [CrossRef] [PubMed]

61. Wang, Y.Y.; Chang, R.B.; Liman, E.R. TRPA1 is a component of the nociceptive response to CO_2. *J. Neurosci.* **2010**, *30*, 12958–12963. [CrossRef] [PubMed]

62. Wang, Y.Y.; Chang, R.B.; Allgood, S.D.; Silver, W.L.; Liman, E.R. A TRPA1-dependent mechanism for the pungent sensation of weak acids. *J. Gen. Physiol.* **2011**, *137*, 493–505. [CrossRef] [PubMed]

63. Macpherson, L.J.; Dubin, A.E.; Evans, M.J.; Marr, F.; Schultz, P.G.; Cravatt, B.F.; Patapoutian, A. Noxious compounds activate TRPA1 ion channels through covalent modification of cysteines. *Nature* **2007**, *445*, 541–545. [PubMed]

64. Macpherson, L.J.; Xiao, B.; Kwan, K.Y.; Petrus, M.J.; Dubin, A.E.; Hwang, S.; Cravatt, B.; Corey, D.P.; Patapoutian, A. An ion channel essential for sensing chemical damage. *J. Neurosci.* **2007**, *27*, 11412–11415. [CrossRef] [PubMed]

65. Viana, F. TRPA1 channels: Molecular sentinels of cellular stress and tissue damage. *J. Physiol.* **2016**, *594*, 4151–4169. [PubMed]

66. Trevisani, M.; Siemens, J.; Materazzi, S.; Bautista, D.M.; Nassini, R.; Campi, B.; Imamachi, N.; Andrè, E.; Patacchini, R.; Cottrell, G.S.; et al. 4-hydroxynonenal, an endogenous aldehyde, causes pain and neurogenic inflammation through activation of the irritant receptor TRPA1. *Proc. Natl. Acad. Sci. USA* **2007**, *104*, 13519–13524. [CrossRef] [PubMed]

67. Miyamoto, T.; Dubin, A.E.; Petrus, M.J.; Patapoutian, A. TRPV1 and TRPA1 mediate peripheral nitric oxide-induced nociception in mice. *PLoS ONE* **2009**, *4*, e7596. [CrossRef] [PubMed]

68. Pozsgai, G.; Hajna, Z.; Bagoly, T.; Boros, M.; Kemény, Á.; Materazzi, S.; Nassini, R.; Helyes, Z.; Szolcsányi, J.; Pintér, E. The role of transient receptor potential ankyrin 1 (TRPA1) receptor activation in hydrogen-sulphide-induced CGRP-release and vasodilation. *Eur. J. Pharmacol.* **2012**, *689*, 56–64. [CrossRef] [PubMed]

69. Eberhardt, M.; Dux, M.; Namer, B.; Miljkovic, J.; Cordasic, N.; Will, C.; Kichko, T.I.; de la Roche, J.; Fischer, M.; Suarez, S.A.; et al. H2S and no cooperatively regulate vascular tone by activating a neuroendocrine HNO-TRPA1-CGRP signalling pathway. *Nat. Commun.* **2014**, *5*, 4381. [CrossRef] [PubMed]

70. Takahashi, N.; Mizuno, Y.; Kozai, D.; Yamamoto, S.; Kiyonaka, S.; Shibata, T.; Uchida, K.; Mori, Y. Molecular characterization of TRPA1 channel activation by cysteine-reactive inflammatory mediators. *Channels* **2008**, *2*, 287–298. [CrossRef] [PubMed]

71. Cruz-Orengo, L.; Dhaka, A.; Heuermann, R.J.; Young, T.J.; Montana, M.C.; Cavanaugh, E.J.; Kim, D.; Story, G.M. Cutaneous nociception evoked by 15-delta PGJ2 via activation of ion channel TRPA1. *Mol. Pain* **2008**, *4*, 30. [CrossRef] [PubMed]

72. Zurborg, S.; Yurgionas, B.; Jira, J.A.; Caspani, O.; Heppenstall, P.A. Direct activation of the ion channel TRPA1 by Ca^{2+}. *Nat. Neurosci.* **2007**, *10*, 277–279. [CrossRef] [PubMed]

73. Brierley, S.M.; Castro, J.; Harrington, A.M.; Hughes, P.A.; Page, A.J.; Rychkov, G.Y.; Blackshaw, L.A. TRPA1 contributes to specific mechanically activated currents and sensory neuron mechanical hypersensitivity. *J. Physiol.* **2011**, *589*, 3575–3593. [CrossRef] [PubMed]

74. Vilceanu, D.; Stucky, C.L. TRPA1 mediates mechanical currents in the plasma membrane of mouse sensory neurons. *PLoS ONE* **2010**, *5*, e12177. [CrossRef] [PubMed]

75. Brierley, S.M.; Hughes, P.A.; Page, A.J.; Kwan, K.Y.; Martin, C.M.; O'Donnell, T.A.; Cooper, N.J.; Harrington, A.M.; Adam, B.; Liebregts, T.; et al. The ion channel TRPA1 is required for normal mechanosensation and is modulated by algesic stimuli. *Gastroenterology* **2009**, *137*, 2084–2095 e2083. [CrossRef] [PubMed]

76. Karashima, Y.; Prenen, J.; Talavera, K.; Janssens, A.; Voets, T.; Nilius, B. Agonist-induced changes in Ca^{2+} permeation through the nociceptor cation channel TRPA1. *Biophys. J.* **2010**, *98*, 773–783. [CrossRef] [PubMed]

77. Shepherd, A.J.; Mohapatra, D.P. Tissue preparation and immunostaining of mouse sensory nerve fibers innervating skin and limb bones. *J. Vis. Exp.* **2012**, *59*, e3485. [CrossRef] [PubMed]

78. Le Pichon, C.E.; Chesler, A.T. The functional and anatomical dissection of somatosensory subpopulations using mouse genetics. *Front. Neuroanat.* **2014**, *8*, 21. [CrossRef] [PubMed]

79. Alessandri-Haber, N.; Dina, O.A.; Joseph, E.K.; Reichling, D.; Levine, J.D. A transient receptor potential vanilloid 4-dependent mechanism of hyperalgesia is engaged by concerted action of inflammatory mediators. *J. Neurosci.* **2006**, *26*, 3864–3874. [CrossRef] [PubMed]

80. Alexander, R.; Kerby, A.; Aubdool, A.A.; Power, A.R.; Grover, S.; Gentry, C.; Grant, A.D. 4alpha-phorbol 12,13-didecanoate activates cultured mouse dorsal root ganglia neurons independently of TRPV4. *Br. J. Pharmacol.* **2013**, *168*, 761–772. [CrossRef] [PubMed]

81. Flegel, C.; Schobel, N.; Altmuller, J.; Becker, C.; Tannapfel, A.; Hatt, H.; Gisselmann, G. RNA-seq analysis of human trigeminal and dorsal root ganglia with a focus on chemoreceptors. *PLoS ONE* **2015**, *10*, e0128951. [CrossRef] [PubMed]

82. Goswami, S.C.; Mishra, S.K.; Maric, D.; Kaszas, K.; Gonnella, G.L.; Clokie, S.J.; Kominsky, H.D.; Gross, J.R.; Keller, J.M.; Mannes, A.J.; et al. Molecular signatures of mouse TRPV1-lineage neurons revealed by RNA-seq transcriptome analysis. *J. Pain* **2014**, *15*, 1338–1359. [CrossRef] [PubMed]

83. Sapio, M.R.; Goswami, S.C.; Gross, J.R.; Mannes, A.J.; Iadarola, M.J. Transcriptomic analyses of genes and tissues in inherited sensory neuropathies. *Exp. Neurol.* **2016**, *283*, 375–395. [CrossRef] [PubMed]

84. Ferrandiz-Huertas, C.; Mathivanan, S.; Wolf, C.J.; Devesa, I.; Ferrer-Montiel, A. Trafficking of thermo-TRP channels. *Membranes* **2014**, *4*, 525–564. [CrossRef] [PubMed]

85. Mickle, A.D.; Shepherd, A.J.; Loo, L.; Mohapatra, D.P. Induction of thermal and mechanical hypersensitivity by parathyroid hormone-related peptide through upregulation of TRPV1 function and trafficking. *Pain* **2015**, *156*, 1620–1636. [CrossRef] [PubMed]

86. Zhang, X.; Huang, J.; McNaughton, P.A. NGF rapidly increases membrane expression of TRPV1 heat-gated ion channels. *EMBO J.* **2005**, *24*, 4211–4223. [CrossRef] [PubMed]

87. Schmidt, M.; Dubin, A.E.; Petrus, M.J.; Earley, T.J.; Patapoutian, A. Nociceptive signals induce trafficking of TRPA1 to the plasma membrane. *Neuron* **2009**, *64*, 498–509. [CrossRef] [PubMed]

88. Meng, J.; Wang, J.; Steinhoff, M.; Dolly, J.O. TNFalpha induces co-trafficking of TRPV1/TRPA1 in VAMP1-containing vesicles to the plasmalemma via Munc18-1/syntaxin1/SNAP-25 mediated fusion. *Sci. Rep.* **2016**, *6*, 21226. [CrossRef] [PubMed]

89. Jin, X.; Morsy, N.; Winston, J.; Pasricha, P.J.; Garrett, K.; Akbarali, H.I. Modulation of TRPV1 by nonreceptor tyrosine kinase, c-Src kinase. *Am. J. Physiol. Cell Physiol.* **2004**, *287*, C558–C563. [CrossRef] [PubMed]

90. Bhave, G.; Hu, H.-J.; Glauner, K.S.; Zhu, W.; Wang, H.; Brasier, D.J.; Oxford, G.S.; Gereau, R.W. Protein kinase c phosphorylation sensitizes but does not activate the capsaicin receptor transient receptor potential vanilloid 1 (TRPV1). *Proc. Natl. Acad. Sci. USA* **2003**, *100*, 12480–12485. [CrossRef] [PubMed]

91. Bhave, G.; Zhu, W.; Wang, H.; Brasier, D.J.; Oxford, G.S.; Gereau Iv, R.W. Camp-dependent protein kinase regulates desensitization of the capsaicin receptor (VR1) by direct phosphorylation. *Neuron* **2002**, *35*, 721–731. [CrossRef]

92. Jung, J.; Shin, J.S.; Lee, S.Y.; Hwang, S.W.; Koo, J.; Cho, H.; Oh, U. Phosphorylation of vanilloid receptor 1 by Ca^{2+}/calmodulin-dependent kinase II regulates its vanilloid binding. *J. Biol. Chem.* **2004**, *279*, 7048–7054. [CrossRef] [PubMed]

93. Numazaki, M.; Tominaga, T.; Toyooka, H.; Tominaga, M. Direct phosphorylation of capsaicin receptor VR1 by protein kinase cepsilon and identification of two target serine residues. *J. Biol. Chem.* **2002**, *277*, 13375–13378. [CrossRef] [PubMed]

94. Vellani, V.; Mapplebeck, S.; Moriondo, A.; Davis, J.B.; McNaughton, P.A. Protein kinase c activation potentiates gating of the vanilloid receptor VR1 by capsaicin, protons, heat and anandamide. *J. Physiol.* **2001**, *534*, 813–825. [CrossRef] [PubMed]

95. Pareek, T.K.; Keller, J.; Kesavapany, S.; Agarwal, N.; Kuner, R.; Pant, H.C.; Iadarola, M.J.; Brady, R.O.; Kulkarni, A.B. Cyclin-dependent kinase 5 modulates nociceptive signaling through direct phosphorylation of transient receptor potential vanilloid 1. *Proc. Natl. Acad. Sci. USA* **2007**, *104*, 660–665. [CrossRef] [PubMed]

96. Mohapatra, D.P.; Nau, C. Desensitization of capsaicin-activated currents in the vanilloid receptor TRPV1 is decreased by the cyclic AMP-dependent protein kinase pathway. *J. Biol. Chem.* **2003**, *278*, 50080–50090. [CrossRef] [PubMed]

97. Mohapatra, D.P.; Nau, C. Regulation of Ca^{2+}-dependent desensitization in the vanilloid receptor TRPV1 by calcineurin and camp-dependent protein kinase. *J. Biol. Chem.* **2005**, *280*, 13424–13432. [CrossRef] [PubMed]

98. Spahn, V.; Stein, C.; Zollner, C. Modulation of transient receptor vanilloid 1 activity by transient receptor potential ankyrin 1. *Mol. Pharmacol.* **2014**, *85*, 335–344. [CrossRef] [PubMed]

99. Chuang, H.H.; Prescott, E.D.; Kong, H.; Shields, S.; Jordt, S.E.; Basbaum, A.I.; Chao, M.V.; Julius, D. Bradykinin and nerve growth factor release the capsaicin receptor from ptdins(4,5)p2-mediated inhibition. *Nature* **2001**, *411*, 957–962. [CrossRef] [PubMed]

100. Lukacs, V.; Yudin, Y.; Hammond, G.R.; Sharma, E.; Fukami, K.; Rohacs, T. Distinctive changes in plasma membrane phosphoinositides underlie differential regulation of TRPV1 in nociceptive neurons. *J. Neurosci.* **2013**, *33*, 11451–11463. [CrossRef] [PubMed]

101. Hanack, C.; Moroni, M.; Lima, W.C.; Wende, H.; Kirchner, M.; Adelfinger, L.; Schrenk-Siemens, K.; Tappe-Theodor, A.; Wetzel, C.; Kuich, P.H.; et al. GABA blocks pathological but not acute TRPV1 pain signals. *Cell* **2015**, *160*, 759–770. [CrossRef] [PubMed]

102. Wang, S.; Dai, Y.; Fukuoka, T.; Yamanaka, H.; Kobayashi, K.; Obata, K.; Cui, X.; Tominaga, M.; Noguchi, K. Phospholipase C and protein kinase A mediate bradykinin sensitization of TRPA1: A molecular mechanism of inflammatory pain. *Brain* **2008**, *131*, 1241–1251. [CrossRef] [PubMed]

103. Kim, D.; Cavanaugh, E.J.; Simkin, D. Inhibition of transient receptor potential A1 channel by phosphatidylinositol-4,5-bisphosphate. *Am. J. Physiol. Cell Physiol.* **2008**, *295*, C92–C99. [CrossRef] [PubMed]

104. Gregus, A.M.; Doolen, S.; Dumlao, D.S.; Buczynski, M.W.; Takasusuki, T.; Fitzsimmons, B.L.; Hua, X.-Y.; Taylor, B.K.; Dennis, E.A.; Yaksh, T.L. Spinal 12-lipoxygenase-derived hepoxilin a3 contributes to inflammatory hyperalgesia via activation of TRPV1 and TRPA1 receptors. *Proc. Natl. Acad. Sci. USA* **2012**, *109*, 6721–6726. [CrossRef] [PubMed]

105. Daniels, R.L.; Takashima, Y.; McKemy, D.D. Activity of the neuronal cold sensor TRPM8 is regulated by phospholipase C via the phospholipid phosphoinositol 4,5-bisphosphate. *J. Biol. Chem.* **2009**, *284*, 1570–1582. [CrossRef] [PubMed]

106. Abe, J.; Hosokawa, H.; Sawada, Y.; Matsumura, K.; Kobayashi, S. Ca^{2+}-dependent PKC activation mediates menthol-induced desensitization of transient receptor potential M8. *Neurosci. Lett.* **2006**, *397*, 140–144. [CrossRef] [PubMed]

107. Premkumar, L.S.; Raisinghani, M.; Pingle, S.C.; Long, C.; Pimentel, F. Downregulation of transient receptor potential melastatin 8 by protein kinase C-mediated dephosphorylation. *J. Neurosci.* **2005**, *25*, 11322–11329. [CrossRef] [PubMed]

108. Yudin, Y.; Lukacs, V.; Cao, C.; Rohacs, T. Decrease in phosphatidylinositol 4,5-bisphosphate levels mediates desensitization of the cold sensor TRPM8 channels. *J. Physiol.* **2011**, *589*, 6007–6027. [CrossRef] [PubMed]

109. De Petrocellis, L.; Starowicz, K.; Moriello, A.S.; Vivese, M.; Orlando, P.; Di Marzo, V. Regulation of transient receptor potential channels of melastatin type 8 (TRPM8): Effect of cAMP, cannabinoid CB(1) receptors and endovanilloids. *Exp. Cell Res.* **2007**, *313*, 1911–1920. [CrossRef] [PubMed]

110. Linte, R.M.; Ciobanu, C.; Reid, G.; Babes, A. Desensitization of cold- and menthol-sensitive rat dorsal root ganglion neurones by inflammatory mediators. *Exp. Br. Res.* **2007**, *178*, 89–98. [CrossRef] [PubMed]

111. Bavencoffe, A.; Gkika, D.; Kondratskyi, A.; Beck, B.; Borowiec, A.S.; Bidaux, G.; Busserolles, J.; Eschalier, A.; Shuba, Y.; Skryma, R.; et al. The transient receptor potential channel trpm8 is inhibited via the alpha 2a adrenoreceptor signaling pathway. *J. Biol. Chem.* **2010**, *285*, 9410–9419. [CrossRef] [PubMed]

112. Sarria, I.; Gu, J. Menthol response and adaptation in nociceptive-like and nonnociceptive-like neurons: Role of protein kinases. *Mol. Pain* **2010**, *6*, 47. [CrossRef] [PubMed]

113. Zhang, X.; Mak, S.; Li, L.; Parra, A.; Denlinger, B.; Belmonte, C.; McNaughton, P.A. Direct inhibition of the cold-activated TRPM8 ion channel by Galpha-q. *Nat. Cell Biol.* **2012**, *14*, 851–858. [CrossRef] [PubMed]

114. De Petrocellis, L.; Vellani, V.; Schiano-Moriello, A.; Marini, P.; Magherini, P.C.; Orlando, P.; Di Marzo, V. Plant-derived cannabinoids modulate the activity of transient receptor potential channels of ankyrin type-1 and melastatin type-8. *J. Pharmacol. Exp. Ther.* **2008**, *325*, 1007–1015. [CrossRef] [PubMed]

115. Andersson, D.A.; Nash, M.; Bevan, S. Modulation of the cold-activated channel TRPM8 by lysophospholipids and polyunsaturated fatty acids. *J. Neurosci.* **2007**, *27*, 3347–3355. [CrossRef] [PubMed]

116. Vanden Abeele, F.; Zholos, A.; Bidaux, G.; Shuba, Y.; Thebault, S.; Beck, B.; Flourakis, M.; Panchin, Y.; Skryma, R.; Prevarskaya, N. Ca^{2+}-independent phospholipase A2-dependent gating of TRPM8 by lysophospholipids. *J. Biol. Chem.* **2006**, *281*, 40174–40182. [CrossRef] [PubMed]

117. Rohacs, T.; Lopes, C.M.; Michailidis, I.; Logothetis, D.E. Pi(4,5)p2 regulates the activation and desensitization of TRPM8 channels through the TRP domain. *Nat. Neurosci.* **2005**, *8*, 626–634. [CrossRef] [PubMed]

118. Liu, B.; Qin, F. Functional control of cold- and menthol-sensitive TRPM8 ion channels by phosphatidylinositol 4,5-bisphosphate. *J. Neurosci.* **2005**, *25*, 1674–1681. [CrossRef] [PubMed]

119. Rohacs, T. Regulation of transient receptor potential channels by the phospholipase C pathway. *Adv. Biol. Regul.* **2013**, *53*, 341–355. [CrossRef] [PubMed]

120. Stokes, A.J.; Shimoda, L.M.; Koblan-Huberson, M.; Adra, C.N.; Turner, H. A TRPV2-PKA signaling module for transduction of physical stimuli in mast cells. *J. Exp. Med.* **2004**, *200*, 137–147. [CrossRef] [PubMed]

121. Alessandri-Haber, N.; Dina, O.A.; Joseph, E.K.; Reichling, D.B.; Levine, J.D. Interaction of transient receptor potential vanilloid 4, integrin, and src tyrosine kinase in mechanical hyperalgesia. *J. Neurosci.* **2008**, *28*, 1046–1057. [CrossRef] [PubMed]

122. Denadai-Souza, A.; Martin, L.; de Paula, M.A.; de Avellar, M.C.; Muscara, M.N.; Vergnolle, N.; Cenac, N. Role of transient receptor potential vanilloid 4 in rat joint inflammation. *Arthritis Rheum.* **2012**, *64*, 1848–1858. [CrossRef] [PubMed]

123. Wegierski, T.; Lewandrowski, U.; Muller, B.; Sickmann, A.; Walz, G. Tyrosine phosphorylation modulates the activity of TRPV4 in response to defined stimuli. *J. Biol. Chem.* **2009**, *284*, 2923–2933. [CrossRef] [PubMed]

124. Melemedjian, O.K.; Tillu, D.V.; Moy, J.K.; Asiedu, M.N.; Mandell, E.K.; Ghosh, S.; Dussor, G.; Price, T.J. Local translation and retrograde axonal transport of CREB regulates IL-6-induced nociceptive plasticity. *Mol. Pain* **2014**, *10*, 45. [CrossRef] [PubMed]

125. Melemedjian, O.K.; Asiedu, M.N.; Tillu, D.V.; Peebles, K.A.; Yan, J.; Ertz, N.; Dussor, G.O.; Price, T.J. IL-6- and NGF-induced rapid control of protein synthesis and nociceptive plasticity via convergent signaling to the eif4f complex. *J. Neurosci.* **2010**, *30*, 15113–15123. [CrossRef] [PubMed]

126. Caterina, M.J.; Leffler, A.; Malmberg, A.B.; Martin, W.J.; Trafton, J.; Petersen-Zeitz, K.R.; Koltzenburg, M.; Basbaum, A.I.; Julius, D. Impaired nociception and pain sensation in mice lacking the capsaicin receptor. *Science* **2000**, *288*, 306–313. [CrossRef] [PubMed]

127. Davis, J.B.; Gray, J.; Gunthorpe, M.J.; Hatcher, J.P.; Davey, P.T.; Overend, P.; Harries, M.H.; Latcham, J.; Clapham, C.; Atkinson, K.; et al. Vanilloid receptor-1 is essential for inflammatory thermal hyperalgesia. *Nature* **2000**, *405*, 183–187. [CrossRef] [PubMed]

128. Eskander, M.A.; Ruparel, S.; Green, D.P.; Chen, P.B.; Por, E.D.; Jeske, N.A.; Gao, X.; Flores, E.R.; Hargreaves, K.M. Persistent nociception triggered by nerve growth factor (NGF) is mediated by TRPV1 and oxidative mechanisms. *J. Neurosci.* **2015**, *35*, 8593–8603. [CrossRef] [PubMed]

129. Hillery, C.A.; Kerstein, P.C.; Vilceanu, D.; Barabas, M.E.; Retherford, D.; Brandow, A.M.; Wandersee, N.J.; Stucky, C.L. Transient receptor potential vanilloid 1 mediates pain in mice with severe sickle cell disease. *Blood* **2011**, *118*, 3376–3383. [CrossRef] [PubMed]

130. Ro, J.Y.; Lee, J.S.; Zhang, Y. Activation of TRPV1 and TRPA1 leads to muscle nociception and mechanical hyperalgesia. *Pain* **2009**, *144*, 270–277. [CrossRef] [PubMed]

131. Shutov, L.P.; Warwick, C.A.; Shi, X.; Gnanasekaran, A.; Shepherd, A.J.; Mohapatra, D.P.; Woodruff, T.M.; Clark, J.D.; Usachev, Y.M. The complement system component C5a produces thermal hyperalgesia via macrophage-to-sensory neuron signaling that requires NGF and TRPV1. *J. Neurosci.* **2016**, *36*, 5055–5070. [CrossRef] [PubMed]

132. Szabo, A.; Helyes, Z.; Sandor, K.; Bite, A.; Pinter, E.; Nemeth, J.; Banvolgyi, A.; Bolcskei, K.; Elekes, K.; Szolcsanyi, J. Role of transient receptor potential vanilloid 1 receptors in adjuvant-induced chronic arthritis: In vivo study using gene-deficient mice. *J. Pharmacol. Exp. Ther.* **2005**, *314*, 111–119. [CrossRef] [PubMed]

133. Walder, R.Y.; Radhakrishnan, R.; Loo, L.; Rasmussen, L.A.; Mohapatra, D.P.; Wilson, S.P.; Sluka, K.A. TRPV1 is important for mechanical and heat sensitivity in uninjured animals and development of heat hypersensitivity after muscle inflammation. *Pain* **2012**, *153*, 1664–1672. [CrossRef] [PubMed]

134. Watanabe, M.; Ueda, T.; Shibata, Y.; Kumamoto, N.; Ugawa, S. The role of TRPV1 channels in carrageenan-induced mechanical hyperalgesia in mice. *Neuroreport* **2015**, *26*, 173–178. [CrossRef] [PubMed]

135. Eid, S.R.; Crown, E.D.; Moore, E.L.; Liang, H.A.; Choong, K.C.; Dima, S.; Henze, D.A.; Kane, S.A.; Urban, M.O. HC-030031, a TRPA1 selective antagonist, attenuates inflammatory- and neuropathy-induced mechanical hypersensitivity. *Mol. Pain* **2008**, *4*, 48. [CrossRef] [PubMed]

136. Petrus, M.; Peier, A.M.; Bandell, M.; Hwang, S.W.; Huynh, T.; Olney, N.; Jegla, T.; Patapoutian, A. A role of TRPA1 in mechanical hyperalgesia is revealed by pharmacological inhibition. *Mol. Pain* **2007**, *3*, 40. [CrossRef] [PubMed]

137. Da Costa, D.S.; Meotti, F.C.; Andrade, E.L.; Leal, P.C.; Motta, E.M.; Calixto, J.B. The involvement of the transient receptor potential a1 (TRPA1) in the maintenance of mechanical and cold hyperalgesia in persistent inflammation. *Pain* **2010**, *148*, 431–437. [CrossRef] [PubMed]

138. Obata, K.; Katsura, H.; Mizushima, T.; Yamanaka, H.; Kobayashi, K.; Dai, Y.; Fukuoka, T.; Tokunaga, A.; Tominaga, M.; Noguchi, K. TRPA1 induced in sensory neurons contributes to cold hyperalgesia after inflammation and nerve injury. *J. Clin. Investig.* **2005**, *115*, 2393–2401. [CrossRef] [PubMed]

139. Liu, B.; Escalera, J.; Balakrishna, S.; Fan, L.; Caceres, A.I.; Robinson, E.; Sui, A.; McKay, M.C.; McAlexander, M.A.; Herrick, C.A.; et al. TRPA1 controls inflammation and pruritogen responses in allergic contact dermatitis. *FASEB J.* **2013**, *27*, 3549–3563. [CrossRef] [PubMed]

140. Than, J.Y.-X.L.; Li, L.; Hasan, R.; Zhang, X. Excitation and modulation of TRPA1, TRPV1, and TRPM8 channel-expressing sensory neurons by the pruritogen chloroquine. *J. Biol. Chem.* **2013**, *288*, 12818–12827. [CrossRef] [PubMed]

141. Wilson, S.R.; Nelson, A.M.; Batia, L.; Morita, T.; Estandian, D.; Owens, D.M.; Lumpkin, E.A.; Bautista, D.M. The ion channel TRPA1 is required for chronic itch. *J. Neurosci.* **2013**, *33*, 9283–9294. [CrossRef] [PubMed]

142. Todaka, H.; Taniguchi, J.; Satoh, J.; Mizuno, A.; Suzuki, M. Warm temperature-sensitive transient receptor potential vanilloid 4 (TRPV4) plays an essential role in thermal hyperalgesia. *J. Biol. Chem.* **2004**, *279*, 35133–35138. [CrossRef] [PubMed]

143. Barton, N.J.; McQueen, D.S.; Thomson, D.; Gauldie, S.D.; Wilson, A.W.; Salter, D.M.; Chessell, I.P. Attenuation of experimental arthritis in TRPV1r knockout mice. *Exp. Mol. Pathol.* **2006**, *81*, 166–170. [CrossRef] [PubMed]

144. Kelly, S.; Chapman, R.J.; Woodhams, S.; Sagar, D.R.; Turner, J.; Burston, J.J.; Bullock, C.; Paton, K.; Huang, J.; Wong, A.; et al. Increased function of pronociceptive TRPV1 at the level of the joint in a rat model of osteoarthritis pain. *Ann. Rheum. Dis.* **2013**. [CrossRef] [PubMed]

145. Fernandes, E.S.; Russell, F.A.; Spina, D.; McDougall, J.J.; Graepel, R.; Gentry, C.; Staniland, A.A.; Mountford, D.M.; Keeble, J.E.; Malcangio, M.; et al. A distinct role for transient receptor potential ankyrin 1, in addition to transient receptor potential vanilloid 1, in tumor necrosis factor α–induced inflammatory hyperalgesia and freund's complete adjuvant–induced monarthritis. *Arthritis Rheum.* **2011**, *63*, 819–829. [CrossRef] [PubMed]

146. Valdes, A.M.; De Wilde, G.; Doherty, S.A.; Lories, R.J.; Vaughn, F.L.; Laslett, L.L.; Maciewicz, R.A.; Soni, A.; Hart, D.J.; Zhang, W.; et al. The ile585val trpv1 variant is involved in risk of painful knee osteoarthritis. *Ann. Rheumatic Dis.* **2011**, *70*, 1556–1561. [CrossRef] [PubMed]

147. Gavva, N.R.; Treanor, J.J.; Garami, A.; Fang, L.; Surapaneni, S.; Akrami, A.; Alvarez, F.; Bak, A.; Darling, M.; Gore, A.; et al. Pharmacological blockade of the vanilloid receptor TRPV1 elicits marked hyperthermia in humans. *Pain* **2008**, *136*, 202–210. [CrossRef] [PubMed]

148. Kym, P.R.; Kort, M.E.; Hutchins, C.W. Analgesic potential of TRPV1 antagonists. *Biochem. Pharmacol.* **2009**, *78*, 211–216. [CrossRef] [PubMed]

149. Kort, M.E.; Kym, P.R. TRPV1 antagonists: Clinical setbacks and prospects for future development. *Prog. Med. Chem.* **2012**, *51*, 57–70. [PubMed]

150. Wong, G.Y.; Gavva, N.R. Therapeutic potential of vanilloid receptor TRPV1 agonists and antagonists as analgesics: Recent advances and setbacks. *Brain Res. Rev.* **2009**, *60*, 267–277. [CrossRef] [PubMed]

151. Rowbotham, M.C.; Nothaft, W.; Duan, W.R.; Wang, Y.; Faltynek, C.; McGaraughty, S.; Chu, K.L.; Svensson, P. Oral and cutaneous thermosensory profile of selective TRPV1 inhibition by ABT-102 in a randomixed healthy volunteer trial. *Pain* **2011**, *152*, 1192–1200. [CrossRef] [PubMed]

152. A Safety, Tolerability and Pharmacokinetic Study of ABT-102 in Healthy Subjects. Clinical Trials.gov 2010. Available online: https://clinicaltrials.gov/ct2/show/NCT00854659?term=ABT102&rank=1 (accessed on 28 October 2016).

153. SB-705498 Dental Pain Study after Tooth Extraction. Clinical Trials.gov 2011. Available online: https://clinicaltrials.gov/ct2/show/NCT00281684?term=SB-705498&rank=8 (accessed on 28 October 2016).
154. SB-705498 Rectal Pain Study. Clinical Trials.gov 2012. Available online: https://clinicaltrials.gov/ct2/show/NCT00461682?term=SB-705498&rank=10 (accessed on 28 October 2016).
155. A Study to Evaluate the Safety and Efficacy of an Investigational Drug in the Treatment of Postoperative Dental Pain (MK-2295-005). Clinical Trials.gov 2015. Available online: https://clinicaltrials.gov/ct2/show/NCT00387140?term=MK2295&rank=1 (accessed on 28 October 2016).
156. Esophageal Hypersensitivity Study in Healthy Volunteers. Clinical Trials.gov 2009. Available online: https://clinicaltrials.gov/ct2/show/NCT00711048?term=AZD1386&rank=11 (accessed on 28 October 2016).
157. Krarup, A.L.; Ny, L.; Astrand, M.; Bajor, A.; Hvid-Jensen, F.; Hansen, M.B.; Simren, M.; Funch-Jensen, P.; Drewes, A.M. Randomised clinical trial: The efficacy of a transient receptor potnetial vanilloid 1 antagonist AZD1386 in human oesophageal pain. *Aliment. Pharmacol. Ther.* **2011**, *33*, 1113–1122. [CrossRef] [PubMed]
158. Study to Investigate the Analgesic Efficacy of a Single Dose of AZD1386. Clinical Trials.gov 2016. Available online: https://clinicaltrials.gov/ct2/show/NCT00672646?term=azd1386&rank=2 (accessed on 28 October 2016).
159. Quiding, H.; Jonzon, B.; Svensson, O.; Webster, L.; Reimfelt, A.; Karin, A.; Karlsten, R.; Segerdahl, M. TRPV1 antagonistic analgesic effect: A randomized study of AZD1386 in pain after third molar extraction. *Pain* **2013**, *154*, 808–812. [CrossRef] [PubMed]
160. Study to Evaluate Efficacy, Safety, Tolerability and Pharmacokinetics of AZD1386 in Patients with Peripheral Neuropathic Pain (AVANT). Clinical Trials.gov 2009. Available online: https://clinicaltrials.gov/ct2/show/NCT00672646?term=azd1386&rank=2 (accessed on 28 October 2016).
161. Study to Evaluate the Efficacy, Safety, Tolerability and Pharmacokinetics of AZD1386 in Patients with Osteoarthritis (OA) of the Knee (OA19). Clinical Trials.gov 2012. Available online: https://clinicaltrials.gov/ct2/show/NCT00672646?term=azd1386&rank=2 (accessed on 28 October 2016).
162. NEO6860, a TRPV1 Antagonist, First in Human Study. Clinical Trials.gov 2016. Available online: https://clinicaltrials.gov/ct2/show/NCT02337543?term=TRPV1&rank=17 (accessed on 28 October 2016).
163. A Proof-of-Concept Study Assessing NEO6860 in Osteoarthritis Pain. Clinical Trials.gov 2016. Available online: https://clinicaltrials.gov/ct2/show/NCT02712957?term=TRPV1&rank=20 (accessed on 28 October 2016).
164. Study of NGX-4010 for the Treatment of Postherpetic Neuralgia. Clinical Trials.gov 2008. Available online: https://www.clinicaltrials.gov/ct2/show/NCT00115310?term=ngx+4010&rank=3 (accessed on 28 October 2016).
165. Mou, J.; Paillard, F.; Trumbull, B.; Trudeau, J.; Stoker, M.; Katz, N.P. Qutenza (capsaicin) 8% patch onset and duration of response and effects of multiple treatments in neuropathic pain patients. *Clin. J. Pain* **2014**, *30*, 286–294. [CrossRef] [PubMed]
166. Study of NGX-4010 for the Treatment of Painful HIV-Associated Neuropathy. Clinical Trials.gov 2011. Available online: https://www.clinicaltrials.gov/ct2/show/results/NCT00321672?term=ngx+4010&rank=1 (accessed on 28 October 2016).
167. Simpson, D.M.; Brown, S.; Tobias, J.K.; Vanhove, G.F.; NGX-4010 C107 Study Group. NGX-4010, a capsaicin 8% dermal patch, for the treatment of HIV-associated distal sensory polyneuropathy: Results of a 52-week open-label study. *Clin. J. Pain* **2014**, *30*, 134–142. [PubMed]
168. Brown, D.C.; Agnello, K.; Iadarola, M.J. Intrathecal resiniferatoxin in a dog model: Efficacy in bone cancer pain. *Pain* **2015**, *156*, 1018–1024. [CrossRef] [PubMed]
169. Resiniferatoxin to Treat Severe Pain Associated with Advanced Cancer. Clinical Trials.gov 2016. Available online: https://clinicaltrials.gov/ct2/show/NCT00804154?term=Resiniferatoxin&rank=1 (accessed on 28 October 2016).
170. Periganglionic Resiniferatoxin for the Treatment of Intractable Pain due to Cancer-Induced Bone Pain. Clinical Trials.gov 2016. Available online: https://clinicaltrials.gov/ct2/show/NCT02522611?term=Resiniferatoxin&rank=2 (accessed on 28 October 2016).
171. Evaluating the Safety and Efficacy of Civamide (Zucapsaicin) in Osteoarthritis (OA) of the Knee(s). Clinical Trials.gov 2011. Available online: https://clinicaltrials.gov/ct2/show/NCT00995306?term=zucapsaicin&rank=2 (accessed on 28 October 2016).

172. Evaluation of Civamide (Zucapsaicin) in Treatment of Postherpetic Neuroalgia and Post-Incisional Neuralgia. Clinical Trials.gov 2014. Available online: https://clinicaltrials.gov/ct2/show/NCT00845923?term=zucapsaicin&rank=4 (accessed on 28 October 2016).

173. A phase III Study of Civamide Nasal Solution (Zucapsaicin) for the Treatment of Episodic Cluster Headache. Clinical Trials.gov 2011. Available online: https://clinicaltrials.gov/ct2/show/NCT00033839?term=zucapsaicin&rank=8 (accessed on 28 October 2016).

174. A Clinical Trial to Study the Effects of GRC 17536 in Patients with Painful Diabetic Peripheral Neuropathy (Painful Extremities due to Peripheral Nerve Damage in Diabetic Patients). Clinical Trials.gov 2014. Available online: https://clinicaltrials.gov/ct2/show/NCT01726413?term=GRC-17536&rank=2 (accessed on 28 October 2016).

175. Efficacy and Safety of SAR292833 Administration for 4 Weeks in Patients with Chronic Peripheral Neuropathic Pain (Alchemilla). Clinical Trials.gov 2016. Available online: https://clinicaltrials.gov/ct2/show/NCT01463397?term=NCT01463397&rank=1 (accessed on 28 October 2016).

176. Winchester, W.J.; Gore, K.; Glatt, S.; Petit, W.; Gardiner, J.C.; Conlon, K.; Postlethwaite, M.; Saintot, P.P.; Roberts, S.; Gosset, J.R.; et al. Inhibition of TRPM8 channels reduces pain in the cold pressor test in humans. *J. Pharmacol. Exp. Ther.* **2014**, *351*, 259–269. [CrossRef] [PubMed]

177. Single dose, Dose Escalation Healthy Volunteers Study of PF-05105679 (Single Dose). Clinical Trials.gov 2011. Available online: https://clinicaltrials.gov/ct2/show/NCT01393652?term=PF-05105679&rank=1 (accessed on 28 October 2016).

178. Kaneko, Y.; Szallasi, A. Transient receptor potnetial (TRP) channels: A clinical perspective. *Br. J. Pharmacol.* **2014**, *171*, 2474–2507. [CrossRef] [PubMed]

179. Reilly, R.M.; McDonald, H.A.; Puttfarcken, P.S.; Joshi, S.K.; Lewis, L.; Pai, M.; Franklin, P.H.; Segreti, J.A.; Neelands, T.R.; Han, P.; et al. Pharmacology of modality-specific transient receptor potential vanilloid-1 antagonists that do not alter body temperature. *J. Pharmacol. Exp. Ther.* **2012**, *342*, 416–428. [CrossRef] [PubMed]

180. Kim, S.; Hwang, S. Emerging roles of TRPA1 in sensation of oxidative stress and its implications in defense and danger. *Arch. Pharm. Res.* **2013**, *36*, 783–791. [CrossRef] [PubMed]

181. Old, E.A.; Nadkarni, S.; Grist, J.; Gentry, C.; Bevan, S.; Kim, K.-W.; Mogg, A.J.; Perretti, M.; Malcangio, M. Monocytes expressing CX3CR1 orchestrate the development of vincristine-induced pain. *J. Clin. Investig.* **2014**, *124*, 2023–2036. [CrossRef] [PubMed]

182. Barrière, D.A.; Rieusset, J.; Chanteranne, D.; Busserolles, J.; Chauvin, M.-A.; Chapuis, L.; Salles, J.; Dubray, C.; Morio, B. Paclitaxel therapy potentiates cold hyperalgesia in streptozotocin-induced diabetic rats through enhanced mitochondrial reactive oxygen species production and TRPA1 sensitization. *Pain* **2012**, *153*, 553–561. [CrossRef] [PubMed]

183. Nassini, R.; Gees, M.; Harrison, S.; De Siena, G.; Materazzi, S.; Moretto, N.; Failli, P.; Preti, D.; Marchetti, N.; Cavazzini, A.; et al. Oxaliplatin elicits mechanical and cold allodynia in rodents via TRPA1 receptor stimulation. *Pain* **2011**, *152*, 1621–1631. [CrossRef] [PubMed]

184. Katsura, H.; Obata, K.; Mizushima, T.; Yamanaka, H.; Kobayashi, K.; Dai, Y.; Fukuoka, T.; Tokunaga, A.; Sakagami, M.; Noguchi, K. Antisense knock down of TRPA1, but not TRPM8, alleviates cold hyperalgesia after spinal nerve ligation in rats. *Exp. Neurol.* **2006**, *200*, 112–123. [CrossRef] [PubMed]

185. Fernández-Peña, C.; Viana, F. Targeting TRPM8 for pain relief. *Open Pain J.* **2013**, *6*, 154–164. [CrossRef]

186. Colburn, R.W.; Lubin, M.L.; Stone, D.J., Jr.; Wang, Y.; Lawrence, D.; D'Andrea, M.R.; Brandt, M.R.; Liu, Y.; Flores, C.M.; Qin, N. Attenuated cold sensitivity in TRPM8 null mice. *Neuron* **2007**, *54*, 379–386. [CrossRef] [PubMed]

187. Rong, W.; Hillsley, K.; Davis, J.B.; Hicks, G.; Winchester, W.J.; Grundy, D. Jejunal afferent nerve sensitivity in wild-type and TRPV11 knockout mice. *J. Physiol.* **2004**, *560*, 867–881. [CrossRef] [PubMed]

188. Kimball, E.S.; Wallace, N.H.; Schneider, C.R.; D'Andrea, M.R.; Hornby, P.J. Vanilloid receptor 1 antagonists attenuate disease severity in dextran sulphate sodium-induced colitis in mice. *Neurogastroenterol. Motil.* **2004**, *16*, 811–818. [CrossRef] [PubMed]

189. Chan, C.L.; Facer, P.; Davis, J.B.; Smith, G.D.; Egerton, J.; Bountra, C.; Williams, N.S.; Anand, P. Sensory fibres expressing capsaicin receptor TRPV1 in patients with rectal hypersensitivity and faecal urgency. *Lancet* **2003**, *361*, 385–391. [CrossRef]

190. Wang, Z.Y.; Wang, P.; Merriam, F.V.; Bjorling, D.E. Lack of TRPV1 inhibits cystitis-induced increased mechanical sensitivity in mice. *Pain* **2008**, *139*, 158–167. [CrossRef] [PubMed]

191. Jones, R.C., 3rd; Xu, L.; Gebhart, G.F. The mechanosensitivity of mouse colon afferent fibers and their sensitization by inflammatory mediators require transient receptor potential vanilloid 1 and acid-sensing ion channel 3. *J. Neurosci.* **2005**, *25*, 10981–10989. [CrossRef] [PubMed]

192. Jones, R.C., 3rd; Otsuka, E.; Wagstrom, E.; Jensen, C.S.; Price, M.P.; Gebhart, G.F. Short-term sensitization of colon mechanoreceptors is associated with long-term hypersensitivity to colon distention in the mouse. *Gastroenterology* **2007**, *133*, 184–194. [CrossRef] [PubMed]

193. Massa, F.; Sibaev, A.; Marsicano, G.; Blaudzun, H.; Storr, M.; Lutz, B. Vanilloid receptor (TRPV1)-deficient mice show increased susceptibility to dinitrobenzene sulfonic acid induced colitis. *J. Mol. Med.* **2006**, *84*, 142–146. [CrossRef] [PubMed]

194. Storr, M. TRPV1 in colitis: Is it a good or a bad receptor?—A viewpoint. *Neurogastroenterol. Motil.* **2007**, *19*, 625–629. [CrossRef] [PubMed]

195. Dang, K.; Bielefeldt, K.; Gebhart, G.F. Differential responses of bladder lumbosacral and thoracolumbar dorsal root ganglion neurons to purinergic agonists, protons, and capsaicin. *J. Neurosci.* **2005**, *25*, 3973–3984. [CrossRef] [PubMed]

196. Cruz, F.; Guimaraes, M.; Silva, C.; Reis, M. Suppression of bladder hyperreflexia by intravesical resiniferatoxin. *Lancet* **1997**, *350*, 640–641. [CrossRef]

197. Premkumar, L.S.; Sikand, P. TRPV1: A target for next generation analgesics. *Curr. Neuropharmacol.* **2008**, *6*, 151–163. [CrossRef] [PubMed]

198. Dinis, P.; Charrua, A.; Avelino, A.; Cruz, F. Intravesical resiniferatoxin decreases spinal c-fos expression and increases bladder volume to reflex micturition in rats with chronic inflamed urinary bladders. *BJU Int.* **2004**, *94*, 153–157. [CrossRef] [PubMed]

199. Ceppa, E.; Cattaruzza, F.; Lyo, V.; Amadesi, S.; Pelayo, J.C.; Poole, D.P.; Vaksman, N.; Liedtke, W.; Cohen, D.M.; Grady, E.F.; et al. Transient receptor potential ion channels V4 and A1 contribute to pancreatitis pain in mice. *Am. J. Physiol. Gastrointest. Liver Physiol.* **2010**, *299*, G556–G571. [CrossRef] [PubMed]

200. D'Aldebert, E.; Cenac, N.; Rousset, P.; Martin, L.; Rolland, C.; Chapman, K.; Selves, J.; Alric, L.; Vinel, J.P.; Vergnolle, N. Transient receptor potential vanilloid 4 activated inflammatory signals by intestinal epithelial cells and colitis in mice. *Gastroenterology* **2011**, *140*, 275–285. [CrossRef] [PubMed]

201. Nakamura, Y.; Une, Y.; Miyano, K.; Abe, H.; Hisaoka, K.; Morioka, N.; Nakata, Y. Activation of transient receptor potential ankyrin 1 evokes nociception through substance p release from primary sensory neurons. *J. Neurochem.* **2012**, *120*, 1036–1047. [CrossRef] [PubMed]

202. Yang, J.; Li, Y.; Zuo, X.; Zhen, Y.; Yu, Y.; Gao, L. Transient receptor potential ankyrin-1 participates in visceral hyperalgesia following experimental colitis. *Neurosci. Lett.* **2008**, *440*, 237–241. [CrossRef] [PubMed]

203. Terada, Y.; Fujimura, M.; Nishimura, S.; Tsubota, M.; Sekiguchi, F.; Nishikawa, H.; Kawabata, A. Contribution of TRPA1 as a downstream signal of proteinase-activated receptor-2 to pancreatic pain. *J. Pharmacol. Sci.* **2013**, *123*, 284–287. [CrossRef] [PubMed]

204. Meseguer, V.; Alpizar, Y.A.; Luis, E.; Tajada, S.; Denlinger, B.; Fajardo, O.; Manenschijn, J.-A.; Fernández-Peña, C.; Talavera, A.; Kichko, T.; et al. TRPA1 channels mediate acute neurogenic inflammation and pain produced by bacterial endotoxins. *Nat. Commun.* **2014**, *5*. [CrossRef] [PubMed]

205. Bessac, B.F.; Sivula, M.; von Hehn, C.A.; Escalera, J.; Cohn, L.; Jordt, S.-E. TRPA1 is a major oxidant sensor in murine airway sensory neurons. *J. Clin. Investig.* **2008**, *118*, 1899–1910. [CrossRef] [PubMed]

206. Andersson, D.A.; Gentry, C.; Alenmyr, L.; Killander, D.; Lewis, S.E.; Andersson, A.; Bucher, B.; Galzi, J.-L.; Sterner, O.; Bevan, S.; et al. TRPA1 mediates spinal antinociception induced by acetaminophen and the cannabinoid δ9-tetrahydrocannabiorcol. *Nat. Commun.* **2011**, *2*, 551. [CrossRef] [PubMed]

207. Van Zanten, S.V. Review: Fibre, antispasmodics, and peppermint oil are all effective for irritable bowel syndrome. *Evid.-Based Med.* **2009**, *14*, 84. [CrossRef] [PubMed]

208. Lashinger, E.S.; Steiginga, M.S.; Hieble, J.P.; Leon, L.A.; Gardner, S.D.; Nagilla, R.; Davenport, E.A.; Hoffman, B.E.; Laping, N.J.; Su, X. AMTB, a TRPM8 channel blocker: Evidence in rats for activity in overactive bladder and painful bladder syndrome. *Am. J. Physiol. Renal Physiol.* **2008**, *295*, F803–F810. [CrossRef] [PubMed]

209. Mantyh, P. Bone cancer pain: Causes, consequences, and therapeutic opportunities. *Pain* **2013**, *154*, S54–S62. [CrossRef] [PubMed]

210. Ghilardi, J.R.; Rohrich, H.; Lindsay, T.H.; Sevcik, M.A.; Schwei, M.J.; Kubota, K.; Halvorson, K.G.; Poblete, J.; Chaplan, S.R.; Dubin, A.E.; et al. Selective blockade of the capsaicin receptor TRPV1 attenuates bone cancer pain. *J. Neurosci.* **2005**, *25*, 3126–3131. [CrossRef] [PubMed]

211. Nieto-Posadas, A.; Picazo-Juarez, G.; Llorente, I.; Jara-Oseguera, A.; Morales-Lazaro, S.; Escalante-Alcalde, D.; Islas, L.D.; Rosenbaum, T. Lysophosphatidic acid directly activates TRPV1 through a c-terminal binding site. *Nat. Chem. Biol.* **2012**, *8*, 78–85. [CrossRef] [PubMed]

212. Pan, H.L.; Zhang, Y.Q.; Zhao, Z.Q. Involvement of lysophosphatidic acid in bone cancer pain by potentiation of TRPV1 via PKC-epsilon pathway in dorsal root ganglion neurons. *Mol. Pain* **2010**, *6*, 85. [CrossRef] [PubMed]

213. Zhao, J.; Pan, H.L.; Li, T.T.; Zhang, Y.Q.; Wei, J.Y.; Zhao, Z.Q. The sensitization of peripheral c-fibers to lysophosphatidic acid in bone cancer pain. *Life Sci.* **2010**, *87*, 120–125. [CrossRef] [PubMed]

214. Brown, D.C.; Iadarola, M.J.; Perkowski, S.Z.; Erin, H.; Shofer, F.; Laszlo, K.J.; Olah, Z.; Mannes, A.J. Physiologic and antinociceptive effects of intrathecal resiniferatoxin in a canine bone cancer model. *Anesthesiology* **2005**, *103*, 1052–1059. [CrossRef] [PubMed]

215. Park, C.K.; Kim, M.S.; Fang, Z.; Li, H.Y.; Jung, S.J.; Choi, S.Y.; Lee, S.J.; Park, K.; Kim, J.S.; Oh, S.B. Functional expression of thermo-transient receptor potential channels in dental primary afferent neurons: Implication for tooth pain. *J. Biol. Chem.* **2006**, *281*, 17304–17311. [CrossRef] [PubMed]

216. Kim, H.Y.; Chung, G.; Jo, H.J.; Kim, Y.S.; Bae, Y.C.; Jung, S.J.; Kim, J.S.; Oh, S.B. Characterization of dental nociceptive neurons. *J. Dent. Res.* **2011**, *90*, 771–776. [CrossRef] [PubMed]

217. Chung, G.; Oh, S.B. TRP channels in dental pain. *Open Pain J.* **2013**, *6*, 31–36. [CrossRef]

218. Chung, M.K.; Lee, J.; Duraes, G.; Ro, J.Y. Lipopolysaccharide-induced pulpitis up-regulates TRPV1 in trigeminal ganglia. *J. Dent. Res.* **2011**, *90*, 1103–1107. [CrossRef] [PubMed]

219. Haas, E.T.; Rowland, K.; Gautam, M. Tooth injury increases expression of the cold sensitive trp channel TRPA1 in trigeminal neurons. *Arch. Oral Biol.* **2011**, *56*, 1604–1609. [CrossRef] [PubMed]

220. Meents, J.E.; Hoffmann, J.; Chaplan, S.R.; Neeb, L.; Schuh-Hofer, S.; Wickenden, A.; Reuter, U. Two TRPV1 receptor antagonists are effective in two different experimental models of migraine. *J. Headache Pain* **2015**, *16*, 57. [CrossRef] [PubMed]

221. Chasman, D.I.; Schurks, M.; Anttila, V.; de Vries, B.; Schminke, U.; Launer, L.J.; Terwindt, G.M.; van den Maagdenberg, A.M.; Fendrich, K.; Volzke, H.; et al. Genome-wide association study reveals three susceptibility loci for common migraine in the general population. *Nat. Genet.* **2011**, *43*, 695–698. [CrossRef] [PubMed]

222. Edelmayer, R.M.; Le, L.N.; Yan, J.; Wei, X.; Nassini, R.; Materazzi, S.; Preti, D.; Appendino, G.; Geppetti, P.; Dodick, D.W.; et al. Activation of TRPA1 on dural afferents: A potential mechanism of headache pain. *Pain* **2012**, *153*, 1949–1958. [CrossRef] [PubMed]

223. Trevisan, G.; Benemei, S.; Materazzi, S.; De Logu, F.; De Siena, G.; Fusi, C.; Fortes Rossato, M.; Coppi, E.; Marone, I.M.; Ferreira, J.; et al. TRPA1 mediates trigeminal neuropathic pain in mice downstream of monocytes/macrophages and oxidative stress. *Brain* **2016**, *139*, 1361–1377. [CrossRef] [PubMed]

224. Cavanaugh, D.J.; Lee, H.; Lo, L.; Shields, S.D.; Zylka, M.J.; Basbaum, A.I.; Anderson, D.J. Distinct subsets of unmyelinated primary sensory fibers mediate behavioral responses to noxious thermal and mechanical stimuli. *Proc. Natl. Acad. Sci. USA* **2009**, *106*, 9075–9080. [CrossRef] [PubMed]

225. Liu, M.G.; Zhuo, M. No requirement of TRPV1 in long-term potentiation or long-term depression in the anterior cingulate cortex. *Mol. Brain* **2014**, *7*, 27. [CrossRef] [PubMed]

226. Geppetti, P.; Materazzi, S.; Nicoletti, P. The transient receptor potential vanilloid 1: Role in airway inflammation and disease. *Eur. J. Pharmacol.* **2006**, *533*, 207–214. [CrossRef] [PubMed]

227. Jia, Y.; McLeod, R.L.; Hey, J.A. TRPV1 receptor: A target for the treatment of pain, cough, airway disease and urinary incontinence. *Drug News Perspect.* **2005**, *18*, 165–171. [CrossRef] [PubMed]

228. Gunthorpe, M.J.; Szallasi, A. Peripheral TRPV1 receptors as targets for drug development: New molecules and mechanisms. *Curr. Pharm. Des.* **2008**, *14*, 32–41. [PubMed]

229. Bhattacharya, A.; Scott, B.P.; Nasser, N.; Ao, H.; Maher, M.P.; Dubin, A.E.; Swanson, D.M.; Shankley, N.P.; Wickenden, A.D.; Chaplan, S.R. Pharmacology and antitussive efficacy of 4-(3-trifluoromethyl-pyridin-2-yl)-piperazine-1-carboxylic acid (5-trifluoromethyl-pyridin-2-yl)-amide (jnj17203212), a transient receptor potential vanilloid 1 antagonist in guinea pigs. *J. Pharmacol. Exp. Ther.* **2007**, *323*, 665–674. [CrossRef] [PubMed]

230. Razavi, R.; Chan, Y.; Afifiyan, F.N.; Liu, X.J.; Wan, X.; Yantha, J.; Tsui, H.; Tang, L.; Tsai, S.; Santamaria, P.; et al. TRPV1+ sensory neurons control beta cell stress and islet inflammation in autoimmune diabetes. *Cell* **2006**, *127*, 1123–1135. [CrossRef] [PubMed]

231. Park, U.; Vastani, N.; Guan, Y.; Raja, S.N.; Koltzenburg, M.; Caterina, M.J. TRP vanilloid 2 knock-out mice are susceptible to perinatal lethality but display normal thermal and mechanical nociception. *J. Neurosci.* **2011**, *31*, 11425–11436. [CrossRef] [PubMed]

232. Link, T.M.; Park, U.; Vonakis, B.M.; Raben, D.M.; Soloski, M.J.; Caterina, M.J. TRPV2 has a pivotal role in macrophage particle binding and phagocytosis. *Nat. Immunol.* **2010**, *11*, 232–239. [CrossRef] [PubMed]

233. Dhaka, A.; Murray, A.N.; Mathur, J.; Earley, T.J.; Petrus, M.J.; Patapoutian, A. TRPM8 is required for cold sensation in mice. *Neuron* **2007**, *54*, 371–378. [CrossRef] [PubMed]

234. Bautista, D.M.; Siemens, J.; Glazer, J.M.; Tsuruda, P.R.; Basbaum, A.I.; Stucky, C.L.; Jordt, S.E.; Julius, D. The menthol receptor TRPM8 is the principal detector of environmental cold. *Nature* **2007**, *448*, 204–208. [CrossRef] [PubMed]

235. Noel, J.; Zimmermann, K.; Busserolles, J.; Deval, E.; Alloui, A.; Diochot, S.; Guy, N.; Borsotto, M.; Reeh, P.; Eschalier, A.; et al. The mechano-activated K+ channels TRAAK and TREK-1 control both warm and cold perception. *EMBO J.* **2009**, *28*, 1308–1318. [CrossRef] [PubMed]

236. Corey, D.P.; Garcia-Anoveros, J.; Holt, J.R.; Kwan, K.Y.; Lin, S.Y.; Vollrath, M.A.; Amalfitano, A.; Cheung, E.L.; Derfler, B.H.; Duggan, A.; et al. TRPA1 is a candidate for the mechanosensitive transduction channel of vertebrate hair cells. *Nature* **2004**, *432*, 723–730. [CrossRef] [PubMed]

237. Nagata, K.; Duggan, A.; Kumar, G.; Garcia-Anoveros, J. Nociceptor and hair cell transducer properties of TRPA1, a channel for pain and hearing. *J. Neurosci.* **2005**, *25*, 4052–4061. [CrossRef] [PubMed]

238. Kwan, K.Y.; Allchorne, A.J.; Vollrath, M.A.; Christensen, A.P.; Zhang, D.S.; Woolf, C.J.; Corey, D.P. TRPA1 contributes to cold, mechanical, and chemical nociception but is not essential for hair-cell transduction. *Neuron* **2006**, *50*, 277–289. [CrossRef] [PubMed]

239. Guimaraes, M.Z.P.; Jordt, S.E. TRPA1: A sensory channel of many talents. In *TRP Ion Channel Function in Sensory Transduction and Cellular Signaling Cascades*; Liedtke, W.B., Heller, S., Eds.; CRC Press: Boca Raton, FL, USA, 2007.

240. Zygmunt, P.M.; Hogestatt, E.D. TRPA1. In *Handbook of Experimental Pharmacology*; Springer: Berlin, Germany, 2014; Volume 222, pp. 583–630.

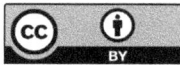

pharmaceuticals

MDPI

Review
TRPV3 in Drug Development

Lisa M. Broad [1,*], Adrian J. Mogg [1], Elizabeth Eberle [2], Marcia Tolley [2], Dominic L. Li [3] and Kelly L. Knopp [3]

[1] Lilly Research Centre, Eli Lilly and Company Ltd., Erl Wood Manor, Windlesham, Surrey GU20 6PH, UK; mogg_adrian@lilly.com

[2] Covance Greenfield Laboratories, Greenfield, Indianapolis, IN 46140, USA; eberle_elizabeth_lutz@network.lilly.com (E.E.); tolley_marcia_k@network.lilly.com (M.T.)

[3] Lilly Research Laboratories, Eli Lilly and Company Inc., Indianapolis, IN 46285, USA; dominic.li5702@gmail.com (D.L.L.); knopp_kelly_l@lilly.com (K.L.K.)

* Correspondance: broad_lisa@lilly.com; Tel.: +44-1276-483-016

Academic Editors: Arpad Szallasi and Susan M. Huang
Received: 1 July 2016; Accepted: 31 August 2016; Published: 9 September 2016

Abstract: Transient receptor potential vanilloid 3 (TRPV3) is a member of the TRP (Transient Receptor Potential) super-family. It is a relatively underexplored member of the thermo-TRP sub-family (Figure 1), however, genetic mutations and use of gene knock-outs and selective pharmacological tools are helping to provide insights into its role and therapeutic potential. TRPV3 is highly expressed in skin, where it is implicated in skin physiology and pathophysiology, thermo-sensing and nociception. Gain of function TRPV3 mutations in rodent and man have enabled the role of TRPV3 in skin health and disease to be particularly well defined. Pre-clinical studies provide some rationale to support development of TRPV3 antagonists for therapeutic application for the treatment of inflammatory skin conditions, itch and pain. However, to date, only one compound directed towards block of the TRPV3 receptor (GRC15300) has progressed into clinical trials. Currently, there are no known clinical trials in progress employing a TRPV3 antagonist.

Keywords: TRPV3; keratinocytes; itch; pain; Olmsted syndrome

1. Introduction

TRPV3 is a non-selective cation channel, displaying relatively high permeability to calcium. It was first cloned in 2002 and displays ~30%–40% sequence homology with other TRPV channels.

Other features in common include the predicted protein structure encompassing six transmembrane spanning domains (1–6), a pore-forming loop between domains 5–6, cytoplasmic amino and carboxyl termini, ankyrin repeats and coiled-coil domains at the amino terminus and several putative phosphorylation sites [1–3] (see Figure 2). The channel is formed from four subunits, with homo-tetrameric TRPV3 receptors being commonly studied. Hetero-tetrameric channels containing TRPV3 and TRPV1, for example, are reported to be able to form by some [3–5], but not all researchers [6]; however, the nature, role and expression of native TRPV3 containing heteromers is far from clear.

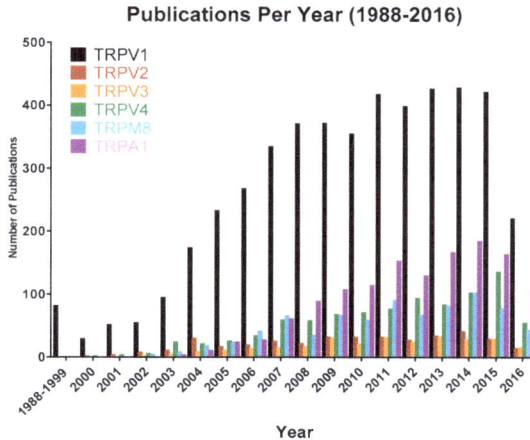

Figure 1. Total publications per year around TRPV3 (orange bars) relative to other thermo-TRPs (TRPV1, TRPV2, TRPV4, TRPM8 and TRPA1). Data as of 25/05/2016. Searches were conducted using PubMed and, where applicable, included alternative nomenclature (e.g., TRPV1 and VR1).

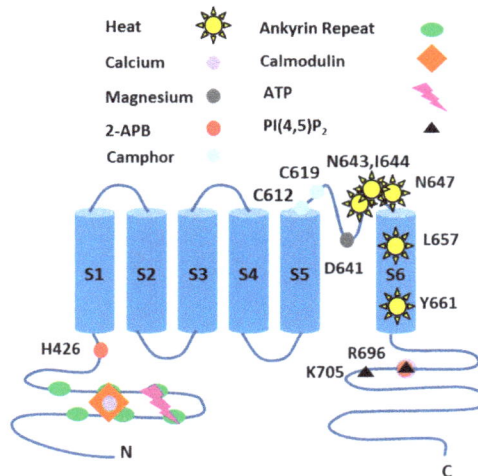

Figure 2. Membrane topology of TRPV3. Residues involved in heat activation (N643, I644, N647, L658 and Y661), activation by 2-APB (H426 and R696), Camphor (C612 and C619) and modulation by phosphatidylinositol 4,5-bisphosphate (PI(4,5)P_2; R696 and K705), ATP (K169 and K174), Mg^{2+} (D641) and Ca^{2+} (R696) are highlighted, in addition to the location of ankyrin repeats [7–13].

In common with other TRP channels, TRPV3 acts as a polymodal signal integrator. It is activated by numerous physical and chemical modulators and by posttranslational modifications, and the impact of individual stimuli is influenced by the presence of other stimuli (see Figure 3 for summary). TRPV3 is activated by innocuous temperature, with the threshold for channel opening at 31–39 °C, and activity is retained over temperatures extending into the noxious range [14]. Chemical agonists include spice extracts (such as camphor and carvacrol), synthetic agents (including 2-aminoethoxy diphenylborate, 2-APB) and endogenous ligand farnesyl pyrophosphate (FPP), [1–3,15,16]. Repeated exposure to heat or chemical agonists leads to sensitization of the receptor [8,17], through hysteresis of gating [14], while co-application of diverse stimuli, such as heat and chemical agonists, is synergistic [17,18]. Activation of G_q coupled GPCRs also sensitizes TRPV3 [19], with key components in the downstream signalling cascade including protein kinase C [20], Ca^{2+}-calmodulin [8,10], phosphatidylinositol 4,5-bisphosphate (PI(4,5)P$_2$) [11] and unsaturated fatty acids [18,20]. Other modulators include voltage [11], ATP [10], Mg^{2+} [12], and intracellular acidification [21,22].

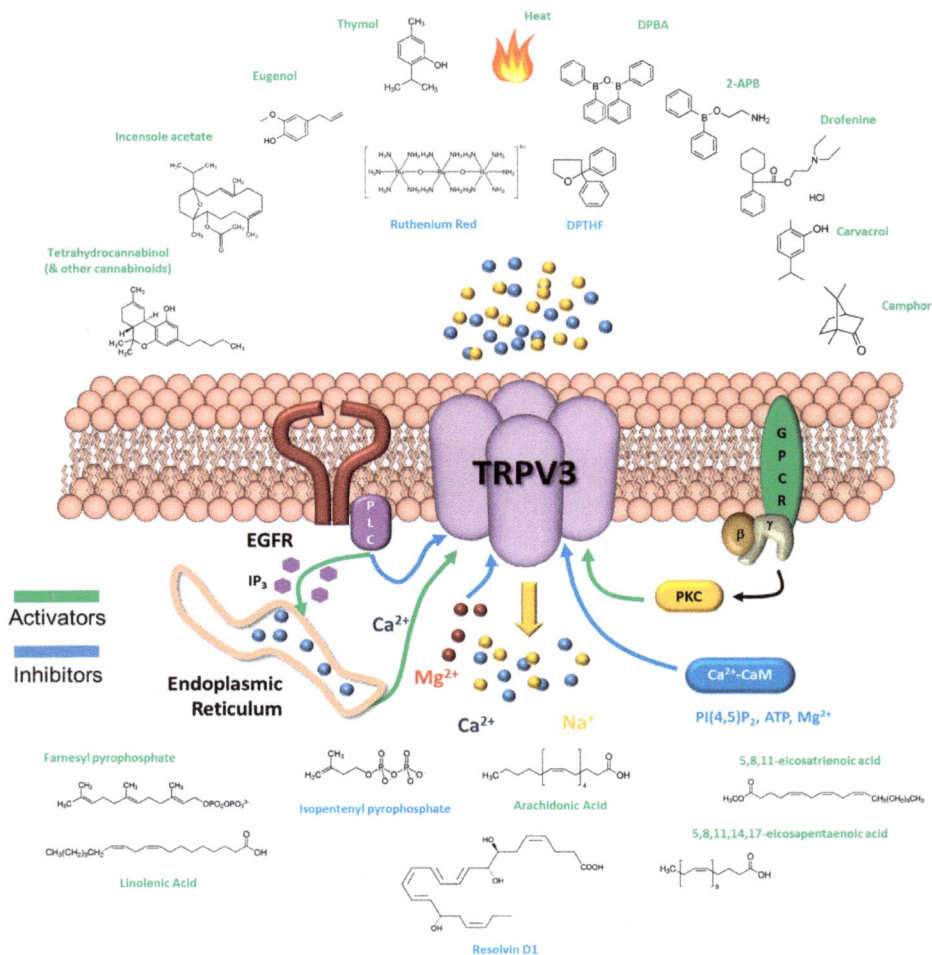

Figure 3. Activators, inhibitors and modulators of TRPV3. Quaternary structure of TRPV3 with compounds and signalling pathways known to activate, inhibit or modulate the receptor. See Introduction for references–additional references [23–26].

The amino acid residues and regions underlying activation of TRPV3 by a number of stimuli have been mapped. Information relating to the mechanism of activation by heat [14,27,28], 2-APB [9] and camphor [13] is available. Likewise, residues involved in mediating modulation by Ca^{2+}/Ca^{2+}-calmodulin; [8,10]; Mg^{2+} [12]; pH [21] and voltage [11] have been defined (Figure 2, see Yang and Zhu for recent detailed review [29]).

2. Expression and Function of TRPV3

In contrast to TRPV1, TRPA1 and TRPM8, a direct role for TRPV3 in the peripheral nervous system is controversial, as expression in sensory neurons is not conserved across species, with minimal detection in rodents [1–3,30]. TRPV3 is however expressed in skin keratinocytes (Figure 4) across species [1,2,31] and in humans, TRPV3 gene expression in skin is the highest of the >50 tissues profiled in the GTEx project [32] (Supplementary Figure S1). TRPV3 expression is also reported in other epithelial cells including oral and nasal epithelium [19,33], distal colon [34] and cornea [35]. In oral epithelia, use of TRPV3 knock mice implicate this channel in wound healing [33]. Likewise, although TRPV3 gene expression in brain overall appears to be very low (Supplementary Figure S1), studies utilising TRPV3 knock-out mice are suggestive of a role for TRPV3 in regulating hippocampal synaptic plasticity [36] and incensole acetate, a reported TRPV3 agonist, broadly modulated brain activity in wild-type, but not TRPV3 knock-out mice [37]. Interestingly, there are several reports detailing TRPV1 channel expression on the endoplasmic reticulum of dorsal root ganglia and sarcoplasmic reticulum of skeletal muscle cells [38,39]. Indeed, it has recently been reported that there is functional expression of TRPV3 on the ER of mouse embryonic stem cells, with the channel having a putative role in controlling cell cycle and cellular proliferation [40]. These novel findings, if confirmed in native adult tissues, may need to be taken into account when developing compounds for TRPV3.

Until recently, reliance on non-selective agonist and antagonist tools, such as Ruthenium Red, has hampered progress in clearly defining a functional role for native TRPV3. For example, evidence for a role of TRPV3 in modulating the CNS dopaminergic system [41,42] and colonic [34] and corneal epithelia responses [35] is largely circumstantial for this very reason. Perhaps unsurprisingly, keratinocytes have been the most commonly utilized preparation for the study of native TRPV3 function by far, and provide the most compelling data package. Early studies in m308 keratinocytes identified whole cell currents, increases in intracellular calcium and release of IL-1α in response to application or co-application of known TRPV3 agonists and modulators, including eugenol, DPBA, camphor, 2-APB and arachidonic acid [19,20]. This work was later extended by Grubisha et al. (2014) [18], who confirmed that these responses could be blocked by a selective TRPV3 antagonist and by shRNA knock-down of TRPV3. In primary cultures of keratinocytes from wild-type mice, whole cell currents, increases in intracellular calcium or production of nitric-oxide were observed in response to TRPV3 agonists, or agonist combinations, including heat, 2-APB, carvacrol and camphor, these responses were sensitized on repeat application [12,17,43–46] and were absent in TRPV3 knock-out mice [17,45,46]. In transgenic mice over-expressing TRPV3 in skin keratinocytes, co-application of heat and 2-APB led to augmented TRPV3 mediated PGE$_2$ release from keratinocytes [30]. In addition, application of 2-APB and carvacrol has been shown to promote TGF-α release from primary cultures of human keratinocytes [45], and in human keratinocyte HaCaT cells, 2-APB and acidic pH promoted whole cell currents blocked by Ruthenium Red [21].

Studies using keratinocytes have provided several insights for how TRPV3 regulates skin function and the function of neighbouring cells (Figure 4). A key protein interaction partner appears to be the epidermal growth factor receptor (EGFR). This receptor is proposed to form a signalling complex with TRPV3, whereby activation of the EGFR results in increased TRPV3 channel activity, stimulation of TGF-α release and epidermal homeostasis [45]. TRPV3 plays a role in maintenance of the skin barrier, as deletion of TRPV3 evokes deleterious changes in epidermal barrier structure. Hair morphogenesis is also disrupted in TRPV3 null mice [17,45]. In cultures of human outer root sheath keratinocytes, activation of TRPV3 induced membrane currents, elevated intracellular calcium, inhibited proliferation, induced apoptosis, inhibited hair shaft elongation and promoted premature hair follicle regression. These cellular effects, including inhibition of hair growth, were blocked by siRNA mediated TRPV3 knock-down [47]. α-Hydroxyl acids, commonly used in the cosmetic industry in chemical peels to promote exfoliation, have also been proposed to exert their effects through activation of keratinocyte TRPV3 [21]. Once again, the suggested mechanism is calcium influx through keratinocyte TRPV3 channels, leading to overload in intracellular calcium and cell death [21]. Of relevance to pain, TRPV3 mediated ATP release from keratinocytes has been shown to activate purinoceptors in dorsal root ganglion neurons [48], thereby influencing nociceptive function. Consistent with this, in transgenic mice over-expressing TRPV3 in skin keratinocytes, increased pain sensitivity was observed [30]. A number of related findings demonstrate that indirect modulation by keratinocytes can strongly influence pain signalling, for example in a recent study in TRPV1-knockout mice selectively expressing TRPV1 in keratinocytes, keratinocyte stimulation was sufficient to evoke acute nociception-related responses [49] and keratinocytes are also reported to induce neuronal excitability after nerve injury [50]. Of note, however, although TRPV3 null mice show disrupted responses to acute noxious heat and innocuous thermal sensation in thermotaxis endpoints [17], responses in other types of pain models are largely unaltered. In addition, the role of TRPV3 in innocuous temperature perception and acute thermal nociception appears to be somewhat dependent on gender and genetic background [46,51], for recent review, see Reference [52].

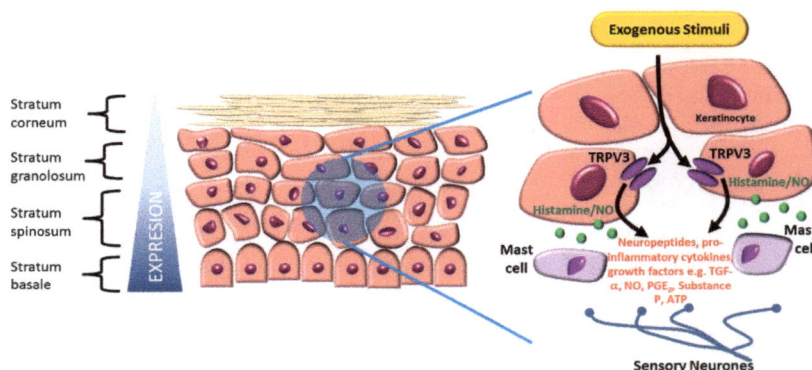

Figure 4. Summary of TRPV3 expression and function in epidermal keratinocytes. TRPV3 protein has been found throughout the epidermis and around hair follicles, with protein elevated under certain inflammatory skin conditions.

Several studies have reported alterations in TRPV3 mRNA and/or protein expression in pathological states, including in the skin of burns victims [53]; in rosacea, a chronic inflammatory skin condition [54]; in psoriasis [55] and in breast tissue biopsies from patients with breast pain [56]. Of note, aberrant TRPV3 function might be anticipated in some pathological states. For example, arachidonic acid, which is a strong potentiator of keratinocyte TRPV3, is present at high concentrations in psoriatic dermatitis (>100 µM; [57]) indicating that TRPV3 activity may be potentiated in psoriatic epidermis. Interestingly, a recent preliminary report describes a mechanistic link between TRPV3 activity in psoriasis through IL-1α and EGFR signalling [55].

3. Insights from Genetic Mutations

Adding further support to the role of TRPV3 in skin physiology and pathology, a TRPV3 gain-of-function G573S/C mutation was identified to underlie the spontaneously hairless, dermatitis phenotype of two rodent strains, DS-Nh mice and WBN/kob-HT rats, used as animal models of atopy [31,58,59]. Development of a TRPV3Gly573Ser transgenic mouse, recapitulated this phenotype, with significantly increased scratching behavior [58]. These transgenic mice also displayed augmented release of NGF in response to heat and significantly increased levels of serum chemokines and interleukins [58]. The increased release of pro-inflammatory and pro-nociceptive factors might be hypothesized to alter nociception, however data from exploration of the pain phenotype of TRPV3 gain-of-function rodents is only just emerging [60].

More recently, similar gain-of-function mutations in TRPV3, including but not limited to the Gly573 mutation, have been identified as the cause of Olmsted syndrome (OS) in humans (for review see [61]). OS is a rare keratinizing disorder characterized by marked thickening of the skin on the soles of the feet and palms of the hands, periorificial keratotic plaques, diffuse alopecia, and pruritus. In a few cases, atypical OS is reported with erythromelalgia. Pain and itching are variable in OS but are reported to be particularly severe in atypical OS patients with erythromelalgia, which leads to acute flares of hyperalgesia and some features of neuropathic pain.

4. TRPV3 Indications

Whilst activation of keratinocyte TRPV3 has been shown to mediate the release of pro-inflammatory and pro-nociceptive mediators and pruritogens, and the gain-of-function mutations implicate TRPV3 in skin conditions where a predominant feature is itch [62], there is a surprising lack of preclinical in vivo data exploring this aspect.

Selective TRPV3 antagonists have recently been introduced by Hydra Biosciences, Glenmark Pharmaceuticals and AbbVie (Section 5), and afford the opportunity to investigate the therapeutic potential of blockade of the TRPV3 channel.

We previously reported that Hydra's FTP-THQ (Figure 5) was a potent and selective in vitro antagonist of recombinant and native TRPV3 receptors, having virtually no activity at TRPV1, TRPV4, TRPM8 and TRPA1 [18]. We have now assessed FTP-THQ in vitro in m308 keratinocytes and confirmed that it can prevent release of ATP and GM-CSF by concentrations of DPBA and 2-APB that are known to selectively activate TRPV3 in these cells ([18]; Figure 6).

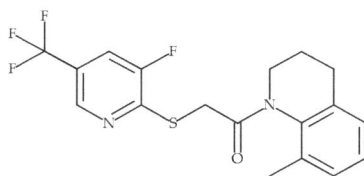

Figure 5. Structure of TRPV3 selective antagonist FTP-THQ [63].

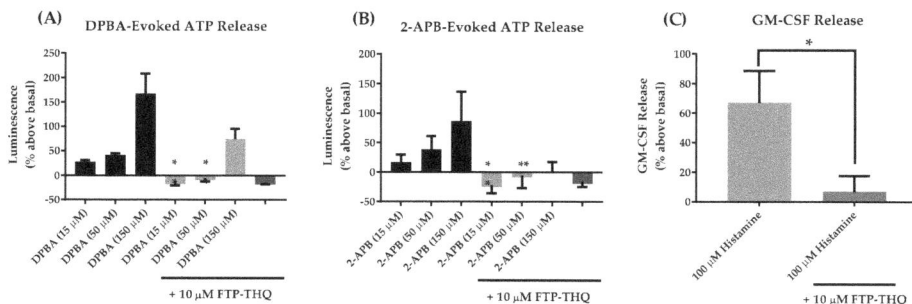

Figure 6. FTP-THQ [1-([3-fluoro-5-(trifluoromethyl)pyridine-2-yl]sulfanylacetyl)-8-methyl-1,2,3,4-tetrahydroquinoline], a potent and selective TRPV3 receptor antagonist blocked TRPV3 mediated release of ATP (**A** & **B**) and GM-CSF (**C**) from mouse keratinocytes in vitro. Results are mean ± SEM of 3 independent experiments. Statistical significance was assessed using the paired Student's *t*-test, * $p < 0.05$, ** $p < 0.001$.

FTP-THQ also has appropriate pharmacokinetic properties to assess its profile in vivo with an in vitro IC_{50} of 117 nM at the rat recombinant receptor and 186 nM at the mouse native receptor [18], and a Brain/Plasma ratio of approximately 7. In mice, after intraperitoneal administration, it dose-dependently blocked histamine-induced itch (Figure 7) with unbound exposure in brain (152 nM) consistent with the in vitro potency value, while the plasma levels where significantly less (37 nM). These data suggest TRPV3 can be pharmacologically modulated in a manner that is consistent with the gain-of-function mutations described in Table 1.

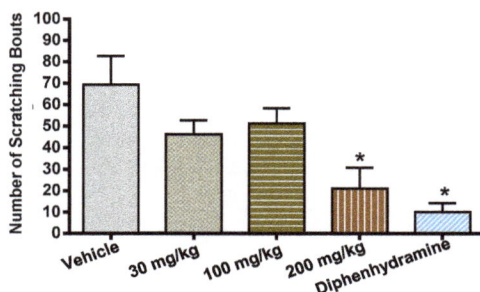

Figure 7. Effects of FTP-THQ on histamine-induced scratching behavior. Harlan CD-1 mice (n = 7–8/treatment group), 4–5 weeks old were acclimated to testing room for 1 h. FTP-THQ was administered at 30, 100, or 200 mg/kg i.p., 1 h prior to histamine, while diphenhyramine was administered at 20 mg/kg, 30 min prior to histamine. Animals were then placed inside a clear plexiglass chamber and the number of scratching bouts was scored for 20 min. Data were collected via Abacus software; one-way ANOVA with post-hoc Dunnett's was used for analysis. * p < 0.05 vs. vehicle control.

From the pain perspective, the genetic data are less compelling, but small molecule manipulation of the receptor with multiple compounds is suggestive of a role in nociceptive processing. For recent reviews, see References [64–66]. The TRPV3 agonist FPP is reported to elicit pain behaviors after intraplantar injection into inflamed animals [16]. The same group has also reported that 17(R)-resolvin D, an endogenous TRPV3 antagonist, is anti-nociceptive in acute and inflammatory pain states [24]. Complementarily, tool antagonist molecules from Hydra, Glenmark and AbbVie described below have attenuated pain behaviors in a number of pre-clinical pain models, including primarily carrageenan and Complete Freund's Adjuvant-induced thermal and/or tactile hypersensitivity, but also in nerve ligation models [63,67,68].

We also evaluated FTP-THQ in a number of pre-clinical pain behavior models and replicated the previous findings in CFA-induced thermal hypersensitivity at the 200 mg/kg dose, and as exemplified in Figure 8, observed effects in the formalin-induced nocifensive responding assay. Interestingly, effects in this assay were observed at lower plasma/brain exposures. Confounding side effects, such as alterations in locomotor activity, were not observed, however, unlike previous reports (see [65]) we did observe a dose-dependent hypothermia with the antagonist. The thermo-sensing TRP channels have collectively been implicated as having the potential to alter normal thermal sensation and temperature regulation, due to findings with TRPV1 antagonists. Our data would suggest, at least in rodents, an alteration in body temperature should be closely monitored. It is unknown if these effects would translate into higher species. Taken together, the collective data indicate that potent and selective TRPV3 antagonists effectively attenuate scratching and pain behavior in pre-clinical animal models, and pharmacological blockade of this target may afford some therapeutic benefit.

By way of summary, Table 1 provides the potential therapeutic utility of TRPV3 modulators. However, as mentioned previously, no current clinical trials are ongoing.

Table 1. Summary of Physiological and Pathophysiological roles of TRPV3.

Potential Roles	Summary of Evidence	Reference(s)
Olmsted Syndrome	Several independent clinical reports identify mutations in the TRPV3 gene as a cause of gain-of-function mutations and recessive Olmsted's Syndrome. Characteristic features include palmoplantar keratoderma, periorificial hyperkeratotic lesions and alopecia. Less common presentations include digit constriction, onychodystrophy and pruritus	[66,69–73]
Olmsted Syndrome with Erythromelalgia	Clinical data of three patients whose disease presentation included intense flares of inflammation, itching, burning pain, vasodilatation, and redness of the extremities consistent with erythromelalgia. Whole exome sequencing identified a de novo heterozygous missense mutation within TRPV3, p.Leu673Phe.	[74,75]
Pruitic and Atopic Dermatitis	Clinical data suggest TRPV3 expression is increased in lesional skin in patients with atopic dermatitis. Preclinical data suggest DS-Nh mice develop allergic and pruitic dermatitis	[58,76]
Psoriasis	Clinical data suggest TRPV3 expression is significantly increased in psoriatic lesions, and that these channels are functional in keratinocytes isolated from lesioned skin. A novel antagonist of TRPV3 dose-dependently inhibited 2APB/carvacrol induced IL–1α release keratinocytes. Similarly, inhibition of EGFR signaling was observed with the antagonist. Inhibitors of both IL–1α release and EGFR signaling have previously attenuated psoriatic symptoms and thus a linkage with TRPV3 is suggested	[55]
Wound Healing	Pre-clinical data suggest higher expression of TRPV3 in mouse oral epithelia versus skin, and expression was upregulated in wounded oral epithelial tissue. TRPV3 activation promoted oral epithelial cell proliferation, which was diminished in TRPV3 knockout mice. Subsequent knock out profiling in a molar tooth extraction model suggest oral wound closure was delayed	[33]
Burn/Post-burn pruritus	Clinical data suggest increased TRPV3 expression in the epidermis of burn scars with pruritus	[29,53]
Hair growth	Pre-clinical data suggest TRPV3 agonists eugenol and 2-aminoethoxydiphenyl borate inhibited hair shaft elongation, suppressed proliferation, and induced apoptosis in human organ-cultured hair follicles. Similarly, functional effects of TRPV3 activation in human ORS keratinocytes were demonstrated as on-target via siRNA	[47]
Skin Barrier Formation	Pre-clinical data suggest TRPV3 forms a direct complex with transglutaminases, thereby regulating growth factor signaling for the formation of the skin barrier	[45]
Rosacea	Clinical data suggest increased TRPV3 expression in epidermal keratinocytes, and dermal labeling was observed in a subset of immune cells and fibroblasts in erythematotelangiectatic rosacea and phymatous rosacea-affected skin. Increased gene expression was also observed in patients with phymatous rosacea	[54]
Cerebral Ischemia	Pre-clinical data suggest the TRPV3 agonist incensole acetate protects against ischemic neuronal damage and reperfusion injury in mice. Reduced infarct volumes, inhibition of TNF-α, IL-1β and TGF-β expression, and NF-κB activation were demonstrated as on-target using TRPV3 knock-out mice	[77,78]
Mastalgia	Clinical data suggest increased expression of TRPV3 in basal keratinocytes that correlated with disease score	[56]
Traumatic Peripheral Nerve Injury	Clinical data suggest increased TRPV3 expression in the DRG neurons of patients with DRG avulsion injury, in the peripheral nerve proximal to the site of brachial plexus injury. However, a decrease in TRPV3 expression was observed in the skin of patients with diabetic neuropathy	[3,79]
Cold - and Heat-evoked Pain	Pre-clinical data showed TRPV3 knockout mice have impaired responses to noxious heat. WBN/Kob-Ht rats, which have a TRPV3 gain-of-function mutation, showed an increased sensitivity to noxious heat and cold stimuli. Multiple antagonists have shown efficacy in inflammatory insult-induced hypersensitivity and nerve ligation-induced hypersensitivity	[45,60,64,65]

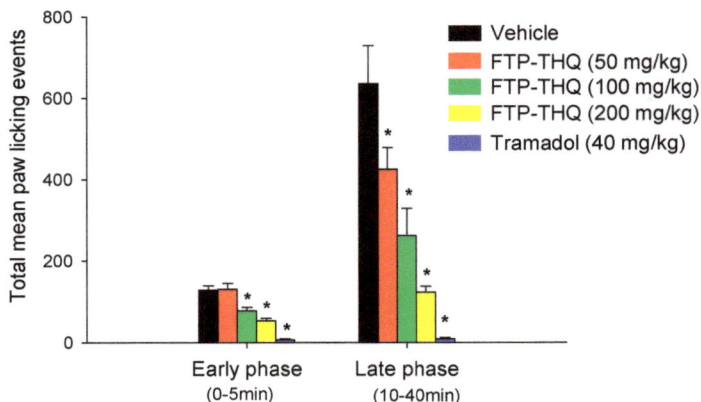

Figure 8. Effects of FTP-THQ on formalin-induced nocifensive behavior. Harlan Sprague Dawley Rats (n = 7–8/treatment group), were acclimated to the testing room for 1 h. FTP-THQ was administered at 50, 100, or 200 mg/kg i.p. 15 min prior to formalin, while the positive control tramadol was administered at 40 mg/kg i.p. 30 min prior to formalin. The animals were placed in Startle Behavior Chambers and behavior events (licking, guarding, flinching) binned in 5-min intervals and plotted as Early and Late Phase. Data were analyzed using 1-way ANOVA, and comparisons of drug treatment groups were compared with control groups using a post-hoc Dunnett's comparison. * $p < 0.05$ vs. vehicle control.

5. TRPV3 Drug Development Overview

Major milestones in the area of TRPV3 drug development are highlighted in Figure 9 and in comparison to TRPV1, the number of patents describing TRPV3 modulators has been modest (Figure 10) with Hydra Biosciences and Glenmark Pharmaceuticals being the main players.

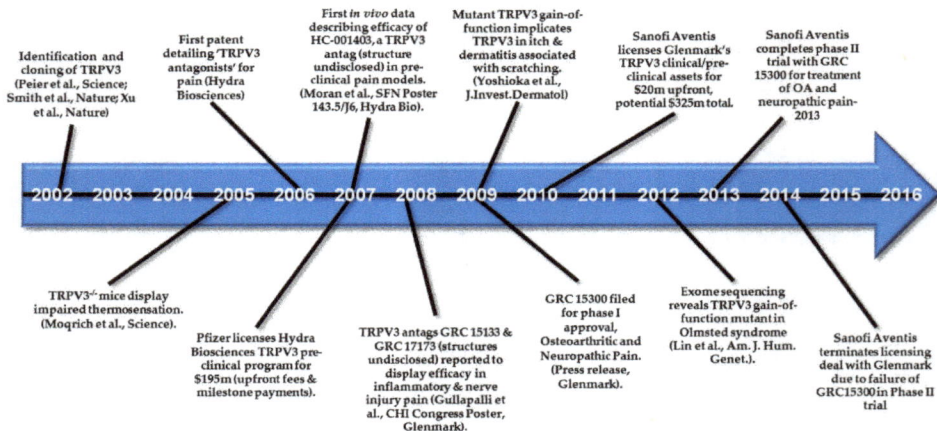

Figure 9. Timeline of major TRPV3 development activities.

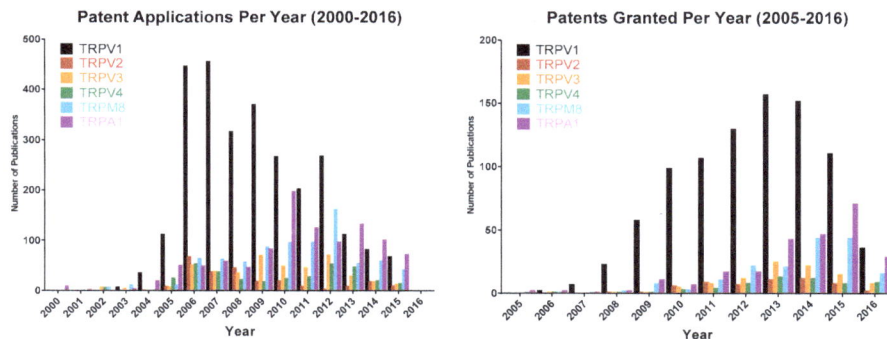

Figure 10. Number of patents applied for and granted per year for each of the thermo-TRPs compared to TRPV3 (orange bars).

5.1. Glenmark Pharmaceuticals Ltd.

Glenmark have patented a range of TRPV3 antagonists [80–84], Figure 11. In 2010, Glenmark entered into an out-licensing agreement with Sanofi Aventis and subsequently progressed their lead molecule (GRC15300, structure unknown) into the clinic for the treatment of osteoarthritic and neuropathic pain. In 2012, GRC15300 entered into Phase II trials for treatment of neuropathic pain; however, by the end of 2013, these trials had been discontinued. The Sanofi-Glenmark agreement was terminated in 2014 and since that date, no further development has been reported.

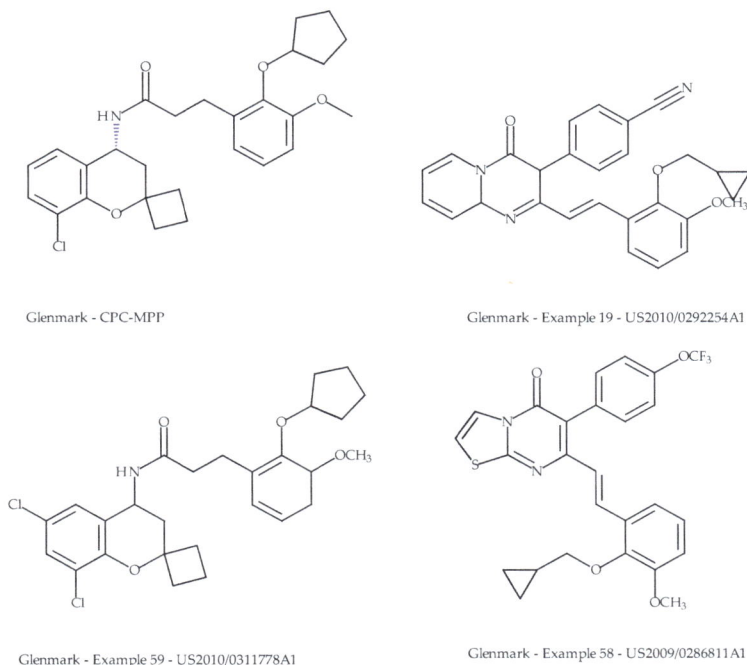

Glenmark - CPC-MPP

Glenmark - Example 19 - US2010/0292254A1

Glenmark - Example 59 - US2010/0311778A1

Glenmark - Example 58 - US2009/0286811A1

Figure 11. Examples of patented TRPV3 antagonists from Glenmark Pharmaceuticals.

5.2. Hydra Biosciences Inc.

Hydra Biosciences have also published several patents and publications on TRPV3 antagonists. In 2007, they entered into a collaboration with Pfizer to develop TRPV3 antagonists for pain. The company web page currently reports an active TRPV3 program directed toward dermatological disorders. In the published patents, there are descriptions of two compounds (Compound 15 and Compound 64 in Reference [68]; Figure 12). Compounds were described as having modest potency (<1 µM) in vitro and were shown to be effective in models of thermal injury, the formalin model, Carrageenan, and CFA. An additional patent [63] discloses FTP-THQ that we have assessed above in a number of in vitro and in vivo assays (Figures 6–8).

5.3. Abbvie Inc.

In recent years, AbbVie have been active in the TRPV3 arena, publishing several patents [85,86] and more recently a paper [67]. They describe a series of compounds, some displaying mid-nanomolar potency in blocking 2-APB-stimulated calcium influx in assays using recombinant human and mouse TRPV3 channels. Their recent publication describes synthesis and biological properties of a series of (Pyridin-2-yl)methanol derivatives, with the lead molecule (Figure 13) having modest in vitro potency (Kb = 0.56 µM) and efficacy in rat models of neuropathic pain (CCI and SNL).

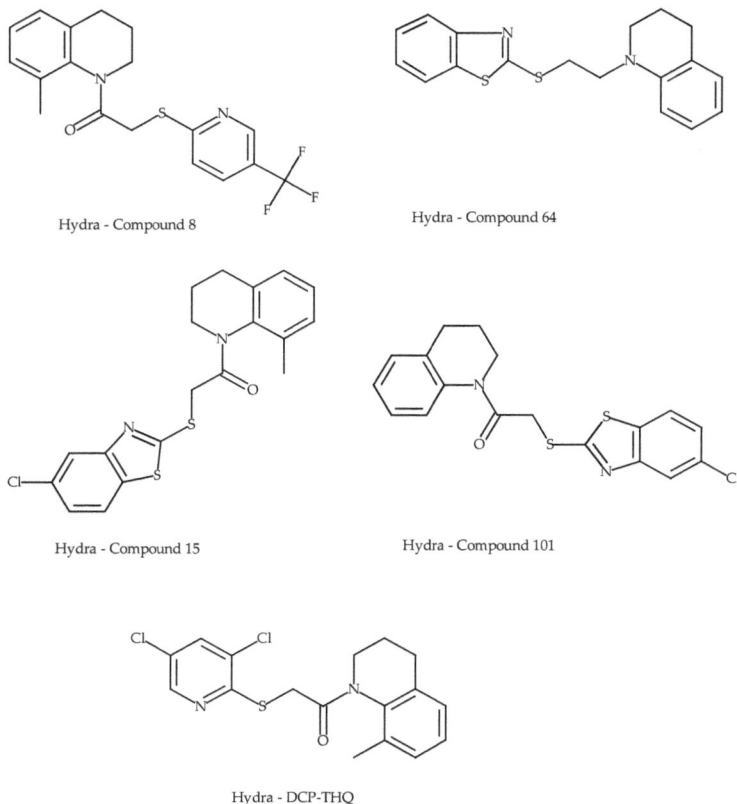

Hydra - Compound 8

Hydra - Compound 64

Hydra - Compound 15

Hydra - Compound 101

Hydra - DCP-THQ

Figure 12. Representatives from Hydra Biosciences patented TRPV3 antagonist series.

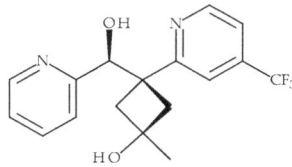

Abbvie - Compound 74a

Figure 13. A leading representative from Abbvie's TRPV3 antagonist series.

5.4. Miscellaneous

Interestingly, there are also several patents detailing the utility of TRPV3 agonists. One describes derivatives of incensole acetate for use as antidepressants [37,87]. Another details TRPV3 agonists for the treatment of TRPV3-associated skin conditions such as acne, psoriasis, dermatitis, and wound healing, and describes the TRPV3 activity of peptides derived from soricidin (a fifty-four amino acid paralytic peptide isolated from the submaxilary saliva gland of the Northern Short-tailed Shrew, *Blanina brevieauda* [88]).

6. Conclusions and Outlook

In summary, we are making headway in understanding the role of TRPV3 in health and disease and this appears to be a promising therapeutic target for itch and skin-related conditions and for the treatment of patients with TRPV3 causally related conditions, such as Olmsted syndrome. To date information from gain of function mutations in rodent and man, coupled with data from gene knock out studies do not provide an overwhelmingly compelling case for targeting TRPV3 as a pain therapeutic; however, pre-clinical data utilizing structurally diverse TRPV3 antagonists do provide some support that blockade of this channel may provide analgesia in chronic pain states. Questions remain however as to how much clinical efficacy for pain can be realized through selectively targeting this mechanism and how results from rodents will translate to humans given the differences in expression in the pain pathway. Given the issues with the side effects associated with targeting other TRP family members, such as TRPV1, including body temperature changes and altered thermal sensitivity, there may be an opportunity to develop topical treatments for TRPV3 given the compelling role in skin.

Supplementary Materials: The following are available online at http://www.mdpi.com/1424-8247/9/3/55/s1, Figure S1: The data used for the analyses described in this manuscript were obtained from: the GTEx Portal on 25 May 2016.

Acknowledgments: We thank Jeff Kennedy for scientific input and Jeff Kennedy and Denise Morrow for early studies evaluating the in vivo efficacy of FTP-THQ in preventing itch related behaviors. We thank Brian Spegal for the body temperature studies conducted with FTP-THQ, Jeff Cramer for pharmacokinetic studies on FTP-THQ and Rosa Simmons for technical assistance with the figures and legends. We thank David Collier and Cara Lee Ann Ruble for inputs relating to the expression profile of TRPV3.

Conflicts of Interest: The authors declare no conflict of interest.

References

1. Peier, A.M.; Reeve, A.J.; Andersson, D.A.; Moqrich, A.; Earley, T.J.; Hergarden, A.C.; Story, G.M.; Colley, S.; Hogenesch, J.B.; McIntyre, P.; et al. A heat-sensitive TRP channel expressed in keratinocytes. *Science* **2002**, *296*, 2046–2049. [CrossRef] [PubMed]
2. Xu, H.; Ramsey, I.S.; Kotecha, S.A.; Moran, M.M.; Chong, J.A.; Lawson, D.; Ge, P.; Lilly, J.; Silos-Santiago, I.; Xie, Y.; et al. TRPV3 is a calcium-permeable temperature-sensitive cation channel. *Nature* **2002**, *418*, 181–186. [CrossRef] [PubMed]

3. Smith, G.D.; Gunthorpe, M.J.; Kelsell, R.E.; Hayes, P.D.; Reilly, P.; Facer, P.; Wright, J.E.; Jerman, J.C.; Walhin, J.-P.; Ooi, L.; et al. TRPV3 is a temperature-sensitive vanilloid receptor-like protein. *Nature* **2002**, *418*, 186–190. [CrossRef] [PubMed]
4. Cheng, W.; Yang, F.; Takanishi, C.L.; Zheng, J. Thermosensitive TRPV channel subunits coassemble into heteromeric channels with intermediate conductance and gating properties. *J. Gen. Physiol.* **2007**, *129*, 16. [CrossRef] [PubMed]
5. Cheng, W.; Yang, F.; Liu, S.; Colton, C.K.; Wang, C.; Cui, Y.; Cao, X.; Zhu, M.X.; Sun, C.; Wang, K.; et al. Heteromeric heat-sensitive transient receptor potential channels exhibit distinct temperature and chemical response. *J. Biol. Chem.* **2012**, *287*, 7279–7288. [CrossRef] [PubMed]
6. Hellwig, N.; Albrecht, N.; Harteneck, C.; Gunter, S.; Schaefer, M. Homo- and heteromeric assembly of TRP channel subunits. *J. Cell. Sci.* **2005**, *118*, 917–928. [CrossRef] [PubMed]
7. Grandl, J.; Hu, H.; Bandell, M.; Bursulaya, B.; Schmidt, M.; Petrus, M.; Patapoutian, A. Pore region of TRPV3 ion channel is specifically required for heat activation. *Nat. Neurosci.* **2008**, *11*, 1007–1013. [CrossRef] [PubMed]
8. Xiao, R.; Tang, J.; Wang, C.; Colton, C.K.; Tian, J.; Zhu, M.X. Calcium plays a central role in the sensitization of TRPV3 channel to repetitive stimulations. *J. Biol. Chem.* **2008**, *283*, 6162–6174. [CrossRef] [PubMed]
9. Hu, H.; Grandl, J.; Bandell, M.; Petrus, M.; Patapoutian, A. Two amino acid residues determine 2-APB sensitivity of the ion channels TRPV3 and TRPV4. *Proc. Natl. Acad. Sci. USA* **2009**, *106*, 1626–1631. [CrossRef] [PubMed]
10. Phelps, C.B.; Wang, R.R.; Choo, S.S.; Gaudet, R. Differential regulation of TRPV1, TRPV3, and TRPV4 sensitivity through a conserved binding site on the ankyrin repeat domain. *J. Biol. Chem.* **2010**, *285*, 731–740. [CrossRef] [PubMed]
11. Doerner, J.F.; Hatt, H.; Ramsey, I.S. Voltage- and temperature-dependent activation of TRPV3 channels is potentiated by receptor-mediated PI(4,5)P2 hydrolysis. *J. Gen. Physiol.* **2011**, *137*, 271–288. [CrossRef] [PubMed]
12. Luo, J.; Stewart, R.; Berdeaux, R.; Hu, H. Tonic inhibition of TRPV3 by Mg^{2+} in mouse epidermal keratinocytes. *J. Investig. Dermatol.* **2012**, *132*, 2158–2165. [CrossRef] [PubMed]
13. Sherkheli, M.A.; Vogt-Eisele, A.K.; Weber, K.; Hatt, H. Camphor modulates TRPV3 cation channels activity by interacting with critical pore-region cysteine residues. *Pak. J. Pharm. Sci.* **2013**, *26*, 431–438. [PubMed]
14. Liu, B.; Yao, J.; Zhu, M.X.; Qin, F. Hysteresis of gating underlines sensitization of TRPV3 channels. *J. Gen. Physiol.* **2011**, *138*, 509–520. [CrossRef] [PubMed]
15. Vogt-Eisele, A.K.; Weber, K.; Sherkheli, M.A.; Vielhaber, G.; Panten, J.; Gisselmann, G.; Hatt, H. Monoterpenoid agonists of TRPV3. *Br. J. Pharmacol.* **2007**, *151*, 530–540. [CrossRef] [PubMed]
16. Bang, S.; Yoo, S.; Yang, T.-J.; Cho, H.; Hwang, S.W. Farnesyl pyrophosphate is a novel pain-producing molecule via specific activation of TRPV3. *J. Biol. Chem.* **2010**, *285*, 19362–19371. [CrossRef] [PubMed]
17. Moqrich, A.; Hwang, S.W.; Earley, T.J.; Petrus, M.J.; Murray, A.N.; Spencer, K.S.R.; Andahazy, M.; Story, G.M.; Patapoutian, A. Impaired thermosensation in mice lacking TRPV3, a heat and camphor sensor in the skin. *Science* **2005**, *307*, 1468–1472. [CrossRef] [PubMed]
18. Grubisha, O.; Mogg, A.J.; Sorge, J.L.; Ball, L.-J.; Sanger, H.; Ruble, C.L.A.; Folly, E.A.; Ursu, D.; Broad, L.M. Pharmacological profiling of the TRPV3 channel in recombinant and native assays. *Br. J. Pharmacol.* **2014**, *171*, 2631–2644. [CrossRef] [PubMed]
19. Xu, H.; Delling, M.; Jun, J.C.; Clapham, D.E. Oregano, thyme and clove-derived flavors and skin sensitizers activate specific TRP channels. *Nat. Neurosci.* **2006**, *9*, 628–635. [CrossRef] [PubMed]
20. Hu, H.-Z.; Xiao, R.; Wang, C.; Gao, N.; Colton, C.K.; Wood, J.D.; Zhu, M.X. Potentiation of TRPV3 channel function by unsaturated fatty acids. *J. Cell. Physiol.* **2006**, *208*, 201–212. [CrossRef] [PubMed]
21. Cao, X.; Yang, F.; Zheng, J.; Wang, K. Intracellular proton-mediated activation of TRPV3 channels accounts for the exfoliation effect of alpha-hydroxyl acids on keratinocytes. *J. Biol. Chem.* **2012**, *287*, 25905–25916. [CrossRef] [PubMed]
22. Gao, L.; Yang, P.; Qin, P.; Lu, Y.; Li, X.; Tian, Q.; Li, Y.; Xie, C.; Tian, J.-B.; Zhang, C.; et al. Selective potentiation of 2-APB-induced activation of TRPV1–3 channels by acid. *Sci. Rep.* **2016**, *6*, 20791. [CrossRef] [PubMed]

23. Bang, S.; Yoo, S.; Yang, T.-J.; Cho, H.; Hwang, S.W. Isopentenyl pyrophosphate is a novel antinociceptive substance that inhibits TRPV3 and TRPA1 ion channels. *Pain* **2011**, *152*, 1156–1164. [CrossRef] [PubMed]

24. Bang, S.; Yoo, S.; Yang, T.J.; Cho, H.; Hwang, S.W. 17(R)-resolvin D1 specifically inhibits transient receptor potential ion channel vanilloid 3 leading to peripheral antinociception. *Br. J. Pharmacol.* **2012**, *165*, 683–692. [CrossRef] [PubMed]

25. de Petrocellis, L.; Orlando, P.; Moriello, A.S.; Aviello, G.; Stott, C.; Izzo, A.A.; di Marzo, V. Cannabinoid actions at TRPV channels: Effects on TRPV3 and TRPV4 and their potential relevance to gastrointestinal inflammation. *Acta Physiol.* **2012**, *204*, 255–266. [CrossRef] [PubMed]

26. Chung, M.-K.; Guler, A.D.; Caterina, M.J. Biphasic currents evoked by chemical or thermal activation of the heat-gated ion channel, TRPV3. *J. Biol. Chem.* **2005**, *280*, 15928–15941. [CrossRef] [PubMed]

27. Grandl, J.; Kim, S.E.; Uzzell, V.; Bursulaya, B.; Petrus, M.; Bandell, M.; Patapoutian, A. Temperature-induced opening of TRPV1 ion channel is stabilized by the pore domain. *Nat. Neurosci.* **2010**, *13*, 708–714. [CrossRef] [PubMed]

28. Kim, S.E.; Patapoutian, A.; Grandl, J. Single residues in the outer pore of TRPV1 and TRPV3 have temperature-dependent conformations. *PLoS ONE* **2013**, *8*, e59593. [CrossRef] [PubMed]

29. Yang, P.; Zhu, M.X. TRPV3. *Handb. Exp. Pharmacol.* **2014**, *222*, 273–291. [PubMed]

30. Huang, S.M.; Lee, H.; Chung, M.-K.; Park, U.; Yu, Y.Y.; Bradshaw, H.B.; Coulombe, P.A.; Walker, J.M.; Caterina, M.J. Overexpressed transient receptor potential vanilloid 3 ion channels in skin keratinocytes modulate pain sensitivity via prostaglandin E2. *J. Neurosci.* **2008**, *28*, 13727–13737. [CrossRef] [PubMed]

31. Asakawa, M.; Yoshioka, T.; Matsutani, T.; Hikita, I.; Suzuki, M.; Oshima, I.; Tsukahara, K.; Arimura, A.; Horikawa, T.; Hirasawa, T.; et al. Association of a mutation in TRPV3 with defective hair growth in rodents. *J. Investig. Dermatol.* **2006**, *126*, 2664–2672. [CrossRef] [PubMed]

32. Lonsdale, J.; Thomas, J.; Salvatore, M.; Phillips, R.; Lo, E.; Shad, S.; Hasz, R.; Walters, G.; Garcia, F.; Young, N.; et al. The genotype-tissue expression (GTEx) project. *Nat. Genet.* **2013**, *45*, 580–585. [CrossRef] [PubMed]

33. Aijima, R.; Wang, B.; Takao, T.; Mihara, H.; Kashio, M.; Ohsaki, Y.; Zhang, J.-Q.; Mizuno, A.; Suzuki, M.; Yamashita, Y.; et al. The thermosensitive TRPV3 channel contributes to rapid wound healing in oral epithelia. *FASEB J.* **2015**, *29*, 182–192. [CrossRef] [PubMed]

34. Ueda, T.; Yamada, T.; Ugawa, S.; Ishida, Y.; Shimada, S. TRPV3, a thermosensitive channel is expressed in mouse distal colon epithelium. *Biochem. Biophys. Res. Commun.* **2009**, *383*, 130–134. [CrossRef] [PubMed]

35. Yamada, T.; Ueda, T.; Ugawa, S.; Ishida, Y.; Imayasu, M.; Koyama, S.; Shimada, S. Functional expression of transient receptor potential vanilloid 3 (TRPV3) in corneal epithelial cells: involvement in thermosensation and wound healing. *Exp. Eye Res.* **2010**, *90*, 121–129. [CrossRef] [PubMed]

36. Brown, T.E.; Chirila, A.M.; Schrank, B.R.; Kauer, J.A. Loss of interneuron LTD and attenuated pyramidal cell LTP in TRPV1 and TRPV3 KO mice. *Hippocampus* **2013**, *23*, 662–671. [CrossRef] [PubMed]

37. Moussaieff, A.; Rimmerman, N.; Bregman, T.; Straiker, A.; Felder, C.C.; Shoham, S.; Kashman, Y.; Huang, S.M.; Lee, H.; Shohami, E.; et al. Incensole acetate, an incense component, elicits psychoactivity by activating TRPV3 channels in the brain. *FASEB J.* **2008**, *22*, 3024–3034. [CrossRef] [PubMed]

38. Gallego-Sandín, S.; Rodríguez-García, A.; Alonso, M.T.; García-Sancho, J. The endoplasmic reticulum of dorsal root ganglion neurons contains functional TRPV1 channels. *J. Biol. Chem.* **2009**, *284*, 32591–32601. [CrossRef] [PubMed]

39. Lotteau, S.; Ducreux, S.; Romestaing, C.; Legrand, C.; Van Coppenolle, F. Characterization of Functional TRPV1 Channels in the Sarcoplasmic Reticulum of Mouse Skeletal Muscle. *PLoS ONE* **2013**, *8*, e58673. [CrossRef] [PubMed]

40. Lo, I.C.; Chan, H.C.; Qi, Z.; Ng, K.L.; So, C.; Tsang, S.Y. TRPV3 channel negatively regulates cell cycle progression and safeguards the pluripotency of embryonic stem cells. *J. Cell. Physiol.* **2016**, *231*, 403–413. [CrossRef] [PubMed]

41. Guatteo, E.; Chung, K.K.H.; Bowala, T.K.; Bernardi, G.; Mercuri, N.B.; Lipski, J. Temperature sensitivity of dopaminergic neurons of the substantia nigra pars compacta: involvement of transient receptor potential channels. *J. Neurophysiol.* **2005**, *94*, 3069–3080. [CrossRef] [PubMed]

42. Singh, U.; Kumar, S.; Shelkar, G.P.; Yadhav, M.; Kokare, D.M.; Goswami, C.; Lechan, R.M.; Singru, P.S. Transient receptor potential vanilloid (TRPV3) in the ventral tegmental area of rat: Role in modulation of the mesolimbic-dopamine reward pathway. *Neuropharmacology* **2016**, *110*, 198–210. [CrossRef] [PubMed]

43. Chung, M.-K.; Lee, H.; Mizuno, A.; Suzuki, M.; Caterina, M.J. 2-aminoethoxydiphenyl borate activates and sensitizes the heat-gated ion channel TRPV3. *J. Neurosci.* **2004**, *24*, 5177–5182. [CrossRef] [PubMed]

44. Chung, M.-K.; Lee, H.; Mizuno, A.; Suzuki, M.; Caterina, M.J. TRPV3 and TRPV4 mediate warmth-evoked currents in primary mouse keratinocytes. *J. Biol. Chem.* **2004**, *279*, 21569–21575. [CrossRef] [PubMed]

45. Cheng, X.; Jin, J.; Hu, L.; Shen, D.; Dong, X.-P.; Samie, M.A.; Knoff, J.; Eisinger, B.; Liu, M.-L.; Huang, S.M.; et al. TRP channel regulates EGFR signaling in hair morphogenesis and skin barrier formation. *Cell* **2010**, *141*, 331–343. [CrossRef] [PubMed]

46. Miyamoto, T.; Petrus, M.J.; Dubin, A.E.; Patapoutian, A. TRPV3 regulates nitric oxide synthase-independent nitric oxide synthesis in the skin. *Nat. Commun.* **2011**, *2*, 369. [CrossRef] [PubMed]

47. Borbíró, I.; Lisztes, E.; Tóth, B.I.; Czifra, G.; Oláh, A.; Szöllosi, A.G.; Szentandrássy, N.; Nánási, P.P.; Péter, Z.; Paus, R.; et al. Activation of transient receptor potential vanilloid-3 inhibits human hair growth. *J. Investig. Dermatol.* **2011**, *131*, 1605–1614. [CrossRef] [PubMed]

48. Mandadi, S.; Sokabe, T.; Shibasaki, K.; Katanosaka, K.; Mizuno, A.; Moqrich, A.; Patapoutian, A.; Fukumi-Tominaga, T.; Mizumura, K.; Tominaga, M. TRPV3 in keratinocytes transmits temperature information to sensory neurons via ATP. *Pflugers Arch. Eur. J. Physiol.* **2009**, *458*, 1093–1102. [CrossRef] [PubMed]

49. Pang, Z.; Sakamoto, T.; Tiwari, V.; Kim, Y.-S.; Yang, F.; Dong, X.; Güler, A.D.; Guan, Y.; Caterina, M.J. Selective keratinocyte stimulation is sufficient to evoke nociception in mice. *Pain* **2015**, *156*, 656–665. [CrossRef] [PubMed]

50. Radtke, C.; Vogt, P.M.; Devor, M.; Kocsis, J.D. Keratinocytes acting on injured afferents induce extreme neuronal hyperexcitability and chronic pain. *Pain* **2010**, *148*, 94–102. [CrossRef] [PubMed]

51. Huang, S.M.; Li, X.; Yu, Y.; Wang, J.; Caterina, M.J. TRPV3 and TRPV4 ion channels are not major contributors to mouse heat sensation. *Mol. Pain* **2011**, *7*, 37. [CrossRef] [PubMed]

52. Nilius, B.; Bíró, T.; Owsianik, G. TRPV3: Time to decipher a poorly understood family member! *J. Physiol.* **2014**, *592*, 295–304. [CrossRef] [PubMed]

53. Yang, Y.S.; Cho, S.I.; Choi, M.G.; Choi, Y.H.; Kwak, I.S.; Park, C.W.; Kim, H.O. Increased expression of three types of transient receptor potential channels (TRPA1, TRPV4 and TRPV3) in burn scars with post-burn pruritus. *Acta Derm. Venereol.* **2015**, *95*, 20–24. [CrossRef] [PubMed]

54. Sulk, M.; Seeliger, S.; Aubert, J.; Schwab, V.D.; Cevikbas, F.; Rivier, M.; Nowak, P.; Voegel, J.J.; Buddenkotte, J.; Steinhoff, M. Distribution and expression of non-neuronal transient receptor potential (TRPV) ion channels in rosacea. *J. Investig. Dermatol.* **2012**, *132*, 1253–1262. [CrossRef] [PubMed]

55. Scott, V.E.; Patel, H.; Wetter, J.; Edlmayer, R.; Neelands, T.; Miller, L.; Huang, S.; Gauld, S.; Todorovic, V.; Gomtsian, A.; et al. Defining a mechanistic link between TRPV3 activity and psoriasis through IL-1α and EGFR signaling pathways. *J. Investig. Dermatol.* **2016**, *136*, S94. [CrossRef]

56. Gopinath, P.; Wan, E.; Holdcroft, A.; Facer, P.; Davis, J.B.; Smith, G.D.; Bountra, C.; Anand, P. Increased capsaicin receptor TRPV1 in skin nerve fibres and related vanilloid receptors TRPV3 and TRPV4 in keratinocytes in human breast pain. *BMC Women's Health* **2005**, *5*, 2. [CrossRef] [PubMed]

57. Brash, A.R. Arachidonic acid as a bioactive molecule. *J. Clin. Investig.* **2001**, *107*, 1339–1345. [CrossRef] [PubMed]

58. Yoshioka, T.; Imura, K.; Asakawa, M.; Suzuki, M.; Oshima, I.; Hirasawa, T.; Sakata, T.; Horikawa, T.; Arimura, A. Impact of the Gly573Ser substitution in TRPV3 on the development of allergic and pruritic dermatitis in mice. *J. Investig. Dermatol.* **2009**, *129*, 714–722. [CrossRef] [PubMed]

59. Xiao, R.; Tian, J.; Tang, J.; Zhu, M.X. The TRPV3 mutation associated with the hairless phenotype in rodents is constitutively active. *Cell Calcium* **2008**, *43*, 334–343. [CrossRef] [PubMed]

60. Maruyama, M.; Sakai, A.; Suzuki, H.; Akimoto, T. Analysis of TRPV3 function in pain sensation using a gain-of-function mutant rat. *Exp. Anim.* **2015**, *64*, S69–S135.

61. Duchatelet, S.; Hovnanian, A. Olmsted syndrome: clinical, molecular and therapeutic aspects. *Orphanet. J. Rare Dis.* **2015**, *10*, 33. [CrossRef] [PubMed]

62. Nilius, B.; Biro, T. TRPV3: A "more than skinny" channel. *Exp. Dermatol.* **2013**, *22*, 447–452. [CrossRef] [PubMed]

63. Moran, M.M.; Chong, J.; Fanger, C.A.; Ripka, A.; Larsen, G.R.; Zhen, X.; Underwood, D.J.; Weigele, M. Compounds for Modulating TRPV3 Function. WO2008033564A1, 2008.

64. Reilly, R.M.; Kym, P.R. Analgesic potential of TRPV3 antagonists. *Curr. Top. Med. Chem.* **2011**, *11*, 2210–2215. [CrossRef] [PubMed]

65. Joshi, N. The TRPV3 Receptor as a Pain Target: A therapeutic promise or just some more new biology? *Open Drug Discov. J.* **2010**, *2*, 89–97. [CrossRef]

66. Huang, S.M.; Chung, M.-K. Targeting TRPV3 for the Development of Novel Analgesics. *Open Pain J.* **2013**, *6*, 119–126. [CrossRef] [PubMed]

67. Gomtsyan, A.R.; Schmidt, R.G.; Bayburt, E.K.; Gfesser, G.A.; Voight, E.A.; Daanen, J.F.; Schmidt, D.L.; Cowart, M.D.; Liu, H.; Altenbach, R.J.; et al. Synthesis and pharmacology of (pyridin-2-yl)methanol derivatives as novel and selective transient receptor potential vanilloid 3 antagonists. *J. Med. Chem.* **2016**, *59*, 4926–4947. [CrossRef] [PubMed]

68. Chong, J.A.; Fanger, C.M.; Larsen, G.R.; Lumma, W.C.; Moran, M.M.; Ripka, A.; Underwood, D.J.; Weigele, M.; Zhen, X. Compounds for Modulating TRPV3 Function. US20060270688A1, 2006.

69. Lin, Z.; Chen, Q.; Lee, M.; Cao, X.; Zhang, J.; Ma, D.; Chen, L.; Hu, X.; Wang, H.; Wang, X.; et al. Exome sequencing reveals mutations in TRPV3 as a cause of Olmsted syndrome. *Am. J. Hum. Genet.* **2012**, *90*, 558–564. [CrossRef] [PubMed]

70. Lai-Cheong, J.E.; Sethuraman, G.; Ramam, M.; Stone, K.; Simpson, M.A.; McGrath, J.A. Recurrent heterozygous missense mutation, p.Gly573Ser, in the TRPV3 gene in an Indian boy with sporadic Olmsted syndrome. *Br. J. Dermatol.* **2012**, *167*, 440–442. [CrossRef] [PubMed]

71. Eytan, O.; Fuchs-Telem, D.; Mevorach, B.; Indelman, M.; Bergman, R.; Sarig, O.; Goldberg, I.; Adir, N.; Sprecher, E. Olmsted syndrome caused by a homozygous recessive mutation in TRPV3. *J. Investig. Dermatol.* **2014**, *134*, 1752–1754. [CrossRef] [PubMed]

72. Ni, C.; Yan, M.; Zhang, J.; Cheng, R.; Liang, J.; Deng, D.; Wang, Z.; Li, M.; Yao, Z. A novel mutation in TRPV3 gene causes atypical familial Olmsted syndrome. *Sci. Rep.* **2016**, *6*, 21815. [CrossRef] [PubMed]

73. Kariminejad, A.; Barzegar, M.; Abdollahimajd, F.; Pramanik, R.; McGrath, J.A. Olmsted syndrome in an Iranian boy with a new de novo mutation in TRPV3. *Clin. Exp. Dermatol.* **2014**, *39*, 492–495. [CrossRef] [PubMed]

74. Duchatelet, S.; Guibbal, L.; de Veer, S.; Fraitag, S.; Nitschke, P.; Zarhrate, M.; Bodemer, C.; Hovnanian, A. Olmsted syndrome with erythromelalgia caused by recessive transient receptor potential vanilloid 3 mutations. *Br. J. Dermatol.* **2014**, *171*, 675–678. [CrossRef] [PubMed]

75. Duchatelet, S.; Pruvost, S.; de Veer, S.; Fraitag, S.; Nitschke, P.; Bole-Feysot, C.; Bodemer, C.; Hovnanian, A. A new TRPV3 missense mutation in a patient with Olmsted syndrome and erythromelalgia. *JAMA Dermatol.* **2014**, *150*, 303–306. [CrossRef] [PubMed]

76. Yamamoto-Kasai, E.; Yasui, K.; Shichijo, M.; Sakata, T.; Yoshioka, T. Impact of TRPV3 on the development of allergic dermatitis as a dendritic cell modulator. *Exp. Dermatol.* **2013**, *22*, 820–824. [CrossRef] [PubMed]

77. Lipski, J.; Park, T.I.H.; Li, D.; Lee, S.C.W.; Trevarton, A.J.; Chung, K.K.H.; Freestone, P.S.; Bai, J.-Z. Involvement of TRP-like channels in the acute ischemic response of hippocampal CA1 neurons in brain slices. *Brain Res.* **2006**, *1077*, 187–199. [CrossRef] [PubMed]

78. Moussaieff, A.; Yu, J.; Zhu, H.; Gattoni-Celli, S.; Shohami, E.; Kindy, M.S. Protective effects of incensole acetate on cerebral ischemic injury. *Brain Res.* **2012**, *1443*, 89–97. [CrossRef] [PubMed]

79. Facer, P.; Casula, M.A.; Smith, G.D.; Benham, C.D.; Chessell, I.P.; Bountra, C.; Sinisi, M.; Birch, R.; Anand, P. Differential expression of the capsaicin receptor TRPV1 and related novel receptors TRPV3, TRPV4 and TRPM8 in normal human tissues and changes in traumatic and diabetic neuropathy. *BMC Neurol.* **2007**, *7*, 11. [CrossRef] [PubMed]

80. Lingam, V.S.P.; Chaudhari, S.S.; Thomas, A.; Khairatkar-Joshi, N.; Kattige, V.G. Fused Pyrimidineone Compounds as TRPV3 Modulators. U.S. Patent 20090286811, 19 November 2009.

81. Lingam, V.S.P.; Thomas, A.; Phatangare, S.K.; Mindhe, A.S.; Khatik, J.Y.; Khairatkar-Joshi, N.; Kattige, V.G. Fused Imidazole Derivatives as TRPV3 Antagonist. U.S. Patent 20110257193, 20 October 2011.

82. Lingam, V.S.P.; Chaudhari, S.S.; Thomas, A.; Khairatkar-Joshi, N.; Kattige, V.G. Fused Pyrimidineone Compounds as TRPV3 Modulators. U.S. Patent 20120115886, 10 May 2012.

83. Lingam, V.S.P.; Thomas, A.; Dattaguru, A.M.; Khatik, J.Y.; Khairatkar-Joshi, N.; Kattige, V.G. Fused Pyramine Derivatives As TRPV3 Modulators. U.S. Patent 20100292254, 18 November 2010.

84. Lingam, V.S.P.; Thomas, A.; Gharat, L.A.; Ukirde, D.V.; Phatangare, S.K.; Mindhe, A.S.; Khairatkar-Joshi, N.; Kattige, V.G. Chromane Derivatives As TRPV3 Modulators. U.S. Patent 20100311778, 9 December 2010.

85. Bayburt, E.K.; Clapham, B.; Cox, P.B.; Daanen, J.F.; Gomtsyan, A.R.; Kort, M.E.; Kym, P.R.; Voight, E.A. Novel TRPV3 Modulators. U.S. Patent 20130150409, 13 June 2013.

86. Bayburt, E.K.; Clapham, B.; Cox, P.B.; Daanen, J.F.; Dart, M.J.; Gfesser, G.A.; Gomtsyan, A.R.; Kort, M.E.; Kym, P.R.; Schmidt, R.G.; et al. Novel TRPV3 Modulators. U.S. Patent 20130131036, 23 May 2009.

87. Moussaieff, A.; Shohami, E.; Kashman, Y.; Fride, E.; Schmitz, M.L.; Renner, F.; Fiebich, B.L.; Munoz, E.; Ben-Neriah, Y.; Mechoulam, R. Incensole acetate, a novel anti-inflammatory compound isolated from Boswellia resin, inhibits nuclear factor-kappa B activation. *Mol. Pharmacol.* **2007**, *72*, 1657–1664. [CrossRef] [PubMed]

88. Stewart, J.M. TRPV3 Agonists for the Treatment of Skin Conditions. U.S. Patent 20150250699, 10 September 2015.

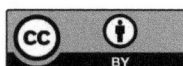

pharmaceuticals

MDPI

Review

TRP Channels in Skin Biology and Pathophysiology

Michael J. Caterina * and Zixuan Pang

Departments of Neurosurgery, Biological Chemistry and Neuroscience, Neurosurgery Pain Research Institute, Johns Hopkins School of Medicine, 725 N. Wolfe St., Baltimore, MD 21205, USA; punfilict@gmail.com
* Correspondence: caterina@jhmi.edu; Tel.: +1-410-502-5457

Academic Editors: Arpad Szallasi and Susan M. Huang
Received: 25 October 2016; Accepted: 9 December 2016; Published: 14 December 2016

Abstract: Ion channels of the Transient Receptor Potential (TRP) family mediate the influx of monovalent and/or divalent cations into cells in response to a host of chemical or physical stimuli. In the skin, TRP channels are expressed in many cell types, including keratinocytes, sensory neurons, melanocytes, and immune/inflammatory cells. Within these diverse cell types, TRP channels participate in physiological processes ranging from sensation to skin homeostasis. In addition, there is a growing body of evidence implicating abnormal TRP channel function, as a product of excessive or deficient channel activity, in pathological skin conditions such as chronic pain and itch, dermatitis, vitiligo, alopecia, wound healing, skin carcinogenesis, and skin barrier compromise. These diverse functions, coupled with the fact that many TRP channels possess pharmacologically accessible sites, make this family of proteins appealing therapeutic targets for skin disorders.

Keywords: transient receptor potential; skin; pain; itch; dermatitis; epidermis

1. Introduction to TRP Channels

Transient Receptor Potential (TRP) channels constitute a large family of ion channels expressed across vertebrate and invertebrate animal species. Mammals express at least 28 different TRP channels that can be divided into six subfamilies, based on their primary amino acid structures: TRPA (ankyrin), TRPC (canonical), TRPM (melastatin), TRPML (mucolipin), TRPP (polycystin) and TRPV (vanilloid) [1–3]. TRP channels are widely distributed across tissues, such that every cell in the body likely expresses one or more subtypes. Furthermore, TRP channels can be gated by an astonishingly diverse array of physical and chemical stimuli, ranging from ions and small molecules to heat, cold, and mechanical force [1–3]. Consequently, TRP channels are important for many aspects of health and disease [4].

Functional TRP channels consist of four subunits surrounding a central channel pore. In most cases, TRP channels are homotetramers of a given subunit, while in others, subunits of two different TRP channel subtypes contribute to a heterotetrameric channel. Although there are some exceptions, as described later in this chapter, each TRP channel subunit possesses six transmembrane domains, interconnected by relatively short loops, plus a relatively long N terminal domain and a somewhat shorter C terminal domain, with the latter two both extending into the cytoplasm (Figure 1). In some, but not all subfamilies, the N terminal domain contains multiple copies of a motif known as the ankyrin repeat that contributes to channel assembly and gating [2]. Recent cryo-electron microscopy studies of TRPV [5–9] and TRPA [10] family members have provided a high-resolution view of the structures of these channels, as well as insights into how their pores can be gated by their respective activators. All known TRP channels are selective for cations, with little or no anion permeability. However, their relative selectivity among cations can vary. Whereas most TRP channels are so-called nonselective cation channels that show permeability to both monovalent cations such as sodium and divalent cations such as calcium and magnesium, a few are highly selective for either calcium or sodium ions [3].

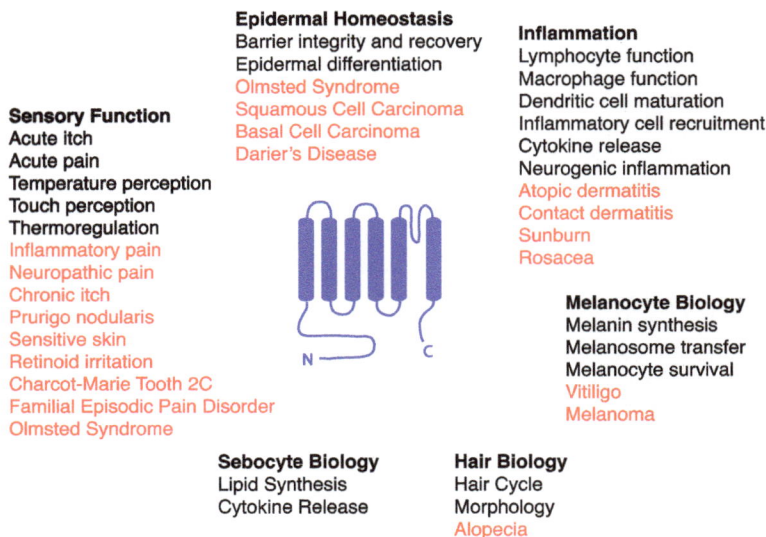

Epidermal Homeostasis
Barrier integrity and recovery
Epidermal differentiation
Olmsted Syndrome
Squamous Cell Carcinoma
Basal Cell Carcinoma
Darier's Disease

Inflammation
Lymphocyte function
Macrophage function
Dendritic cell maturation
Inflammatory cell recruitment
Cytokine release
Neurogenic inflammation
Atopic dermatitis
Contact dermatitis
Sunburn
Rosacea

Sensory Function
Acute itch
Acute pain
Temperature perception
Touch perception
Thermoregulation
Inflammatory pain
Neuropathic pain
Chronic itch
Prurigo nodularis
Sensitive skin
Retinoid irritation
Charcot-Marie Tooth 2C
Familial Episodic Pain Disorder
Olmsted Syndrome

Melanocyte Biology
Melanin synthesis
Melanosome transfer
Melanocyte survival
Vitiligo
Melanoma

Sebocyte Biology
Lipid Synthesis
Cytokine Release

Hair Biology
Hair Cycle
Morphology
Alopecia

Figure 1. Summary of physiological (black) and pathophysiological (red) processes to which Transient Receptor Potential (TRP) channels contribute in various skin cell types. Topological diagram of a TRP channel subunit is shown at center, with amino (N) and carboxyl (C) termini labeled. Extracellular domain is at top.

Like other tissues, the skin expresses an abundance of TRP channel subtypes that significantly affect its development, integrity, and function under healthy conditions and in disease states [11,12]. There are a number of fundamental mechanisms, described in greater detail throughout this review, through which this occurs. Most notably, the ability of many TRP channels to mediate calcium influx into cutaneous neurons, keratinocytes, melanocytes, or immune cells provides a mechanism by which these channels influence cellular proliferation, differentiation, secretion of paracrine/autocrine factors, cytotoxicity, cell migration, and a host of other processes relevant to skin health and disease. Calcium is of particular importance to keratinocytes, since the skin exhibits a gradient of extracellular calcium from relatively low levels in the basal epidermis to relatively high levels in more mature epidermal layers. This gradient, in part, helps to drive the progressive differentiation of epidermal keratinocytes as they are displaced apically by proliferating basal cells [13]. Dysregulation of calcium homeostasis, as occurs in conditions such as Hailey-Hailey disease [14] or Darier's disease [15], results in abnormal epidermal differentiation, keratosis, poor adhesion between keratinocytes, and other abnormalities. Another important output of TRP channels is membrane depolarization. In cutaneous sensory neurons, TRP channel-mediated depolarization in response to a host of chemical, thermal, and mechanical stimuli triggers action potential firing, eventually leading to sensations of temperature, pain, or itch [16]. The effects of TRP channel-mediated depolarization, moreover, are not confined to neurons, since membrane depolarization in nonexcitable cells like keratinocytes or lymphocytes can affect cellular processes such as ATP release [17] or calcium flux through Orai family channels [18]. Finally, a growing list of protein interactors has been identified for TRP channels, further expanding the potential signaling repertoire of these molecules [19,20]. In this chapter, we will provide an overview of TRP channel expression in various cell types in the skin, as well as the physiological and pathological cutaneous processes to which they contribute. A summary of these diverse processes is presented in Figure 1, highlighting multiple opportunities for therapeutic targeting of TRP channels in skin.

2. Contributions of TRP Channels to Skin Biology and Pathophysiology

2.1. TRPC Channels and Skin

2.1.1. TRPC Channels and Keratinocyte Differentiation

Expression of nearly every TRPC channel subtype, including TRPC1, TRPC3, TRPC4, TRPC5, and TRPC6, has been reported in human keratinocytes. TRPC1 and TRPC4 are both upregulated during keratinocyte differentiation in vitro. This expression level change appears to be functionally important, since knockdown of either TRPC1 or TRPC4 in keratinocytes in vitro was shown to reduce the level of store-operated calcium entry and to inhibit keratinocyte differentiation [21,22]. TRPC6 has also been shown to be required for normal human keratinocyte differentiation in vitro [23]. In addition, small molecules of the triterpine family have been shown to promote keratinocyte differentiation both in vitro and in vivo through a mechanism that appears to involve TRPC6 [24].

2.1.2. TRPC Channels in Darier's Disease

Darier's Disease, also known as Darier-White disease, is a rare autosomal dominant dermatological disease initially discovered by the French dermatologist Ferdinard-Jean Darier in 1889. It is characterized by keratotic papules that may occur throughout the body [25]. Darier's Disease is caused by heterozygous loss of the endoplasmic reticulum calcium pump protein SERCA2b, which is encoded by the gene ATP2A2 located on 12q23-24.1 [26]. In addition to skin papules, patients with this disorder often suffer from neuropsychiatric symptoms [27]. There have also been reports of bone cysts [28]. Because SERCA2b is the only SERCA pump expressed in keratinocytes, this defect results in failure to sequester calcium in the ER lumen and the consequent accumulation of excess cytoplasmic calcium. Interestingly, examination of TRP channel expression in keratinocytes from heterozygous SERCA knockout mice revealed a compensatory upregulation of TRPC1 [29]. Although this change might a priori be predicted to worsen calcium overload in these cells, it was found that TRPC1 upregulation somehow enhanced keratinocyte resistance to apoptosis [29]. Whether compensatory TRPC1 expression ameliorates or exacerbates the Darier's Disease phenotype in intact skin, however, remains unclear. It also remains to be determined whether other syndromic features of Darier's disease involve alterations in TRP channel-mediated calcium signaling in skeletal or nervous tissues similar to those proposed for keratinocytes.

2.1.3. TRPC Channels and Sensory Function

There are numerous connections between TRPC channels and cutaneous sensory function. Although TRPC channels are expressed in most cell types, TRPC1, TRPC3, TRPC5 and TRPC6 are the subfamily members characterized most extensively in sensory neurons. Based on pharmacological studies with the relatively nonselective TRPC channel antagonist, SKF-96365, TRPC channels might also contribute to pain and hyperalgesia caused by the bee venom component, mellitin [30]. TRPC3 is expressed in small- to medium-diameter nociceptors [31–33], and has been shown to be important for store-operated calcium entry responses downstream of G protein-coupled receptors for purines and proteases [32], providing a potential mechanism for the involvement of this channel in some forms of inflammatory hyperalgesia. TRPC3 has further been implicated in nociceptor activation by IgG immune complexes and thus might be a contributor to pain in allergic contact dermatitis [34]. It has also been shown that TRPC1 and TRPC6, which are co-expressed in sensory neurons with TRPV4, facilitate hyperalgesic responses mediated by the latter channel, through mechanisms that have not been clearly resolved [31]. Further evidence for a role for TRPC1 in sensory function comes from the observation that this channel is required for normal mechanically evoked responses in two subpopulations of mechanosensory cutaneous neurons (Aδ-low threshold mechanoreceptors and slowly-adapting Aβ-low threshold mechanoreceptors) and for behavioral responses to very gentle mechanical stimuli [35]. Finally, TRPC5, which is also expressed in a subpopulation of peripheral sensory neurons that innervate the skin, can be activated by mildly cold temperatures. However, no obvious defects in cold detection were observed in mice lacking this channel [33].

2.2. TRPV1 and Skin

TRPV1 is among the most extensively characterized mammalian TRP channels. Upon gating, this channel produces multiple cellular signals, including membrane depolarization and an increase in cytoplasmic calcium. TRPV1 is expressed at the highest level in a subpopulation of peptidergic peripheral sensory neurons involved in the perception of pain. When overexpressed recombinantly in cell lines, TRPV1 can be activated by capsaicin, the major pungent ingredient in chili peppers, or by related chemical compounds that share a vanilloid chemical group, thus providing the "transient receptor vanilloid" subfamily its name [1]. TRPV1 can alternatively be activated by extracellular protons, by certain small lipophilic molecules, including endogenous cannabinoid lipids such as anandamide and N-arachidonoyl dopamine [1], or by a number of other chemical agonists such as 2-aminoethoxydiphenyl borate (2-APB), which had previously been recognized as a dose dependent activator and inhibitor of IP3 receptors and store-operated calcium channels [36]. In addition, TRPV1 was the first recognized molecular thermoreceptor, as it can be activated in the absence of chemical ligands by painfully hot temperatures ($>42 \,^{\circ}\mathrm{C}$) [1]. This polymodal chemo-thermo sensitivity likely accounts for the perception of "heat" experienced during consumption of chili peppers, and has led TRPV1 to receive substantial attention as a candidate target for pain control [37].

2.2.1. TRPV1 in Pain, Itch, and Neurogenic Inflammation

Gene knockout studies in mice, as well as administration of TRPV1 antagonists to mice, rats, and humans, have confirmed roles for this channel in pain sensation. For example, mice lacking TRPV1 are insensitive to capsaicin and show partially diminished heat-evoked pain at baseline and a virtual absence of inflammation-induced thermal hyperalgesia [38,39]. Reductions in heat pain [40], inflammatory pain [41,42] and cancer pain [43,44] sensitivity have also been observed in rodents and/or human treated with TRPV1-selective antagonists. Furthermore, a number of phase I and II clinical trials of TRPV1 antagonists have been conducted to examine their potential analgesic utility [45,46]. Studies using TRPV1 antagonists have also provided evidence for a role of TRPV1 molecules located at the central terminals of primary sensory neurons in certain forms of mechanical hypersensitivity, though the cellular mechanisms underlying such roles remain to be elucidated [47].

Beyond the perception of pain, TRPV1 has been shown to participate in other neuronal functions relevant to the skin. For example, TRPV1 null mice exhibit reduced itch-related scratching behavior in response to interleukin 31 (IL31) [48] or histamine [49]. TRPV1 also facilitates the function of TRPV4 in itch perception [50]. In addition, capsaicin-induced neurogenic inflammation (i.e., inflammation produced by the neuronal release of vasoactive peptides) is suppressed in the absence of TRPV1 [1,51]. Therefore, the interaction of neuronally-expressed TRPV1 with the skin is bidirectional, involving both sensory and efferent activities.

2.2.2. TRPV1 Expression in Keratinocytes

Aside from the functional importance of neuronally-expressed TRPV1, there is considerable evidence to suggest that TRPV1 may participate more directly in epidermal biology by virtue of its expression in keratinocytes. Evidence for such expression is strongest in human keratinocytes. Inoue et al. [52] first reported the existence of TRPV1-like immunoreactivity and TRPV1 mRNA in cultured human keratinocytes. They also showed that in these keratinocyte cell cultures, capsaicin or protons could evoke an influx of calcium that was inhibited by the TRPV1 antagonist, capsazepine. In contrast, whereas primary neonatal mouse keratinocytes and the mouse 308 keratinocyte cell line were shown to express TRPV1 mRNA, they did not respond to capsaicin in physiological assays [53,54]. Immunological, mRNA, and calcium imaging-based evidence for TRPV1 expression was also reported in the human HaCaT keratinocyte cell line [55]. In these cells, capsaicin could evoke the release of IL8 and prostaglandin E2 (PGE2) and upregulate the expression of cyclooxygenase 2 (COX2), providing evidence for potential proinflammatory activities. TRPV1 agonist-mediated calcium influx was also observed in human NHEK keratinocytes, and these responses, as well, could be blocked by either capsazepine or another TRPV1 antagonist, PAC-14028 [56]. Furthermore, heat shock was shown to trigger matrix metalloproteinase 1 (MMP-1) transcription in both HaCaT and NHK keratinocytes, in a manner apparently dependent on TRPV1 [57]. There is additional evidence that TRPV1 may be expressed in keratinocytes in intact healthy human skin. For example, Stander et al. [58] observed TRPV1-like immunoreactivity in keratinocytes of the stratum basalis and stratum granularis, as well as in dermal mast cells, hair follicles, sebaceous gland epithelial cells, and cutaneous sensory nerve terminals. A common problem with many human skin immunostaining studies is the absence of definitive controls for antibody specificity. However, the possibility of intrinsic cutaneous TRPV1 expression in that same study was corroborated by polymerase chain reaction detection of TRPV1 mRNA.

2.2.3. TRPV1 in Epidermal Homeostasis and Dermatitis

Despite the challenges of definitive demonstration of TRPV1 expression in rodent keratinocytes, multiple studies in rodents have suggested TRPV1 involvement in epidermal barrier function and the regulation of dermatitis. In hairless mice, capsaicin delays epidermal barrier recovery following tape-stripping and the TRPV1 antagonist capsazepine accelerates such recovery [59]. A potential role for heat as a mediator of this effect arose indirectly from the observation that barrier recovery is accelerated at relatively warm skin temperatures (36 °C–40 °C), compared with cooler temperatures. Agonists of two other warmth-sensitive TRP channels found in keratinocytes, TRPV3 and TRPV4 (see below), failed to recapitulate the effects of heat. In a series of studies [56,60,61], a TRPV1 antagonist, PAC-14028, was shown to accelerate skin barrier recovery either following tape stripping or in two models of atopic dermatitis: *Dermatophagoides farina* (Df) challenge in a susceptible mouse strain and challenge with the small molecule hapten oxazolone in previously sensitized mice. PAC-14028 also reduced rises in serum immunoglobulins, skin thickening, mast cell degranulation, and scratching behavior following repetitive Df administration. However, the apparent direction of TRPV1 effects on epidermal homeostasis and dermatitis has not been uniform across studies. In one study, oxazolone induced ear edema was increased in mice lacking TRPV1 or in wild-type mice in which TRPV1-expressing neurons were desensitized with vanilloid compounds [62]. The authors of that study postulated that anti-inflammatory agents released by TRPV1 expressing neurons accounted for the apparently anti-dermatitic effects of this channel. Although the reasons for discrepancies among these studies remain unclear, they might include the use of immunologically distinct mouse strains or off-target effects of some of the TRPV1 modulating agents used. Furthermore, a definitive dissection of the functions of neuronal vs. non-neuronal TRPV1 function in these models remains to be performed.

2.2.4. TRPV1 and Ultraviolet Radiation

Lee et al. [63] demonstrated that ultraviolet B (UVB) light could induce a calcium influx in HaCaT cells that was sensitive to TRPV1 antagonists, as well as an increase in MMP1 expression that was suppressed by TRPV1 antagonists and TRPV1 siRNA knockdown and facilitated by capsaicin. This study also reported a UVB-induced increase in TRPV1 western blot signal in HaCaT cells and a UVB induced increase in TRPV1 immunostaining in human skin. Based on their findings, the authors of this study speculated on a potential role for TRPV1 in UVB induced skin aging. Consistent with human keratinocyte studies, in hairless mice, the TRPV1 antagonist, iodo-resiniferatoxin, could suppress UVB induced skin thickening and expression of MMP, COX2, and p53 [64]. However, whether that effect was keratinocyte-intrinsic or neuronally mediated was again not definitively established.

2.2.5. TRPV1 Epidermal Upregulation in Human Skin Diseases

Elevations in either epidermal TRPV1-like immunostaining or skin TRPV1 mRNA expression have been reported in several different human skin diseases, including prurigo nodularis [58], rosacea [65], and herpes zoster infection [66]. In addition, there may be a link between TRPV1 and sensitive skin, as defined by augmented sensitivity in the lactic acid stinging test [67]. TRPV1 mRNA and keratinocyte TRPV1-like immunostaining were elevated in patients with positive responses in this psychophysical test [67]. These patients are presumed to have either an impaired skin barrier and/or alterations in their neurovascular responsiveness [67]. Interestingly, TRPV1 immunoreactivity was lower in individuals with darker skin, suggesting that melanin might interfere with those factors that promote TRPV1 upregulation [67]. Perhaps related to these findings, the skin irritant phenoxyethanol was found to increase calcium influx into HaCaT cells in a manner inhibitable by TRPV1 antagonists [68]. Furthermore, it has been shown that retinoids evoke pain behavior in rodents by acting at TRPV1, presumably in neurons. This might explain the burning sensation reported for these compounds in humans [69].

2.2.6. TRPV1 and Skin Cancer

Some studies have provided evidence suggestive of a connection between TRPV1 and skin cancer. However, these findings have often been indirect and relied upon pharmacological tools. For example, capsaicin was shown to be co-carcinogenic in rodent skin [70] and the TRPV1 antagonist AMG9810 was shown to act as a tumor promoter [71] However, in the former study, the effects of capsaicin turned out to be mediated by EGFR signaling, independent of TRPV1, while in the latter study, the TRPV1 dependence of the AMG9810 effects, which also somehow involved EGFR signaling, was not directly addressed. Thus, no role for TRPV1 in skin cancer has yet been definitively established.

2.2.7. TRPV1 in Skin Appendages

In human hair follicles, TRPV1-like immunoreactivity was observed in specific epithelial subcompartments, including the outer root sheath and hair matrix [58,72]. In organ cultures of these hair follicles, activation of TRPV1 suppressed epithelial proliferation and hair shaft elongation and promoted hair follicle regression [72]. TRPV1-like immunoreactivity has also been reported in epithelial compartments of mouse hair follicles, and examination of hair cycle in TRPV1 knockout mice revealed a delayed catagen phase [73].

There is also evidence for TRPV1 expression in human sebocytes, the major constituents of cutaneous sebaceous glands. In these cells, TRPV1 stimulation with capsaicin suppresses lipid synthesis and the release of proinflammatory cytokines [74].

2.3. TRPV2 and Skin

TRPV2 was originally discovered as a calcium-permeable channel that could be regulated by insulin-like growth factor I signaling [75], and in parallel, as a channel that could be activated by extremely high temperatures (>52 °C) [76]. TRPV2 was subsequently found to be capable of being activated by a range of stimuli, including PI3 kinase signaling [77], certain cannabinoid compounds (Δ9-tetrahydrocannabinol, cannabidiol) [78], probenecid [79], 2-APB [36], hypoosmolarity [80], and mechanical cell stretch [81]. In the skin, TRPV2 is most highly expressed in two categories of cells: sensory neurons and immune/inflammatory cells.

2.3.1. TRPV2 and Sensory Function

The contribution of TRPV2 to sensory function remains enigmatic. Although rodent TRPV2 has been shown to be activated by heat [76], mice lacking TRPV2 showed no detectable defects in noxious heat sensation, even if the potentially confounding activity of TRPV1 was eliminated [82]. Furthermore, heat sensitivity appears not to be conserved in human TRPV2 [83]. There is evidence that TRPV2 plays a role in neurite outgrowth, particularly in response to mechanical stretch of neurons [81] or nerve growth factor stimulation [84]. Whether this has implications for nerve regeneration in the skin has yet to be explored.

2.3.2. TRPV2 and Immune Cell Function

TRPV2 expression has been reported in a range of immune/inflammatory cell types, including macrophages, mast cells, natural killer cells, dendritic cells and lymphocytes [85]. Within these cell types, TRPV2 has been implicated in regulating diverse functions that include cytokine release [86], chemotaxis [87,88], phagocytosis [87], endocytosis [89], inflammasome activity [90], and podosome assembly [91]. In human skin, elevated TRPV2-like immunoreactivity was observed in both macrophages and mast cells in the setting of rosacea [65]. Aberrant TRPV2 expression has also been reported in hematological tumors and cell lines, including those derived from mantle cell lymphoma, multiple myeloma, Burkitt lymphoma, acute myeloid leukemia, and myelodysplastic syndrome [92,93].

2.4. TRPV3 and Skin

The cloning of TRPV3 was reported almost simultaneously by three groups [94–96]. TRPV3 mRNA and protein were shown to be expressed prominently in skin keratinocytes [94,96]. Like several other TRPV channels, TRPV3 can be activated by thermal or chemical stimuli. TRPV3 exhibits a temperature-dependent rise in activity at temperatures exceeding 33 $^{\circ}$C–39 $^{\circ}$C, with the specific apparent threshold varying among studies [94–96]. Reported chemical agonists of TRPV3 include 2-APB [36,97], farnesyl Pyrophosphate [98], and various plant-derived compounds, including camphor [99], carvacrol, eugenol, and thymol [100]. TRPV3 responses agonist stimulation can be further potentiated by several factors, including unsaturated fatty acids [101], repetitive heat stimulation [96], or cholesterol [102]. Conversely, factors that suppress TRPV3 activity include oxygen-dependent hydroxylation of TRPV3 by Factor-inhibiting-hypoxia inducible factor [103].

2.4.1. TRPV3 and Cutaneous Temperature Sensation

The robust expression of TRPV3 in keratinocytes, as well as this channel's heat-responsiveness, led a number of labs to investigate potential roles for this channel in skin temperature sensation. In vitro experiments in both the mouse 308 keratinocyte cell line and primary keratinocytes demonstrated warmth-evoked currents that resembled those mediated by recombinantly expressed TRPV3 [54]. Accordingly, these TRPV3-like currents were lost in keratinocytes isolated from TRPV3 knock out mice [99]. In contrast, TRPV3 protein proved difficult to detect in sensory neurons [99]. Together, these findings suggested that TRPV3 might participate in an "indirect" mechanism of heat sensation involving skin keratinocyte communication with sensory neurons. Consistent with this notion, TRPV3 was shown to mediate the heat-evoked release of a number of mediators with the capability to influence neuronal activity. For example, in keratinocyte-sensory neuron cocultures, heat activation was reported to produce a rise in keratinocyte calcium levels, followed by a delayed calcium influx response in the neurons, an effect that was apparently mediated by ATP signaling and dependent on keratinocyte TRPV3 [104]. It was also demonstrated that in keratinocytes, heat evokes the release of nitric oxide through a mechanism that is independent of nitric oxide synthase, and that this response is dependent on TRPV3 [105]. Similarly, keratinocytes cultured from mice overexpressing TRPV3 selectively in keratinocytes showed augmented release of prostaglandin E2 (PGE2) in response to both heat and 2-APB stimulation [106]. Together, these findings provided evidence that TRPV3 may serve as an important role in keratinocyte-neuron communication.

At the whole-animal level, there is also evidence that TRPV3 might contribute, under some circumstances, to heat perception. The original description of TRPV3 knockout mice reported that these mice exhibited deficits in both thermal preference behavior and heat-evoked nociception [99]. However, subsequent studies of these behaviors in TRPV3 knockout mice on more homogeneous genetic backgrounds yielded a more complex picture. Although the absence of TRPV3 on a pure C57Bl6 background produced no detectable change in thermally-evoked behavior, in two separate studies, TRPV3 knockout on the 129/S6 [107], or 129S1/SvImJ [105] backgrounds resulted in subtle alterations in thermal preference behavior. Interestingly, in one of these studies [105], the TRPV3 phenotype was sex dependent, occurring only in females. It should be noted that all these observations were made in global TRPV3 knockout mice, in which the channel was absent from all tissues throughout life. It is possible that a more definitive conclusion about the role of TRPV3 might be obtained from analysis of inducible keratinocyte- or neuron-selective TRPV3 knockout in adults. Mice lacking both TRPV3 and TRPV4 (see below) exhibited virtually normal thermal preference behavior and only a slight deficit in heat-evoked nociception [107]. However, in another study, it was demonstrated that while in mice lacking TRPV1 alone, a dynamic hotplate evoked an unusual escape behavior, this phenotype was abolished in mice lacking both TRPV1 and TRPV3 [108]. Thus, while TRPV3 might be a partial contributor to heat sensation under specific conditions, these genetic studies suggest that it is not a major participant in this process.

2.4.2. TRPV3 and Epidermal Homeostasis and Hair Development

A number of studies have implicated TRPV3 in epidermal homeostasis and hair growth. Global TRPV3 knockout in mice was originally reported to produce transient alterations in abdominal hair morphology [99]. Subsequently, selective knockout of TRPV3 in mouse keratinocytes was found to produce several skin phenotypes, including perinatal skin barrier defects and abnormal epidermal maturation that appeared to resolve spontaneously and curly body hair and whiskers [109]. Similarities to reported effects of perturbations in EGFR signaling led the investigators of this latter paper to explore a potential relationship between these two signaling proteins. Indeed, they found that activation of TRPV3 in keratinocytes triggers the protease-mediated shedding of the EGFR ligand, TGF-α. They also found that TRPV3 could promote transglutaminase activity in keratinocytes, providing a potential explanation for the skin barrier defects in TRPV3 knockout mice. At least one human study also implicated TRPV3 in the regulation of hair growth [110]. These authors showed that application of the TRPV3 agonists eugenol or 2-APB to either cultured human hair follicles or outer root sheath (ORS) keratinocytes, produced a dose-dependent suppression of proliferation and induction of apoptosis in both systems.

2.4.3. TRPV3 and Skin Pathology

There is also a growing body of evidence suggesting that TRPV3 is a key contributor to epidermal homeostasis and skin sensory function in certain pathological conditions. For example, although published studies are limited, there are reports in the patent literature that TRPV3 antagonists can suppress certain forms of mechanical hypersensitivity in rats after nerve injury [111]. In addition, it was reported that, in the mouse acetone-ether-water model of chronic dry skin, the genetic absence of TRPV3 resulted in reduced scratching behavior [112]. TRPV3-like immunoreactivity was also noted to be upregulated in the skin of breast surgery patients who reported postsurgical pain [113]. Similarly, TRPV3 mRNA was found to be upregulated in keratinocytes derived from patients with hypertrophic post burn scars who also reported itching [114]. Moreover, mouse studies have linked TRPV3 to epithelial wound healing in skin and oral mucosa [105,115].

The most compelling association between TRPV3 and skin pathology has come from the study of naturally occurring mutations in the gene encoding this channel. The earliest indications of this link came from rodent studies, where two TRPV3 mutations at the same residue (Gly573Ser and Gly573Cys, respectively) were found to be the causes of alopecia in two different rodent lines, the DS-Nh mouse and the WBN/Kob-Ht rat [116]. Further research by the same group [117] indicated that epidermal sheets derived from Ds-Nh mice exhibited elevated intracellular calcium levels. This finding is consistent with the subsequent finding that both the Gly573Ser and Gly 573Cys mutations confer a high level of constitutive activity on recombinant TRPV3 [118]. Additional examination of the in vivo consequences of these same TRPV3 mutations, resulted in additional skin phenotypes that included enhanced predilection towards evoked allergic contact dermatitis or, in some cases, spontaneous dermatitis [116,119]. The development of these dermatitis phenotypes was quite variable between studies and even within a study, between mice crossed onto different genetic backgrounds or housed under different conditions. This variable penetrance suggests the existence of both intrinsic and environmental modifiers of the dermatitis phenotype.

It is especially noteworthy that pathological gain-of-function mutations in TRPV3 are not confined to rodents. In 2012, whole-exome sequencing of six patients with Olmsted Syndrome revealed a TRPV3 mutation is strongly associated with this disease [120]. Olmsted Syndrome is a severe dermatological disease characterized by bilateral palmoplantar and periorificial keratoderma as well as severe itching or pain. Remarkably, the mutations discovered in Olmsted patients were homologous to those observed previously the Ds-Nh mice. The discovery of the link between Olmsted Syndrome and TRPV3 led to additional genetic studies in this condition. As a result, an increasing number of Olmsted patients were found to have TRPV3 mutations. Thus far, 10 TRPV3 mutations have been associated with approximately 20 Olmsted patients [121]. In addition, investigators recently discovered a gain-of-function mutation in a Chinese family that appears to be the cause of focal palmoplantar keratoderma [122] and another that was linked to another form of hereditary palmoplantar keratoderma without associated perioreficial lesions [121].

2.5. TRPV4 and Skin

TRPV4 was originally identified as a widely-expressed TRP channel that could be activated by changes in extracellular osmolarity [123–125]. Subsequently, it was shown that this channel could be activated by a range of physical and chemical stimuli, including cytochrome P450 metabolites of arachidonic acid [126], and warm temperatures [127]. Consistent with its expression pattern and wide range of activators, TRPV4 has been implicated in numerous processes in health and disease, many of which involve the skin.

2.5.1. TRPV4 and Epidermal Barrier Function

TRPV4 is abundantly expressed in skin keratinocytes [127]. A role for this channel in epidermal barrier homeostasis comes from the observations that activation of this channel increases intracellular calcium in human keratinocytes and promotes cell-cell junction formation between these cells, and that knockdown of TRPV4 expression impairs development of high transepithelial resistance in cultured human keratinocytes [128]. Furthermore, warm temperatures and chemical agonists of TRPV4 accelerate barrier recovery in explanted human skin tissues after stratum corneum removal [129].

2.5.2. TRPV4 and Skin Cancer

TRPV4 mRNA and immunohistochemical staining are reduced in premalignant skin lesions and in basal and squamous cell carcinomas [130]. Whether there is a functional role for TRPV4 in tumorigenesis has yet to be determined.

2.5.3. TRPV4 and Sensory Function

Multiple studies have provided evidence for roles for TRPV4 in sensory processes. In some cases, these functions are attributable to keratinocyte-expressed TRPV4, while in others TRPV4 channels expressed in neurons may be the more relevant pool. TRPV4 has been shown to participate in osmotically-evoked pain behaviors [131,132] and also in acute mechanical nociception [133,134] and in mechanical hyperalgesia in certain models of inflammatory [135–137] and neuropathic [138–140] pain. In some chemotherapy induced neuropathy models, mechanical hyperalgesia appears to involve alterations in the interactions between TRPV4, $\alpha2\beta1$ integrin, and src kinase [138]. Certain pro-algesic agents, such as agonists of the protease-activate receptor PAR2, also produce mechanical hyperalgesia through a process that involves TRPV4 [141]. TRPV4 has also been implicated in sunburn-associated hyperalgesia. TRPV4 mediates the release of the nociceptive/pruriceptive peptide, endothelin-1 from keratinocytes in response to UVB irradiation [142]. Moreover, mice lacking TRPV4 or treated with TRPV4 antagonists exhibited reduced UVB induced inflammation and mechanical and thermal hyperalgesia [142]. This effect is partially keratinocyte-autonomous, since it was observed in keratinocyte conditional TRPV4 knockout animals, and since TRPV4 mediates calcium entry into cultured mouse keratinocytes upon UVB exposure [142]. Consistent with these findings in mouse, TRPV4-like immunoreactivity was found to be elevated in human skin following UVB exposure [142].

There is a growing body of evidence implicating TRPV4 in itch perception. TRPV4 appears to play a role in itch perception in response to some, but not all pruritogens [143,144]. This is attributable at least in part to TRPV4 function in keratinocytes, where calcium influx through this channel triggers ERK phosphorylation. Scratching behaviors evoked by several pruritogens, including histamine, compound 48/80, and endothelin-1, but not that evoked by chloroquine, were partially suppressed in mice in which TRPV4 was deleted from keratinocytes [144]. However, contributions from sensory neuron-expressed TRPV4 to itch perception cannot be excluded. In both histaminergic and non-histaminergic itch, the contribution of TRPV4 appears to be facilitated by TRPV1 [50].

TRPV4 has also been implicated in innocuous warmth sensation, although the effect of TRPV4 knockout on this function is modest and condition-dependent. For example, whereas mice lacking TRPV4 were originally reported to show a shift in thermal preference on a thermal gradient towards slightly warmer temperatures [145], in later studies, as indicated above, mice lacking both TRPV4 and TRPV3 showed apparently normal thermal selection behavior, with only a slightly delayed withdrawal response to painful heat [107].

Numerous point mutations in TRPV4 have been shown to produce Charcot Marie Tooth disease type 2C [146–148]. Although not a skin disease per se, CMT2C is a sensorimotor degenerative disease that can include mild sensory loss.

2.6. TRPV6 and Skin

TRPV6 and Keratinocyte Differentiation

TRPV6, one of the most calcium-selective of mammalian TRP channels, is expressed in keratinocytes, where it plays important roles in epidermal differentiation [23]. Two different stimuli that are known to promote keratinocyte differentiation, elevations in extracellular calcium and 1, 25, dihydroxyvitamin D3, both upregulate transcription of TRPV6 [23]. This channel, in turn, mediates calcium influx to elevate basal intracellular levels [23]. As evidence of the importance of this process, in vitro siRNA silencing of TRPV6 suppresses the differentiation of keratinocytes in response to a calcium switch [23]. Moreover, one form of thermal spring water was shown to augment human keratinocyte differentiation in vitro through a mechanism that appeared to involve TRPV6 [149]. In addition, mice lacking TRPV6 exhibit an abnormally thin stratum corneum and a defective epidermal calcium gradient [150]. Although elevated TRPV6 expression has been associated with increased aggressiveness of prostate cancer [151], a potential link between TRPV6 and skin cancer has not been explored.

2.7. TRPA1 and Skin

TRPA1 is a nonselective cation channel that is abundantly expressed in a subpopulation of nociceptive sensory neurons, in addition to numerous other cell types. This channel is noteworthy for its direct and indirect responsiveness to an astoundingly diverse range of chemical, thermal, and mechanical stimuli. One large class of chemical TRPA1 activators includes electrophillic agents such as allyl isothiocyanate (mustard oil), cinnamaldehyde, acrolein, tear gas constituents, formaldehyde, and certain prostaglandins such as 15-deoxy-Δ12,14-prostaglandin J2. These electrophiles activate TRPA1 by covalent modification of specific cysteine residues located in the channel's cytoplasmic N-terminus. Many non-electrophillic chemicals, including certain anesthetics (e.g., propophol, isofluorane, lidocaine), fenamate nonsteroidal anti-inflammatory drugs, cannabinoids (e.g., Δ(9)-Tetrahydrocannabinol), cooling agents (e.g., icillin), and intracellular calcium ions can also activate TRPA1, presumably via more conventional ligand-receptor interactions. Its regulation by intracellular Ca^{2+} makes TRPA1 an effective integrator of other excitatory signaling pathways [152]. TRPA1 also exhibits a complex and species-specific pattern of thermosensitivity. In certain invertebrate and reptile species, TRPA1 can be activated directly or indirectly by warm temperatures and is essential for the detection of these temperatures in vivo [153–155]. Massive overexpression of TRPA1 in trigeminal sensory neurons likely accounts for the exquisite sensitivity of pit vipers to their warm prey [156]. In mammals, conversely, TRPA1 was originally reported to be activated by intense cold [157], a phenomenon that was recapitulated in some [158] but not all subsequent studies. Warm temperatures were shown to suppress and desensitize rat TRPA1 [159]. However, it was also recently shown that human TRPA1 exhibits a U-shaped temperature-response profile, with activation by both cold and heat. The complexity of this thermosensory behavior may in part be a consequence of strong TRPA1 regulation by modulating factors such as redox state [160]. TRPA1 proline hydroxylation analogously mediates changes in TRPA1 cold sensitivity in response to intracellular oxygen concentrations [161]. TRPA1 can also be activated in response to certain pathogen-associated molecular patterns and host-derived damage-associated molecular patterns. These effects can be either direct (e.g., lipopolysaccharide [162]) or indirect (e.g., let-7 miRNA acting via TLR7 [163]). Finally, TRPA1 has been implicated in mechanosensory processes [164–166]. However, this may reflect indirect mechanisms, rather than direct mechanical activation of the channel. Indeed, whereas classical mechanically-activated currents have not been reported in excised patches from cells expressing TRPA1, hypertonic stimuli can activate this channel in heterologous expression systems [167].

2.7.1. TRPA1 and Cutaneous Pain Sensation

The complex pattern of direct and indirect response characteristics described above renders TRPA1 an active participant in a host of sensory and non-sensory processes in both health and disease, many of which involve the skin. For example, studies employing knockout mice or TRPA1 selective antagonists have revealed essential functions for TRPA1 in multiple aspects of cutaneous pain sensation, including pain evoked by electrophilic chemicals (e.g., mustard oil, formalin) or mechanical stimulation [165,168,169]. In the case of cold-evoked pain, the importance of TRPA1 is less evident under baseline conditions, but becomes exaggerated in the setting of tissue injury or inflammation [170]. TRPA1 is also a key participant in two common models of pathological chronic pain, streptozotocin-induced diabetic neuropathy [171] and chemotherapy-induced neuropathy [172]. At least part of the acute pain component in the former model is attributable to activation of TRPA1 by streptozotocin-generated peroxynitrite [173]. However, even later stages of neuropathic pain, including the loss of peripheral nerve fibers, are inhibited by the inhibition of TRPA1 [174]. Moreover, methylglyoxal, a metabolic byproduct of diabetic hyperglycemia, is an electrophillic TRPA1 activator [171]. In the case of chemotherapy-induced neuropathy, TRPA1 appears to be activated indirectly by platin-induced alteration of redox state [172]. Mutations or polymorphisms in TRPA1 have also been linked to human pain. Patients bearing an N855S gain-of-function mutation in this channel are afflicted with Familial Episodic Pain Disorder, a condition associated with upper body pain that can be triggered by stressful stimuli such as fatigue, cold, or fasting [175]. Reactive oxygen species acting at TRPA1 may also be responsible for the augmented cutaneous sensitivity to ambient light in patients with porphyria, a potential contributor to pain in that condition [176].

2.7.2. TRPA1 and Itch

Multiple studies have shown that TRPA1 is also an important mediator of acute and chronic itch perception. Acute responses to non-histaminergic pruritogens (e.g., chloroquine, endothelin-1, compound 48/80) in the mouse are defective in the absence of TRPA1, owing to the positioning of this channel downstream of signaling by two pruritogen-sensing G protein-coupled receptors, MrgA3 and MrgC11 [177]. Endogenous pruritogens can also produce scratching behavior through TRPA1. For example, thymic stromal lymphopoietin (TSLP), which is released by keratinocytes in response to histaminergic signaling, activates neuronal TRPA1 downstream of the TSLP receptor [178]. Similarly, itch produced in response to bile acids, as might occur in the context of biliary obstruction, appears to be TRPA1 dependent, with the channel acting downstream of G protein-coupled bile receptors such as TGR5 [179]. The absence of TRPA1 has also been shown to reduce scratching behaviors in the acetone-ether-water mouse model of dry skin and chronic itch [180]. In addition, TRPA1 was upregulated in sensory neurons and TRPA1 antagonists reduced itch behavior in an interleukin 13-overexpressing transgenic model of atopic dermatitis [181]. Consistent with this observation, IL31 receptors were found to be colocalized with both TRPA1 and TRPV1 in sensory neurons, and genetic elimination of either channel reduced IL31-induced itch [48]. TRPA1 has also been shown to be an important contributor to the pruritis associated with contact dermatitis evoked by any of several different haptens [182]. This latter role might involve, among other mechanisms, direct action of TRPA1 by haptens, since 2,4-dinitrochlorobenzene and oxazolone, commonly used haptens for contact hypersensitivity experiments, have been shown to activate recombinant TRPA1 [182,183].

2.7.3. TRPA1 and Inflammation

As a nonselective cation channel expressed in nociceptive and pruriceptive sensory neurons, TRPA1 is ideally suited to trigger the membrane depolarization necessary for the pain and itch sensations ascribed to it in the previous sections. However, evidence from a variety of studies indicates that the participation of TRPA1 in pathological processes related to itch and pain extends beyond its sensory function to include an active role in inflammation. For example, in the acetone-ether-water model of chronic dry skin [180] and in several different models of contact hypersensitivity [182], mice lacking TRPA1 showed reduced epidermal thickening, a suppressed cytokine response, and reductions in other hallmarks of inflammation. A similar proinflammatory role for TRPA1 has also been observed in other tissues, such as the lungs of mice with allergen-induced asthma [184].

2.7.4. TRPA1 and Barrier Function

Although TRPA1 knockout mice have not been reported to exhibit any alterations in epidermal barrier function, there is pharmacological data to suggest that this channel can modulate barrier restoration. In hairless mice, cinnamaldehyde, mustard oil, and bradykinin all accelerated barrier recovery following tape stripping, and these effects could be blocked by a selective TRPA1 antagonist. Similarly, cooling of skin could accelerate barrier recovery, again in a manner inhibitable by the TRPA1 antagonist [185]. Given that TRPA1 and TRPV1 produce similar effects of cellular depolarization and calcium influx, it is interesting to compare these effects of TRPA1 activation with those described above for TRPV1, where channel activation appears to delay barrier recovery. Whether the apparently opposite consequences of activating these functionally similar channels relates to differential coupling to downstream signaling pathways, differential expression patterns, a complex consequence of channel activation and desensitization, or some other distinction remains to be determined.

2.7.5. Loci of TRPA1 Action in Its Cutaneous Functions

Within neurons, the apparent sites at which TRPA1 might mediate its sensory functions include not only the peripheral terminals, where TRPA1 triggers action potential firing, but also their cell bodies and their central terminals in the spinal cord dorsal horn, where TRPA1 can modulate neurotransmitter release onto spinal circuits [186]. At least a component of the pro-inflammatory roles of TRPA1 in skin and in other tissues such as lung might also be attributable to its expression in sensory neurons. When stimulated, many of the sensory neurons expressing TRPA1 release pro-inflammatory neuropeptides such as substance P (SP) and calcitonin gene-related polypeptide (CGRP) into their target tissues, with consequent vasodilation and plasma extravasation [51]. Moreover, pharmacological or genetic blockade of SP signaling was shown to attenuate the inflammatory response associated with contact dermatitis [182]. However, the relationship between neuronal peptide release and inflammation is not entirely straightforward, since the neurogenic release of SP and CGRP has been shown to paradoxically suppress recruitment of immune cells to sites of bacterial infection [187] and since these neurons might also release anti-inflammatory peptides such as somatostatin [188].

As with many other TRP channels, TRPA1 expression in the skin is not confined to neurons. For example, expression of this channel has also been observed in cutaneous mast cells, where it is upregulated in the interleukin 13 overexpression mouse model of atopic dermatitis [181].

There is also evidence for TRPA1 expression in keratinocytes, although again this finding might differ between species. While it was originally reported that TRPA1 is expressed directly in mouse keratinocytes, a recent study, called this finding into question [189]. Although this leaves the function of TRPA1 in mouse keratinocytes unclear, transient expression of TRPA1 in keratin 14-lineage cells and consequent roles in the establishment of mechanosensory circuits cannot be excluded as a possibility. By comparison, TRPA1 expression in human keratinocytes is more strongly supported. In human scalp skin-derived cultures, TRPA1 mRNA and a TRPA1-like Western blot band were observed in primary keratinocytes. TRPA1-like immunoreactivity was also observed in basal epidermal and hair follicle keratinocytes in skin biopsies [181].

TRPA1 mRNA and protein were also detected in human scalp skin-derived melanocytes, and fibroblasts [181]. Moreover, by means of its responsiveness to ROS, TRPA1 mediates the earliest component of the bimodal hyperpigmentation response of melanocytes to Ultraviolet A (UVA) irradiation [190]. Several human melanoma-derived cell lines were also shown to express TRPA1 and to exhibit calcium responses to TRPA1 agonists that could be suppressed by a TRPA1 selective antagonist. However, in the same study, TRPA1 agonist-induced changes in cellular proliferation were insensitive to this same antagonist, potentially arguing against a clear role for this channel as a target of melanoma therapy [191]. Given these findings, additional tools and experiments will be required to precisely define the sites at which TRPA1 produces its effects on skin biology and the mechanisms by which it does so.

2.8. TRPM1 and Skin

2.8.1. TRPM1 and Melanocytes

TRPM1 is prominently expressed in melanocytes, where it appears to participate in the generation of the photoprotective pigment, melanin, presumably by increasing intracellular Ca^{2+} levels [192]. Regulation of TRPM1 in melanocytes occurs at multiple levels, including transcription of TRPM1 mRNA [193], generation of different TRPM1 splice variants [194], TRPM1 activation downstream of G protein-coupled receptors such as metabotropic glutamate receptor 6 [195], and, possibly, miRNA regulation of TRPM1 mRNA stability or translation [196]. An early clue that TRPM1 was functionally important in melanogenesis came from the observation that mutations in the TRPM1 gene with incomplete dominance results in so-called "leopard spotting", the patchy loss of pigmentation in the skin of Apalloosa horses [197]. In humans, TRPM1 expression levels are correlated with melanin content, with greater levels of TRPM1 in populations with more heavily pigmented skin [198]. The contribution of TRPM1 to pigmentation might be relevant to the pathogenesis of human vitiligo. Lesional skin in patients with either localized or generalized vitiligo shows significantly reduced levels of TRPM1 mRNA expression [196]. Within melanocytic nevii, TRPM1 expression drops as the melanocytes progress towards a less-differentiated melanoblast phenotype that does not produce melanin [194]. TRPM1 might also be involved in UV induced changes in skin pigmentation, though this link has not been explicitly confirmed [192]. One barrier to better defining the biological functions of TRPM1 in this process is that mice lack epidermal melanocytes, and thus do not exhibit UVB induced pigmentation changes. However, experiments involving humanized mouse skin might help overcome this limitation [199].

2.8.2. TRPM1 and Melanoma

TRPM1 has also long been linked to melanoma, where reduced levels of TRPM1 expression and the appearance of alternatively spliced forms of TRPM1 mRNA are correlated with a less differentiated and more malignant phenotype [192,194]. While it is possible that TRPM1 activity, per se, contributes to melanoma progression and invasiveness, a more likely mechanism arises from the fact that miRNA 211, a tumor suppressor miRNA, is encoded in one of the introns of the TRPM1 gene and its transcription is co-regulated with that of TRPM1 [200].

2.9. TRPM2 and Skin

2.9.1. TRPM2 and Cutaneous Pain Sensation

TRPM2 is a widely expressed channel that can be activated by two types of stimuli: reactive oxygen species (e.g., H_2O_2) and warm temperatures. It was recently demonstrated that this channel is required for normal behavioral responses of mice to innocuous warm temperatures [201]. Consistent with this requirement, TRPM2 is expressed in a subpopulation of peripheral sensory neurons, and genetic elimination of TRPM2 results in an apparent reduction in the proportion of sensory neurons responsive to warm temperatures but not to other chemical agonists of heat-sensitive TRP channels. Curiously, however, the proportion of cells that express TRPM2 mRNA is far greater than that responsive to warmth. The basis of this discrepancy is unclear, but it might reflect inefficient translation or trafficking of TRPM2 protein or a requirement for other components for full thermal responsiveness.

2.9.2. TRPM2 and Melanoma

TRPM2 is also expressed in melanocytes and its activity can be suppressed by an endogenous dominant negative splice variant, TRPM2-TE. This splice variant is upregulated in melanoma, and either prevention of its synthesis or exogenous overexpression of full-length TRPM2 renders melanoma cells more susceptible to apoptosis and necrosis [194].

2.10. TRPM3 and Skin

TRPM3 and Cutaneous Pain Sensation

TRPM3 is expressed in a wide range of cell types, including a subpopulation of small to medium diameter sensory neurons. Like several other TRP channels expressed in this latter cell type, TRPM3 can be activated by painfully hot temperatures. It can alternatively be activated by chemical agonists, including the neurosteroid, pregnenolone sulfate and sphingolipids such as D-erythro-sphingosine [202]. Another curious feature of TRPM3 is that, in addition to a conventional nonselective cation pore, when this channel is stimulated with a combination of PS and clotrimazole, it exhibits a second, parallel ion permeation path, selective for small monovalent cations [203]. The physiological significance of this secondary conduction pathway, which resembles the "omega current" observed in some mutant voltage-gated sodium channels, has yet to be determined. Nevertheless, there is strong evidence supporting the physiological importance of TRPM3 to cutaneous sensory function. Neurons derived from mice lacking TRPM3 show defects in acute responsiveness to either PS or painful heat. Accordingly, these mice show behavioral deficits in response to these agonists, as well as defective heat hyperalgesia following inflammation with complete Freund's adjuvant [202].

2.11. TRPM4 and Skin

TRPM4 and Lymphocytes

Although TRPM4 expression has not been demonstrated in either keratinocytes or sensory neurons, it is expressed in various immune cell populations, including T lymphocytes. Comparison of TH2 and TH1 cells has revealed a higher TRPM4 expression level in the former cells [18]. Inhibition of

TRPM4 expression in TH2 cells leads to an elevation in intracellular calcium levels, with associated alterations in cytokine release profile. This seemingly paradoxical finding likely stems from the fact that TRPM4 is monovalent cation-selective, and activation of this channel depolarizes the membrane without associated calcium flux. That depolarization, moreover, reduces the electrochemical driving force for calcium influx through Orai channels. Thus, TRPM4 is poised to regulate T cell polarization and inflammatory responses in the skin.

2.12. TRPM7 and Skin

TRPM7 and Melanocytes

Although TRPM7 has not been studied extensively in mammalian skin, studies in zebrafish illustrate an important role for this channel in melanocytes. Melanocytes in mutant zebrafish lacking TRPM7 undergo death by necrosis [204]. This phenotype could be ameliorated by prevention of melanin synthesis, suggesting that the importance of TRPM7 is to facilitate chemical detoxification of intermediates of melanin synthesis.

2.13. TRPM8 and Skin

2.13.1. TRPM8 and Cutaneous Cold and Pain Sensation

TRPM8 was originally identified as a protein differentially expressed in prostate cancer cell lines. However, it was subsequently "rediscovered" as a receptor for cold-mimetic compounds such as menthol and icilin, as well as a channel that could be gated by mildly cold temperatures, themselves. TRPM8 is robustly expressed by a subpopulation of primary sensory neurons that are responsive to these same stimuli. Consistent with this expression pattern, genetic knockout experiments have shown convincingly that TRPM8 is required for normal responsiveness of sensory neurons to mild cold and, even more strikingly, for mouse behavioral avoidance of uncomfortably cool temperatures [205–207]. By comparison, the relationship of TRPM8 to pain is more complex. On the one hand, TRPM8 expression in a population of nociceptive neurons that also express TRPV1 appears to contribute to hypersensitivity to cold under conditions of inflammation or nerve injury. On the other hand, behavioral avoidance of intense cold is largely unaffected in TRPM8 knockout mice and under certain circumstances, TRPM8 stimulation (presumably in TRPM8-only neurons) actually suppresses pain sensitivity [208]. This cross-modal suppression is analogous to that observed between cold and itch perception [209], and is probably mediated by central nervous system circuits. At the same time, within sensory neurons, activation of mu opiate receptors leads to internalization of TRPM8 protein, providing a possible mechanism for opioid induced cold analgesia [210].

Another, recently identified TRPM8 activator is testosterone [211,212]. Androgen-dependent upregulation of TRPM8 gene expression has long been recognized in androgen-dependent prostate tumors [213]. However, in addition to its conventional transcription-mediated mechanisms of action, testosterone appears to activate TRPM8 by directly binding to the extracellular domain of the channel. In a recent human psychophysical study, testosterone application to the skin produced a cooling sensation, followed by a mild stinging sensation. This dual response was greater in female subjects than in males. Based on these findings, the authors speculated that testosterone acts as a natural cold-mimetic agent, but that high endogenous testosterone levels in males might desensitize TRPM8 over time. If true, this might account, in part, for the enhanced sensitivity of females to cold. Further experiments will be necessary to evaluate this provocative notion.

2.13.2. TRPM8 and Epidermal Homeostasis

With respect to non-thermosensory cutaneous functions for TRPM8, the earliest studies of TRPM8 knockout mice yielded no obvious epidermal phenotypes [205–207]. However, according to a more recent study [214], this lack of phenotype might have been a consequence of the specific strategies used to generate those mice, since those early strategies were based on disrupting exons encoding the TRPM8 amino terminus. Full-length TRPM8, which contains this domain, is not prominently expressed in keratinocytes. However, the authors of this recent study found that both human and mouse keratinocytes express an N terminally truncated TRPM8 splice variant lacking the N terminus and the first two transmembrane domains. They named this splice variant epithelial TRPM8 (eTRPM8). Genetically ablating the pore region shared by all TRPM8 isoforms, including eTRPM8, resulted in mice with an epidermal homeostasis phenotype. Specifically, these "pan-TRPM8 knockouts" exhibited a reduced proliferative cell number in the basal epidermis, an increase in superficial, late stage epidermal differentiation, and a reduction in the thickness of the stratum corneum. Unlike full-length TRPM8, eTRPM8 protein is confined to the endoplasmic reticulum, where it functions as a calcium release channel that facilitates elevations in calcium within adjacent mitochondria in response to canonical TRPM8 stimuli such as icilin, menthol, or cold. The authors of this study outlined two potential mechanisms by which this response might alter keratinocyte biology. First, mitochondrial calcium influx enhances synthesis of adenosine triphosphate, which when released from keratinocytes might alter their proliferation and differentiation in an autocrine manner. Second, in response to mildly cold stimuli, eTRPM8 augments production of superoxide, another candidate modulator of epidermal proliferation/differentiation. While these are certainly plausible explanations for the pan-TRPM8 knockout epidermal phenotype, additional cell type-specific knockout experiments will be required to determine whether the phenotype is truly a keratinocyte-autonomous phenomenon, or whether neuronal TRPM8 is also a contributor.

Other studies have provided additional links between TRPM8 and epidermal homeostasis. For example, TRPM8 agonists, like TRPA1 agonists, have been shown to accelerate barrier recovery following tape stripping of the skin and to reduce the epithelial proliferation response of the skin to barrier disruption [215]. It has also been reported that either chemical or thermal TRPM8 activation can reduce PGE2 release from human keratinocytes in response to UVB irradiation [216]. Whether these effects are mediated by full-length TRPM8 and/or eTRPM8 has not yet been established.

2.13.3. TRPM8 and Melanoma

TRPM8 expression has been observed in human melanoma cells, where its activation results in elevations in intracellular calcium and reduced cell viability [217,218]. This finding suggests that TRPM8 agonists might serve as candidate therapeutics for melanoma.

2.14. TRPML3 and Skin

TRPML3 and Melanocytes

Members of the TRP-mucolipin (TRPML) channel subfamily are most notable for their functions not at the plasma membrane, but rather within intracellular organelles. One member of this family, TRPML3, has been shown to be especially important for normal melanocyte differentiation [219]. TRPML3 is highly expressed in healthy melanocytes. However, a gain-of-function mutation in the TRPML3 gene is responsible for the phenotypic traits of varitint-waddler mutant mice, which exhibit a combination of a vestibular defect and coat pigmentation defects. The pigmentation defect appears to result from the constitutive elevation of intracellular calcium in the melanocytes of these animals, and their subsequent cell death.

3. Conclusions

In summary, numerous TRP channels are expressed in the cell types that constitute the skin, and they contribute in multiple ways to skin physiology under healthy conditions and to the pathological changes that occur in the setting of skin disease. Consequently, strategies aimed at this functionally diverse family of ion channels might provide useful means of combatting disorders of cutaneous homeostasis, sensation, and neoplasia.

Acknowledgments: Supported by the Neurosurgery Pain Research Institute at Johns Hopkins School of Medicine.

Author Contributions: Z.P. and M.J.C. both contributed to the writing of the manuscript.

Conflicts of Interest: M.J.C. is an inventor on a patent related to TRPV1 and TRPV2 that is licensed through The University of California, San Francisco and Merck, and may be entitled to royalties on that patent. He has also previously served on the Scientific Advisory Board of Hydra Biosciences, which works on products related to TRP Channels. These conflicts are being managed by the Johns Hopkins Office of Policy Coordination. No one beyond the authors of this review played a role in the writing of the manuscript or the decision to publish the results.

References

1. Caterina, M.J.; Julius, D. The vanilloid receptor: A molecular gateway to the pain pathway. *Annu. Rev. Neurosci.* **2001**, *24*, 487–517. [CrossRef] [PubMed]
2. Montell, C.; Birnbaumer, L.; Flockerzi, V.; Bindels, R.J.; Bruford, E.A.; Caterina, M.J.; Clapham, D.E.; Harteneck, C.; Heller, S.; Julius, D.; et al. A unified nomenclature for the superfamily of TRP cation channels. *Mol. Cell* **2002**, *9*, 229–231. [CrossRef]
3. Ramsey, I.S.; Delling, M.; Clapham, D.E. An introduction to TRP channels. *Annu. Rev. Physiol.* **2006**, *68*, 619–647. [CrossRef] [PubMed]
4. Nilius, B.; Owsianik, G.; Voets, T.; Peters, J.A. Transient receptor potential cation channels in disease. *Physiol. Rev.* **2007**, *87*, 165–217. [CrossRef] [PubMed]
5. Agarwala, M.K.; George, R.; Pramanik, R.; McGrath, J.A. Olmsted syndrome in an Indian male with a new de novo mutation in TRPV3. *Br. J. Dermatol.* **2016**, *174*, 209–211. [CrossRef] [PubMed]
6. Cao, E.; Liao, M.; Cheng, Y.; Julius, D. TRPV1 structures in distinct conformations reveal activation mechanisms. *Nature* **2013**, *504*, 113–118. [CrossRef] [PubMed]
7. Huynh, K.W.; Cohen, M.R.; Jiang, J.; Samanta, A.; Lodowski, D.T.; Zhou, Z.H.; Moiseenkova-Bell, V.Y. Structure of the full-length TRPV2 channel by cryo-EM. *Nat. Commun.* **2016**, *7*, 11130. [CrossRef] [PubMed]
8. Liao, M.; Cao, E.; Julius, D.; Cheng, Y. Structure of the TRPV1 ion channel determined by electron cryo-microscopy. *Nature* **2013**, *504*, 107–112. [CrossRef] [PubMed]
9. Zubcevic, L.; Herzik, M.A., Jr.; Chung, B.C.; Liu, Z.; Lander, G.C.; Lee, S.Y. Cryo-electron microscopy structure of the TRPV2 ion channel. *Nat. Struct. Mol. Biol.* **2016**, *23*, 180–186. [CrossRef] [PubMed]
10. Paulsen, C.E.; Armache, J.P.; Gao, Y.; Cheng, Y.; Julius, D. Structure of the TRPA1 ion channel suggests regulatory mechanisms. *Nature* **2015**, *525*, 552. [CrossRef] [PubMed]
11. Caterina, M.J. TRP channel cannabinoid receptors in skin sensation, homeostasis, and inflammation. *ACS Chem. Neurosci.* **2014**, *5*, 1107–1116. [CrossRef] [PubMed]
12. Lumpkin, E.A.; Caterina, M.J. Mechanisms of sensory transduction in the skin. *Nature* **2007**, *445*, 858–865. [CrossRef] [PubMed]
13. Yuspa, S.H.; Hennings, H.; Tucker, R.W.; Jaken, S.; Kilkenny, A.E.; Roop, D.R. Signal transduction for proliferation and differentiation in keratinocytes. *Ann. N. Y. Acad. Sci.* **1988**, *548*, 191–196. [CrossRef] [PubMed]
14. Hu, Z.; Bonifas, J.M.; Beech, J.; Bench, G.; Shigihara, T.; Ogawa, H.; Ikeda, S.; Mauro, T.; Epstein, E.H., Jr. Mutations in ATP2C1, encoding a calcium pump, cause Hailey-Hailey disease. *Nat. Genet.* **2000**, *24*, 61–65. [CrossRef] [PubMed]
15. Sakuntabhai, A.; Dhitavat, J.; Burge, S.; Hovnanian, A. Mosaicism for ATP2A2 mutations causes segmental darier's disease. *J. Investig. Dermatol.* **2000**, *115*, 1144–1147. [CrossRef] [PubMed]
16. Basbaum, A.I.; Bautista, D.M.; Scherrer, G.; Julius, D. Cellular and molecular mechanisms of pain. *Cell* **2009**, *139*, 267–284. [CrossRef] [PubMed]
17. Zhao, P.; Barr, T.P.; Hou, Q.; Dib-Hajj, S.D.; Black, J.A.; Albrecht, P.J.; Petersen, K.; Eisenberg, E.; Wymer, J.P.; Rice, F.L.; et al. Voltage-gated sodium channel expression in rat and human epidermal keratinocytes: Evidence for a role in pain. *Pain* **2008**, *139*, 90–105. [CrossRef] [PubMed]
18. Weber, K.S.; Hildner, K.; Murphy, K.M.; Allen, P.M. TRPM4 differentially regulates Th1 and Th2 function by altering calcium signaling and NFAT localization. *J. Immunol.* **2010**, *185*, 2836–2846. [CrossRef] [PubMed]
19. Hanack, C.; Moroni, M.; Lima, W.C.; Wende, H.; Kirchner, M.; Adelfinger, L.; Schrenk-Siemens, K.; Tappe-Theodor, A.; Wetzel, C.; Kuich, P.H.; et al. GABA blocks pathological but not acute TRPV1 pain signals. *Cell* **2015**, *160*, 759–770. [CrossRef] [PubMed]

20. Kiselyov, K.; Shin, D.M.; Kim, J.Y.; Yuan, J.P.; Muallem, S. TRPC channels: Interacting proteins. *Handb. Exp. Pharmacol.* **2007**, 559–574. [CrossRef]

21. Beck, B.; Lehen'kyi, V.; Roudbaraki, M.; Flourakis, M.; Charveron, M.; Bordat, P.; Polakowska, R.; Prevarskaya, N.; Skryma, R. TRPC channels determine human keratinocyte differentiation: New insight into basal cell carcinoma. *Cell Calcium* **2008**, *43*, 492–505. [CrossRef] [PubMed]

22. Cai, S.; Fatherazi, S.; Presland, R.B.; Belton, C.M.; Izutsu, K.T. TRPC channel expression during calcium-induced differentiation of human gingival keratinocytes. *J. Dermatol. Sci.* **2005**, *40*, 21–28. [CrossRef] [PubMed]

23. Lehen'kyi, V.; Beck, B.; Polakowska, R.; Charveron, M.; Bordat, P.; Skryma, R.; Prevarskaya, N. TRPV6 is a Ca^{2+} entry channel essential for Ca^{2+}-induced differentiation of human keratinocytes. *J. Biol. Chem.* **2007**, *282*, 22582–22591. [CrossRef] [PubMed]

24. Woelfle, U.; Laszczyk, M.N.; Kraus, M.; Leuner, K.; Kersten, A.; Simon-Haarhaus, B.; Scheffler, A.; Martin, S.F.; Muller, W.E.; Nashan, D.; et al. Triterpenes promote keratinocyte differentiation in vitro, ex vivo and in vivo: A role for the transient receptor potential canonical (subtype) 6. *J. Investig. Dermatol.* **2010**, *130*, 113–123. [CrossRef] [PubMed]

25. Takagi, A.; Kamijo, M.; Ikeda, S. Darier disease. *J. Dermatol.* **2016**, *43*, 275–279. [CrossRef] [PubMed]

26. Sakuntabhai, A.; Ruiz-Perez, V.; Carter, S.; Jacobsen, N.; Burge, S.; Monk, S.; Smith, M.; Munro, C.S.; O'Donovan, M.; Craddock, N.; et al. Mutations in ATP2A2, encoding a Ca^{2+} pump, cause darier disease. *Nat. Genet.* **1999**, *21*, 271–277. [PubMed]

27. Gordon-Smith, K.; Jones, L.A.; Burge, S.M.; Munro, C.S.; Tavadia, S.; Craddock, N. The neuropsychiatric phenotype in darier disease. *Br. J. Dermatol.* **2010**, *163*, 515–522. [CrossRef] [PubMed]

28. Castori, M.; Barboni, L.; Duncan, P.J.; Paradisi, M.; Laino, L.; De Bernardo, C.; Robinson, D.O.; Grammatico, P. Darier disease, multiple bone cysts, and aniridia due to double de novo heterozygous mutations in ATP2A2 and PAX6. *Am. J. Med. Genet. A* **2009**, *149A*, 1768–1772. [CrossRef] [PubMed]

29. Pani, B.; Cornatzer, E.; Cornatzer, W.; Shin, D.M.; Pittelkow, M.R.; Hovnanian, A.; Ambudkar, I.S.; Singh, B.B. Up-regulation of transient receptor potential canonical 1 (TRPC1) following sarco(endo)plasmic reticulum Ca^{2+} ATPase 2 gene silencing promotes cell survival: A potential role for TRPC1 in darier's disease. *Mol. Biol. Cell* **2006**, *17*, 4446–4458. [CrossRef] [PubMed]

30. Ding, J.; Zhang, J.R.; Wang, Y.; Li, C.L.; Lu, D.; Guan, S.M.; Chen, J. Effects of a non-selective TRPC channel blocker, SKF-96365, on melittin-induced spontaneous persistent nociception and inflammatory pain hypersensitivity. *Neurosci. Bull.* **2012**, *28*, 173–181. [CrossRef] [PubMed]

31. Alessandri-Haber, N.; Dina, O.A.; Chen, X.; Levine, J.D. TRPC1 and TRPC6 channels cooperate with TRPV4 to mediate mechanical hyperalgesia and nociceptor sensitization. *J. Neurosci.* **2009**, *29*, 6217–6228. [CrossRef] [PubMed]

32. Alkhani, H.; Ase, A.R.; Grant, R.; O'Donnell, D.; Groschner, K.; Seguela, P. Contribution of TRPC3 to store-operated calcium entry and inflammatory transductions in primary nociceptors. *Mol. Pain* **2014**, *10*, 43. [CrossRef] [PubMed]

33. Zimmermann, K.; Lennerz, J.K.; Hein, A.; Link, A.S.; Kaczmarek, J.S.; Delling, M.; Uysal, S.; Pfeifer, J.D.; Riccio, A.; Clapham, D.E. Transient receptor potential cation channel, subfamily C, member 5 (TRPC5) is a cold-transducer in the peripheral nervous system. *Proc. Natl. Acad. Sci. USA* **2011**, *108*, 18114–18119. [CrossRef] [PubMed]

34. Qu, L.; Li, Y.; Pan, X.; Zhang, P.; LaMotte, R.H.; Ma, C. Transient receptor potential canonical 3 (TRPC3) is required for IgG immune complex-induced excitation of the rat dorsal root ganglion neurons. *J. Neurosci.* **2012**, *32*, 9554–9562. [CrossRef] [PubMed]

35. Garrison, S.R.; Dietrich, A.; Stucky, C.L. TRPC1 contributes to light-touch sensation and mechanical responses in low-threshold cutaneous sensory neurons. *J. Neurophysiol.* **2012**, *107*, 913–922. [CrossRef] [PubMed]

36. Hu, H.Z.; Gu, Q.; Wang, C.; Colton, C.K.; Tang, J.; Kinoshita-Kawada, M.; Lee, L.Y.; Wood, J.D.; Zhu, M.X. 2-aminoethoxydiphenyl borate is a common activator of TRPV1, TRPV2, and TRPV3. *J. Biol. Chem.* **2004**, *279*, 35741–35748. [CrossRef] [PubMed]

37. Gunthorpe, M.J.; Chizh, B.A. Clinical development of TRPV1 antagonists: Targeting a pivotal point in the pain pathway. *Drug Discov. Today* **2009**, *14*, 56–67. [CrossRef] [PubMed]

38. Caterina, M.J.; Leffler, A.; Malmberg, A.B.; Martin, W.J.; Trafton, J.; Petersen-Zeitz, K.R.; Koltzenburg, M.; Basbaum, A.I.; Julius, D. Impaired nociception and pain sensation in mice lacking the capsaicin receptor. *Science* **2000**, *288*, 306–313. [CrossRef] [PubMed]

39. Davis, J.B.; Gray, J.; Gunthorpe, M.J.; Hatcher, J.P.; Davey, P.T.; Overend, P.; Harries, M.H.; Latcham, J.; Clapham, C.; Atkinson, K.; et al. Vanilloid receptor-1 is essential for inflammatory thermal hyperalgesia. *Nature* **2000**, *405*, 183–187. [CrossRef] [PubMed]

40. Chizh, B.A.; O'Donnell, M.B.; Napolitano, A.; Wang, J.; Brooke, A.C.; Aylott, M.C.; Bullman, J.N.; Gray, E.J.; Lai, R.Y.; Williams, P.M.; et al. The effects of the TRPV1 antagonist SB-705498 on TRPV1 receptor-mediated activity and inflammatory hyperalgesia in humans. *Pain* **2007**, *132*, 132–141. [CrossRef] [PubMed]

41. Gavva, N.R.; Tamir, R.; Qu, Y.; Klionsky, L.; Zhang, T.J.; Immke, D.; Wang, J.; Zhu, D.; Vanderah, T.W.; Porreca, F.; et al. AMG 9810 [(*E*)-3-(4-*t*-butylphenyl)-*N*-(2,3-dihydrobenzo[b][1,4] dioxin-6-yl)acrylamide], a novel vanilloid receptor 1 (TRPV1) antagonist with antihyperalgesic properties. *J. Pharmacol. Exp. Ther.* **2005**, *313*, 474–484. [CrossRef] [PubMed]

42. Puttfarcken, P.S.; Han, P.; Joshi, S.K.; Neelands, T.R.; Gauvin, D.M.; Baker, S.J.; Lewis, L.G.; Bianchi, B.R.; Mikusa, J.P.; Koenig, J.R.; et al. A-995662 [(*R*)-8-(4-methyl-5-(4-(trifluoromethyl)phenyl)oxazol-2-ylamino)-1,2,3,4-tetrahydr onaphthalen-2-ol], a novel, selective TRPV1 receptor antagonist, reduces spinal release of glutamate and CGRP in a rat knee joint pain model. *Pain* **2010**, *150*, 319–326. [CrossRef] [PubMed]

43. Ghilardi, J.R.; Rohrich, H.; Lindsay, T.H.; Sevcik, M.A.; Schwei, M.J.; Kubota, K.; Halvorson, K.G.; Poblete, J.; Chaplan, S.R.; Dubin, A.E.; et al. Selective blockade of the capsaicin receptor TRPV1 attenuates bone cancer pain. *J. Neurosci.* **2005**, *25*, 3126–3131. [CrossRef] [PubMed]

44. Niiyama, Y.; Kawamata, T.; Yamamoto, J.; Furuse, S.; Namiki, A. SB366791, a TRPV1 antagonist, potentiates analgesic effects of systemic morphine in a murine model of bone cancer pain. *Br. J. Anaesth.* **2009**, *102*, 251–258. [CrossRef] [PubMed]

45. Lee, Y.; Hong, S.; Cui, M.; Sharma, P.K.; Lee, J.; Choi, S. Transient receptor potential vanilloid type 1 antagonists: A patent review (2011–2014). *Expert Opin. Ther. Pat.* **2015**, *25*, 291–318. [CrossRef] [PubMed]

46. Rami, H.K.; Gunthorpe, M.J. The therapeutic potential of TRPV1 (VR1) antagonists: Clinical answers await. *Drug Disc. Today Ther. Strateg.* **2004**. [CrossRef]

47. McGaraughty, S.; Chu, K.L.; Faltynek, C.R.; Jarvis, M.F. Systemic and site-specific effects of a-425619, a selective TRPV1 receptor antagonist, on wide dynamic range neurons in CFA-treated and uninjured rats. *J. Neurophysiol.* **2006**, *95*, 18–25. [CrossRef] [PubMed]

48. Cevikbas, F.; Wang, X.; Akiyama, T.; Kempkes, C.; Savinko, T.; Antal, A.; Kukova, G.; Buhl, T.; Ikoma, A.; Buddenkotte, J.; et al. A sensory neuron-expressed IL-31 receptor mediates T helper cell-dependent itch: Involvement of TRPV1 and TRPA1. *J. Allergy Clin. Immunol.* **2014**, *133*, 448–460. [CrossRef] [PubMed]

49. Shim, W.S.; Tak, M.H.; Lee, M.H.; Kim, M.; Kim, M.; Koo, J.Y.; Lee, C.H.; Kim, M.; Oh, U. TRPV1 mediates histamine-induced itching via the activation of phospholipase A2 and 12-lipoxygenase. *J. Neurosci.* **2007**, *27*, 2331–2337. [CrossRef] [PubMed]

50. Kim, S.; Barry, D.M.; Liu, X.Y.; Yin, S.; Munanairi, A.; Meng, Q.T.; Cheng, W.; Mo, P.; Wan, L.; Liu, S.B.; et al. Facilitation of TRPV4 by TRPV1 is required for itch transmission in some sensory neuron populations. *Sci. Signal.* **2016**, *9*, ra71. [CrossRef] [PubMed]

51. Geppetti, P.; Nassini, R.; Materazzi, S.; Benemei, S. The concept of neurogenic inflammation. *BJU Int.* **2008**, *101* (Suppl. 3), 2–6. [CrossRef] [PubMed]

52. Inoue, K.; Koizumi, S.; Fuziwara, S.; Denda, S.; Inoue, K.; Denda, M. Functional vanilloid receptors in cultured normal human epidermal keratinocytes. *Biochem. Biophys. Res. Commun.* **2002**, *291*, 124–129. [CrossRef] [PubMed]

53. Chung, M.K.; Lee, H.; Caterina, M.J. Warm temperatures activate TRPV4 in mouse 308 keratinocytes. *J. Biol. Chem.* **2003**, *278*, 32037–32046. [CrossRef] [PubMed]

54. Chung, M.K.; Lee, H.; Mizuno, A.; Suzuki, M.; Caterina, M.J. TRPV3 and TRPV4 mediate warmth-evoked currents in primary mouse keratinocytes. *J. Biol. Chem.* **2004**, *279*, 21569–21575. [CrossRef] [PubMed]

55. Southall, M.D.; Li, T.; Gharibova, L.S.; Pei, Y.; Nicol, G.D.; Travers, J.B. Activation of epidermal vanilloid receptor-1 induces release of proinflammatory mediators in human keratinocytes. *J. Pharmacol. Exp. Ther.* **2003**, *304*, 217–222. [CrossRef] [PubMed]

56. Yun, J.W.; Seo, J.A.; Jeong, Y.S.; Bae, I.H.; Jang, W.H.; Lee, J.; Kim, S.Y.; Shin, S.S.; Woo, B.Y.; Lee, K.W.; et al. TRPV1 antagonist can suppress the atopic dermatitis-like symptoms by accelerating skin barrier recovery. *J. Dermatol. Sci* **2011**, *62*, 8–15. [CrossRef] [PubMed]

57. Li, W.H.; Lee, Y.M.; Kim, J.Y.; Kang, S.; Kim, S.; Kim, K.H.; Park, C.H.; Chung, J.H. Transient receptor potential vanilloid-1 mediates heat-shock-induced matrix metalloproteinase-1 expression in human epidermal keratinocytes. *J. Investig. Dermatol.* **2007**, *127*, 2328–2335. [CrossRef] [PubMed]

58. Stander, S.; Moormann, C.; Schumacher, M.; Buddenkotte, J.; Artuc, M.; Shpacovitch, V.; Brzoska, T.; Lippert, U.; Henz, B.M.; Luger, T.A.; et al. Expression of vanilloid receptor subtype 1 in cutaneous sensory nerve fibers, mast cells, and epithelial cells of appendage structures. *Exp. Dermatol.* **2004**, *13*, 129–139. [CrossRef] [PubMed]

59. Denda, M.; Sokabe, T.; Fukumi-Tominaga, T.; Tominaga, M. Effects of skin surface temperature on epidermal permeability barrier homeostasis. *J. Investig. Dermatol.* **2007**, *127*, 654–659. [CrossRef] [PubMed]

60. Lim, K.M.; Park, Y.H. Development of PAC-14028, a novel transient receptor potential vanilloid type 1 (TRPV1) channel antagonist as a new drug for refractory skin diseases. *Arch. Pharm. Res.* **2012**, *35*, 393–396. [CrossRef] [PubMed]

61. Yun, J.W.; Seo, J.A.; Jang, W.H.; Koh, H.J.; Bae, I.H.; Park, Y.H.; Lim, K.M. Antipruritic effects of TRPV1 antagonist in murine atopic dermatitis and itching models. *J. Investig. Dermatol.* **2011**, *131*, 1576–1579. [CrossRef] [PubMed]

62. Banvolgyi, A.; Palinkas, L.; Berki, T.; Clark, N.; Grant, A.D.; Helyes, Z.; Pozsgai, G.; Szolcsanyi, J.; Brain, S.D.; Pinter, E. Evidence for a novel protective role of the vanilloid TRPV1 receptor in a cutaneous contact allergic dermatitis model. *J. Neuroimmunol.* **2005**, *169*, 86–96. [CrossRef] [PubMed]

63. Lee, Y.M.; Kim, Y.K.; Kim, K.H.; Park, S.J.; Kim, S.J.; Chung, J.H. A novel role for the TRPV1 channel in UV-induced matrix metalloproteinase (MMP)-1 expression in HaCaT cells. *J. Cell. Physiol.* **2009**, *219*, 766–775. [CrossRef] [PubMed]

64. Lee, Y.M.; Kang, S.M.; Lee, S.R.; Kong, K.H.; Lee, J.Y.; Kim, E.J.; Chung, J.H. Inhibitory effects of TRPV1 blocker on UV-induced responses in the hairless mice. *Arch. Dermatol. Res.* **2011**, *303*, 727–736. [CrossRef] [PubMed]

65. Sulk, M.; Seeliger, S.; Aubert, J.; Schwab, V.D.; Cevikbas, F.; Rivier, M.; Nowak, P.; Voegel, J.J.; Buddenkotte, J.; Steinhoff, M. Distribution and expression of non-neuronal transient receptor potential (TRPV) ion channels in rosacea. *J. Investig. Dermatol.* **2012**, *132*, 1253–1262. [CrossRef] [PubMed]

66. Han, S.B.; Kim, H.; Cho, S.H.; Lee, J.D.; Chung, J.H.; Kim, H.S. Transient receptor potential vanilloid-1 in epidermal keratinocytes may contribute to acute pain in herpes zoster. *Acta Derm. Venereol.* **2016**, *96*, 319–322. [CrossRef] [PubMed]

67. Ehnis-Perez, A.; Torres-Alvarez, B.; Cortes-Garcia, D.; Hernandez-Blanco, D.; Fuentes-Ahumada, C.; Castanedo-Cazares, J.P. Relationship between transient receptor potential vanilloid-1 expression and the intensity of sensitive skin symptoms. *J. Cosmet. Dermatol.* **2016**, *15*, 231–237. [CrossRef] [PubMed]

68. Li, D.G.; Du, H.Y.; Gerhard, S.; Imke, M.; Liu, W. Inhibition of TRPV1 prevented skin irritancy induced by phenoxyethanol. A preliminary in vitro and in vivo study. *Int. J. Cosmet. Sci.* **2016**. [CrossRef]

69. Yin, S.; Luo, J.; Qian, A.; Du, J.; Yang, Q.; Zhou, S.; Yu, W.; Du, G.; Clark, R.B.; Walters, E.T.; et al. Retinoids activate the irritant receptor TRPV1 and produce sensory hypersensitivity. *J. Clin. Investig.* **2013**, *123*, 3941–3951. [CrossRef] [PubMed]

70. Hwang, M.K.; Bode, A.M.; Byun, S.; Song, N.R.; Lee, H.J.; Lee, K.W.; Dong, Z. Cocarcinogenic effect of capsaicin involves activation of EGFR signaling but not TRPV1. *Cancer Res.* **2010**, *70*, 6859–6869. [CrossRef] [PubMed]

71. Li, S.; Bode, A.M.; Zhu, F.; Liu, K.; Zhang, J.; Kim, M.O.; Reddy, K.; Zykova, T.; Ma, W.Y.; Carper, A.L.; et al. TRPV1-antagonist AMG9810 promotes mouse skin tumorigenesis through EGFR/akt signaling. *Carcinogenesis* **2011**, *32*, 779–785. [CrossRef] [PubMed]

72. Bodo, E.; Biro, T.; Telek, A.; Czifra, G.; Griger, Z.; Toth, B.I.; Mescalchin, A.; Ito, T.; Bettermann, A.; Kovacs, L.; et al. A hot new twist to hair biology: Involvement of vanilloid receptor-1 (VR1/TRPV1) signaling in human hair growth control. *Am. J. Pathol.* **2005**, *166*, 985–998. [CrossRef]

73. Biro, T.; Bodo, E.; Telek, A.; Geczy, T.; Tychsen, B.; Kovacs, L.; Paus, R. Hair cycle control by vanilloid receptor-1 (TRPV1): Evidence from TRPV1 knockout mice. *J. Investig. Dermatol.* **2006**, *126*, 1909–1912. [CrossRef] [PubMed]

74. Toth, B.I.; Benko, S.; Szollosi, A.G.; Kovacs, L.; Rajnavolgyi, E.; Biro, T. Transient receptor potential vanilloid-1 signaling inhibits differentiation and activation of human dendritic cells. *FEBS Lett.* **2009**, *583*, 1619–1624. [CrossRef] [PubMed]

75. Kanzaki, M.; Zhang, Y.Q.; Mashima, H.; Li, L.; Shibata, H.; Kojima, I. Translocation of a calcium-permeable cation channel induced by insulin-like growth factor-i. *Nat. Cell Biol.* **1999**, *1*, 165–170. [PubMed]

76. Caterina, M.J.; Rosen, T.A.; Tominaga, M.; Brake, A.J.; Julius, D. A capsaicin receptor homologue with a high threshold for noxious heat. *Nature* **1999**, *398*, 436–441. [PubMed]

77. Penna, A.; Juvin, V.; Chemin, J.; Compan, V.; Monet, M.; Rassendren, F.A. Pi3-kinase promotes TRPV2 activity independently of channel translocation to the plasma membrane. *Cell Calcium* **2006**, *39*, 495–507. [CrossRef] [PubMed]

78. Qin, N.; Neeper, M.P.; Liu, Y.; Hutchinson, T.L.; Lubin, M.L.; Flores, C.M. TRPV2 is activated by cannabidiol and mediates CGRP release in cultured rat dorsal root ganglion neurons. *J. Neurosci.* **2008**, *28*, 6231–6238. [CrossRef] [PubMed]

79. Bang, S.; Kim, K.Y.; Yoo, S.; Lee, S.H.; Hwang, S.W. Transient receptor potential V2 expressed in sensory neurons is activated by probenecid. *Neurosci. Lett.* **2007**, *425*, 120–125. [CrossRef] [PubMed]

80. Muraki, K.; Iwata, Y.; Katanosaka, Y.; Ito, T.; Ohya, S.; Shigekawa, M.; Imaizumi, Y. TRPV2 is a component of osmotically sensitive cation channels in murine aortic myocytes. *Circ. Res.* **2003**, *93*, 829–838. [CrossRef] [PubMed]

81. Shibasaki, K.; Murayama, N.; Ono, K.; Ishizaki, Y.; Tominaga, M. TRPV2 enhances axon outgrowth through its activation by membrane stretch in developing sensory and motor neurons. *J. Neurosci.* **2010**, *30*, 4601–4612. [CrossRef] [PubMed]

82. Park, U.; Vastani, N.; Guan, Y.; Raja, S.N.; Koltzenburg, M.; Caterina, M.J. TRP vanilloid 2 knock-out mice are susceptible to perinatal lethality but display normal thermal and mechanical nociception. *J. Neurosci.* **2011**, *31*, 11425–11436. [CrossRef] [PubMed]

83. Neeper, M.P.; Liu, Y.; Hutchinson, T.L.; Wang, Y.; Flores, C.M.; Qin, N. Activation properties of heterologously expressed mammalian TRPV2: Evidence for species dependence. *J. Biol. Chem.* **2007**, *282*, 15894–15902. [CrossRef] [PubMed]

84. Cohen, M.R.; Johnson, W.M.; Pilat, J.M.; Kiselar, J.; DeFrancesco-Lisowitz, A.; Zigmond, R.E.; Moiseenkova-Bell, V.Y. Nerve growth factor regulates transient receptor potential vanilloid 2 via extracellular signal-regulated kinase signaling to enhance neurite outgrowth in developing neurons. *Mol. Cell. Biol.* **2015**, *35*, 4238–4252. [CrossRef] [PubMed]

85. Santoni, G.; Farfariello, V.; Liberati, S.; Morelli, M.B.; Nabissi, M.; Santoni, M.; Amantini, C. The role of transient receptor potential vanilloid type-2 ion channels in innate and adaptive immune responses. *Front. Immunol.* **2013**, *4*, 34. [CrossRef] [PubMed]

86. Yamashiro, K.; Sasano, T.; Tojo, K.; Namekata, I.; Kurokawa, J.; Sawada, N.; Suganami, T.; Kamei, Y.; Tanaka, H.; Tajima, N.; et al. Role of transient receptor potential vanilloid 2 in LPS-induced cytokine production in macrophages. *Biochem. Biophys. Res. Commun.* **2010**, *398*, 284–289. [CrossRef] [PubMed]

87. Link, T.M.; Park, U.; Vonakis, B.M.; Raben, D.M.; Soloski, M.J.; Caterina, M.J. TRPV2 has a pivotal role in macrophage particle binding and phagocytosis. *Nat. Immunol.* **2010**, *11*, 232–239. [CrossRef] [PubMed]

88. Nagasawa, M.; Nakagawa, Y.; Tanaka, S.; Kojima, I. Chemotactic peptide fmetleuphe induces translocation of the TRPV2 channel in macrophages. *J. Cell. Physiol.* **2007**, *210*, 692–702. [CrossRef] [PubMed]

89. Szollosi, A.G.; Olah, A.; Toth, I.B.; Papp, F.; Czifra, G.; Panyi, G.; Biro, T. Transient receptor potential vanilloid-2 mediates the effects of transient heat shock on endocytosis of human monocyte-derived dendritic cells. *FEBS Lett.* **2013**, *587*, 1440–1445. [CrossRef] [PubMed]

90. Compan, V.; Baroja-Mazo, A.; Lopez-Castejon, G.; Gomez, A.I.; Martinez, C.M.; Angosto, D.; Montero, M.T.; Herranz, A.S.; Bazan, E.; Reimers, D.; et al. Cell volume regulation modulates NLRP3 inflammasome activation. *Immunity* **2012**, *37*, 487–500. [CrossRef] [PubMed]

91. Nagasawa, M.; Kojima, I. Translocation of calcium-permeable TRPV2 channel to the podosome: Its role in the regulation of podosome assembly. *Cell Calcium* **2012**, *51*, 186–193. [CrossRef] [PubMed]

92. Liberati, S.; Morelli, M.B.; Amantini, C.; Farfariello, V.; Santoni, M.; Conti, A.; Nabissi, M.; Cascinu, S.; Santoni, G. Loss of TRPV2 homeostatic control of cell proliferation drives tumor progression. *Cells* **2014**, *3*, 112–128. [CrossRef] [PubMed]

93. Morelli, M.B.; Liberati, S.; Amantini, C.; Nabiss, M.; Santoni, M.; Farfariello, V.; Santoni, G. Expression and function of the transient receptor potential ion channel family in the hematologic malignancies. *Curr. Mol. Pharmacol.* **2013**, *6*, 137–148. [CrossRef] [PubMed]

94. Peier, A.M.; Reeve, A.J.; Andersson, D.A.; Moqrich, A.; Earley, T.J.; Hergarden, A.C.; Story, G.M.; Colley, S.; Hogenesch, J.B.; McIntyre, P.; et al. A heat-sensitive TRP channel expressed in keratinocytes. *Science* **2002**, *296*, 2046–2049. [CrossRef] [PubMed]

95. Smith, G.D.; Gunthorpe, M.J.; Kelsell, R.E.; Hayes, P.D.; Reilly, P.; Facer, P.; Wright, J.E.; Jerman, J.C.; Walhin, J.P.; Ooi, L.; et al. TRPV3 is a temperature-sensitive vanilloid receptor-like protein. *Nature* **2002**, *418*, 186–190. [CrossRef] [PubMed]

96. Xu, H.; Ramsey, I.S.; Kotecha, S.A.; Moran, M.M.; Chong, J.A.; Lawson, D.; Ge, P.; Lilly, J.; Silos-Santiago, I.; Xie, Y.; et al. TRPV3 is a calcium-permeable temperature-sensitive cation channel. *Nature* **2002**, *418*, 181–186. [CrossRef] [PubMed]

97. Chung, M.K.; Lee, H.; Mizuno, A.; Suzuki, M.; Caterina, M.J. 2-aminoethoxydiphenyl borate activates and sensitizes the heat-gated ion channel TRPV3. *J. Neurosci.* **2004**, *24*, 5177–5182. [CrossRef] [PubMed]

98. Bang, S.; Yoo, S.; Yang, T.J.; Cho, H.; Hwang, S.W. Farnesyl pyrophosphate is a novel pain-producing molecule via specific activation of TRPV3. *J. Biol. Chem.* **2010**, *285*, 19362–19371. [CrossRef] [PubMed]

99. Moqrich, A.; Hwang, S.W.; Earley, T.J.; Petrus, M.J.; Murray, A.N.; Spencer, K.S.; Andahazy, M.; Story, G.M.; Patapoutian, A. Impaired thermosensation in mice lacking TRPV3, a heat and camphor sensor in the skin. *Science* **2005**, *307*, 1468–1472. [CrossRef] [PubMed]

100. Xu, H.; Delling, M.; Jun, J.C.; Clapham, D.E. Oregano, thyme and clove-derived flavors and skin sensitizers activate specific TRP channels. *Nat. Neurosci.* **2006**, *9*, 628–635. [CrossRef] [PubMed]

101. Hu, H.Z.; Xiao, R.; Wang, C.; Gao, N.; Colton, C.K.; Wood, J.D.; Zhu, M.X. Potentiation of TRPV3 channel function by unsaturated fatty acids. *J. Cell. Physiol.* **2006**, *208*, 201–212. [CrossRef] [PubMed]

102. Klein, A.S.; Tannert, A.; Schaefer, M. Cholesterol sensitises the transient receptor potential channel TRPV3 to lower temperatures and activator concentrations. *Cell Calcium* **2014**, *55*, 59–68. [CrossRef] [PubMed]

103. Karttunen, S.; Duffield, M.; Scrimgeour, N.R.; Squires, L.; Lim, W.L.; Dallas, M.L.; Scragg, J.L.; Chicher, J.; Dave, K.A.; Whitelaw, M.L.; et al. Oxygen-dependent hydroxylation by fih regulates the TRPV3 ion channel. *J. Cell Sci.* **2015**, *128*, 225–231. [CrossRef] [PubMed]

104. Mandadi, S.; Sokabe, T.; Shibasaki, K.; Katanosaka, K.; Mizuno, A.; Moqrich, A.; Patapoutian, A.; Fukumi-Tominaga, T.; Mizumura, K.; Tominaga, M. TRPV3 in keratinocytes transmits temperature information to sensory neurons via atp. *Pflugers Arch.* **2009**, *458*, 1093–1102. [CrossRef] [PubMed]

105. Miyamoto, T.; Petrus, M.J.; Dubin, A.E.; Patapoutian, A. TRPV3 regulates nitric oxide synthase-independent nitric oxide synthesis in the skin. *Nat. Commun.* **2011**, *2*, 369. [CrossRef] [PubMed]

106. Huang, S.M.; Lee, H.; Chung, M.K.; Park, U.; Yu, Y.Y.; Bradshaw, H.B.; Coulombe, P.A.; Walker, J.M.; Caterina, M.J. Overexpressed transient receptor potential vanilloid 3 ion channels in skin keratinocytes modulate pain sensitivity via prostaglandin E2. *J. Neurosci.* **2008**, *28*, 13727–13737. [CrossRef] [PubMed]

107. Huang, S.M.; Li, X.; Yu, Y.; Wang, J.; Caterina, M.J. TRPV3 and TRPV4 ion channels are not major contributors to mouse heat sensation. *Mol. Pain* **2011**, *7*, 37. [CrossRef] [PubMed]

108. Marics, I.; Malapert, P.; Reynders, A.; Gaillard, S.; Moqrich, A. Acute heat-evoked temperature sensation is impaired but not abolished in mice lacking TRPV1 and TRPV3 channels. *PLoS ONE* **2014**, *9*, e99828. [CrossRef] [PubMed]

109. Cheng, X.; Jin, J.; Hu, L.; Shen, D.; Dong, X.P.; Samie, M.A.; Knoff, J.; Eisinger, B.; Liu, M.L.; Huang, S.M.; et al. TRP channel regulates EGFR signaling in hair morphogenesis and skin barrier formation. *Cell* **2010**, *141*, 331–343. [CrossRef] [PubMed]

110. Borbiro, I.; Lisztes, E.; Toth, B.I.; Czifra, G.; Olah, A.; Szollosi, A.G.; Szentandrassy, N.; Nanasi, P.P.; Peter, Z.; Paus, R.; et al. Activation of transient receptor potential vanilloid-3 inhibits human hair growth. *J. Investig. Dermatol.* **2011**, *131*, 1605–1614. [CrossRef] [PubMed]

111. Broad, L.M.; Mogg, A.J.; Eberle, E.; Tolley, M.; Li, D.L.; Knopp, K.L. TRPV3 in drug development. *Pharmaceuticals* **2016**, *9*. [CrossRef] [PubMed]

112. Yamamoto-Kasai, E.; Imura, K.; Yasui, K.; Shichijou, M.; Oshima, I.; Hirasawa, T.; Sakata, T.; Yoshioka, T. TRPV3 as a therapeutic target for itch. *J. Investig. Dermatol.* **2012**, *132*, 2109–2112. [CrossRef] [PubMed]

113. Gopinath, P.; Wan, E.; Holdcroft, A.; Facer, P.; Davis, J.B.; Smith, G.D.; Bountra, C.; Anand, P. Increased capsaicin receptor TRPV1 in skin nerve fibres and related vanilloid receptors TRPV3 and TRPV4 in keratinocytes in human breast pain. *BMC Womens Health* **2005**, *5*, 2. [CrossRef] [PubMed]

114. Kim, H.O.; Cho, Y.S.; Park, S.Y.; Kwak, I.S.; Choi, M.G.; Chung, B.Y.; Park, C.W.; Lee, J.Y. Increased activity of TRPV3 in keratinocytes in hypertrophic burn scars with postburn pruritus. *Wound Repair Regen.* **2016**, *24*, 841–850. [CrossRef] [PubMed]

115. Aijima, R.; Wang, B.; Takao, T.; Mihara, H.; Kashio, M.; Ohsaki, Y.; Zhang, J.Q.; Mizuno, A.; Suzuki, M.; Yamashita, Y.; et al. The thermosensitive TRPV3 channel contributes to rapid wound healing in oral epithelia. *FASEB J.* **2015**, *29*, 182–192. [CrossRef] [PubMed]

116. Asakawa, M.; Yoshioka, T.; Matsutani, T.; Hikita, I.; Suzuki, M.; Oshima, I.; Tsukahara, K.; Arimura, A.; Horikawa, T.; Hirasawa, T.; et al. Association of a mutation in TRPV3 with defective hair growth in rodents. *J. Investig. Dermatol.* **2006**, *126*, 2664–2672. [CrossRef] [PubMed]

117. Imura, K.; Yoshioka, T.; Hikita, I.; Tsukahara, K.; Hirasawa, T.; Higashino, K.; Gahara, Y.; Arimura, A.; Sakata, T. Influence of TRPV3 mutation on hair growth cycle in mice. *Biochem. Biophys. Res. Commun.* **2007**, *363*, 479–483. [CrossRef] [PubMed]

118. Xiao, R.; Tian, J.; Tang, J.; Zhu, M.X. The TRPV3 mutation associated with the hairless phenotype in rodents is constitutively active. *Cell Calcium* **2008**, *43*, 334–343. [CrossRef] [PubMed]

119. Imura, K.; Yoshioka, T.; Hirasawa, T.; Sakata, T. Role of TRPV3 in immune response to development of dermatitis. *J. Inflamm. (Lond.)* **2009**, *6*, 17. [CrossRef] [PubMed]

120. Lin, Z.; Chen, Q.; Lee, M.; Cao, X.; Zhang, J.; Ma, D.; Chen, L.; Hu, X.; Wang, H.; Wang, X.; et al. Exome sequencing reveals mutations in TRPV3 as a cause of olmsted syndrome. *Am. J. Hum. Genet.* **2012**, *90*, 558–564. [CrossRef] [PubMed]

121. Wilson, N.J.; Cole, C.; Milstone, L.M.; Kiszewski, A.E.; Hansen, C.D.; O'Toole, E.A.; Schwartz, M.E.; McLean, W.H.; Smith, F.J. Expanding the phenotypic spectrum of olmsted syndrome. *J. Investig. Dermatol.* **2015**, *135*, 2879–2883. [CrossRef] [PubMed]

122. He, Y.; Zeng, K.; Zhang, X.; Chen, Q.; Wu, J.; Li, H.; Zhou, Y.; Glusman, G.; Roach, J.; Etheridge, A.; et al. A gain-of-function mutation in TRPV3 causes focal palmoplantar keratoderma in a Chinese family. *J. Investig. Dermatol.* **2015**, *135*, 907–909. [CrossRef] [PubMed]

123. Liedtke, W.; Choe, Y.; Marti-Renom, M.A.; Bell, A.M.; Denis, C.S.; Sali, A.; Hudspeth, A.J.; Friedman, J.M.; Heller, S. Vanilloid receptor-related osmotically activated channel (VR-OAC), a candidate vertebrate osmoreceptor. *Cell* **2000**, *103*, 525–535. [CrossRef]

124. Strotmann, R.; Harteneck, C.; Nunnenmacher, K.; Schultz, G.; Plant, T.D. OTRPC4, a nonselective cation channel that confers sensitivity to extracellular osmolarity. *Nat. Cell Biol.* **2000**, *2*, 695–702. [PubMed]

125. Wissenbach, U.; Bodding, M.; Freichel, M.; Flockerzi, V. TRP12, a novel TRP related protein from kidney. *FEBS Lett.* **2000**, *485*, 127–134. [CrossRef]

126. Watanabe, H.; Vriens, J.; Prenen, J.; Droogmans, G.; Voets, T.; Nilius, B. Anandamide and arachidonic acid use epoxyeicosatrienoic acids to activate TRPV4 channels. *Nature* **2003**, *424*, 434–438. [CrossRef] [PubMed]

127. Guler, A.D.; Lee, H.; Iida, T.; Shimizu, I.; Tominaga, M.; Caterina, M. Heat-evoked activation of the ion channel, TRPV4. *J. Neurosci.* **2002**, *22*, 6408–6414. [PubMed]

128. Kida, N.; Sokabe, T.; Kashio, M.; Haruna, K.; Mizuno, Y.; Suga, Y.; Nishikawa, K.; Kanamaru, A.; Hongo, M.; Oba, A.; et al. Importance of transient receptor potential vanilloid 4 (TRPV4) in epidermal barrier function in human skin keratinocytes. *Pflugers Arch.* **2012**, *463*, 715–725. [CrossRef] [PubMed]

129. Akazawa, Y.; Yuki, T.; Yoshida, H.; Sugiyama, Y.; Inoue, S. Activation of TRPV4 strengthens the tight-junction barrier in human epidermal keratinocytes. *Skin Pharmacol. Physiol.* **2013**, *26*, 15–21. [CrossRef] [PubMed]

130. Fusi, C.; Materazzi, S.; Minocci, D.; Maio, V.; Oranges, T.; Massi, D.; Nassini, R. Transient receptor potential vanilloid 4 (TRPV4) is downregulated in keratinocytes in human non-melanoma skin cancer. *J. Investig. Dermatol.* **2014**, *134*, 2408–2417. [CrossRef] [PubMed]

131. Alessandri-Haber, N.; Joseph, E.; Dina, O.A.; Liedtke, W.; Levine, J.D. TRPV4 mediates pain-related behavior induced by mild hypertonic stimuli in the presence of inflammatory mediator. *Pain* **2005**, *118*, 70–79. [CrossRef] [PubMed]

132. Alessandri-Haber, N.; Yeh, J.J.; Boyd, A.E.; Parada, C.A.; Chen, X.; Reichling, D.B.; Levine, J.D. Hypotonicity induces TRPV4-mediated nociception in rat. *Neuron* **2003**, *39*, 497–511. [CrossRef]

133. Liedtke, W.; Friedman, J.M. Abnormal osmotic regulation in TRPV4 −/− mice. *Proc. Natl. Acad. Sci. USA* **2003**, *100*, 13698–13703. [CrossRef] [PubMed]

134. Suzuki, M.; Mizuno, A.; Kodaira, K.; Imai, M. Impaired pressure sensation in mice lacking TRPV4. *J. Biol. Chem.* **2003**, *278*, 22664–22668. [CrossRef] [PubMed]

135. Chen, Y.; Kanju, P.; Fang, Q.; Lee, S.H.; Parekh, P.K.; Lee, W.; Moore, C.; Brenner, D.; Gereau, R.W.T.; Wang, F.; et al. TRPV4 is necessary for trigeminal irritant pain and functions as a cellular formalin receptor. *Pain* **2014**, *155*, 2662–2672. [CrossRef] [PubMed]

136. Chen, Y.; Williams, S.H.; McNulty, A.L.; Hong, J.H.; Lee, S.H.; Rothfusz, N.E.; Parekh, P.K.; Moore, C.; Gereau, R.W., IV; Taylor, A.B.; et al. Temporomandibular joint pain: A critical role for TRPV4 in the trigeminal ganglion. *Pain* **2013**, *154*, 1295–1304. [CrossRef] [PubMed]

137. Segond von Banchet, G.; Boettger, M.K.; Konig, C.; Iwakura, Y.; Brauer, R.; Schaible, H.G. Neuronal IL-17 receptor upregulates TRPV4 but not TRPV1 receptors in DRG neurons and mediates mechanical but not thermal hyperalgesia. *Mol. Cell. Neurosci.* **2013**, *52*, 152–160. [CrossRef] [PubMed]

138. Alessandri-Haber, N.; Dina, O.A.; Yeh, J.J.; Parada, C.A.; Reichling, D.B.; Levine, J.D. Transient receptor potential vanilloid 4 is essential in chemotherapy-induced neuropathic pain in the rat. *J. Neurosci.* **2004**, *24*, 4444–4452. [CrossRef] [PubMed]

139. Chen, Y.; Yang, C.; Wang, Z.J. Proteinase-activated receptor 2 sensitizes transient receptor potential vanilloid 1, transient receptor potential vanilloid 4, and transient receptor potential ankyrin 1 in paclitaxel-induced neuropathic pain. *Neuroscience* **2011**, *193*, 440–451. [CrossRef] [PubMed]

140. Ding, X.L.; Wang, Y.H.; Ning, L.P.; Zhang, Y.; Ge, H.Y.; Jiang, H.; Wang, R.; Yue, S.W. Involvement of TRPV4-NO-cGMP-PKG pathways in the development of thermal hyperalgesia following chronic compression of the dorsal root ganglion in rats. *Behav. Brain Res.* **2010**, *208*, 194–201. [CrossRef] [PubMed]

141. Grant, A.D.; Cottrell, G.S.; Amadesi, S.; Trevisani, M.; Nicoletti, P.; Materazzi, S.; Altier, C.; Cenac, N.; Zamponi, G.W.; Bautista-Cruz, F.; et al. Protease-activated receptor 2 sensitizes the transient receptor potential vanilloid 4 ion channel to cause mechanical hyperalgesia in mice. *J. Physiol.* **2007**, *578 Pt 3*, 715–733. [CrossRef] [PubMed]

142. Moore, C.; Cevikbas, F.; Pasolli, H.A.; Chen, Y.; Kong, W.; Kempkes, C.; Parekh, P.; Lee, S.H.; Kontchou, N.A.; Yeh, I.; et al. Uvb radiation generates sunburn pain and affects skin by activating epidermal TRPV4 ion channels and triggering endothelin-1 signaling. *Proc. Natl. Acad. Sci. USA* **2013**, *110*, E3225–3234. [CrossRef] [PubMed]

143. Akiyama, T.; Ivanov, M.; Nagamine, M.; Davoodi, A.; Carstens, M.I.; Ikoma, A.; Cevikbas, F.; Kempkes, C.; Buddenkotte, J.; Steinhoff, M.; et al. Involvement of TRPV4 in serotonin-evoked scratching. *J. Investig. Dermatol.* **2016**, *136*, 154–160. [CrossRef] [PubMed]

144. Chen, Y.; Fang, Q.; Wang, Z.; Zhang, J.Y.; MacLeod, A.S.; Hall, R.P.; Liedtke, W.B. Transient receptor potential vanilloid 4 ion channel functions as a pruriceptor in epidermal keratinocytes to evoke histaminergic itch. *J. Biol. Chem.* **2016**, *291*, 10252–10262. [CrossRef] [PubMed]

145. Lee, H.; Iida, T.; Mizuno, A.; Suzuki, M.; Caterina, M.J. Altered thermal selection behavior in mice lacking transient receptor potential vanilloid 4. *J. Neurosci.* **2005**, *25*, 1304–1310. [CrossRef] [PubMed]

146. Auer-Grumbach, M.; Olschewski, A.; Papic, L.; Kremer, H.; McEntagart, M.E.; Uhrig, S.; Fischer, C.; Frohlich, E.; Balint, Z.; Tang, B.; et al. Alterations in the ankyrin domain of TRPV4 cause congenital distal SMA, scapuloperoneal SMA and HMSN2C. *Nat. Genet.* **2010**, *42*, 160–164. [CrossRef] [PubMed]

147. Deng, H.X.; Klein, C.J.; Yan, J.; Shi, Y.; Wu, Y.; Fecto, F.; Yau, H.J.; Yang, Y.; Zhai, H.; Siddique, N.; et al. Scapuloperoneal spinal muscular atrophy and CMT2C are allelic disorders caused by alterations in TRPV4. *Nat. Genet.* **2010**, *42*, 165–169. [CrossRef] [PubMed]

148. Landoure, G.; Zdebik, A.A.; Martinez, T.L.; Burnett, B.G.; Stanescu, H.C.; Inada, H.; Shi, Y.; Taye, A.A.; Kong, L.; Munns, C.H.; et al. Mutations in TRPV4 cause charcot-marie-tooth disease type 2C. *Nat. Genet.* **2010**, *42*, 170–174. [CrossRef] [PubMed]

149. Lehen'kyi, V.; Vandenberghe, M.; Belaubre, F.; Julie, S.; Castex-Rizzi, N.; Skryma, R.; Prevarskaya, N. Acceleration of keratinocyte differentiation by transient receptor potential vanilloid (TRPV6) channel activation. *J. Eur. Acad. Dermatol. Venereol.* **2011**, *25* (Suppl. 1), 12–18. [CrossRef] [PubMed]

150. Bianco, S.D.; Peng, J.B.; Takanaga, H.; Suzuki, Y.; Crescenzi, A.; Kos, C.H.; Zhuang, L.; Freeman, M.R.; Gouveia, C.H.; Wu, J.; et al. Marked disturbance of calcium homeostasis in mice with targeted disruption of the TRPV6 calcium channel gene. *J. Bone Miner. Res.* **2007**, *22*, 274–285. [CrossRef] [PubMed]

151. Peng, J.B.; Zhuang, L.; Berger, U.V.; Adam, R.M.; Williams, B.J.; Brown, E.M.; Hediger, M.A.; Freeman, M.R. CAT1 expression correlates with tumor grade in prostate cancer. *Biochem. Biophys. Res. Commun.* **2001**, *282*, 729–734. [CrossRef] [PubMed]

152. Nilius, B.; Appendino, G.; Owsianik, G. The transient receptor potential channel TRPA1: From gene to pathophysiology. *Pflugers Arch.* **2012**, *464*, 425–458. [CrossRef] [PubMed]

153. Kwon, Y.; Shim, H.S.; Wang, X.; Montell, C. Control of thermotactic behavior via coupling of a TRP channel to a phospholipase C signaling cascade. *Nat. Neurosci.* **2008**, *11*, 871–873. [CrossRef] [PubMed]

154. Rosenzweig, M.; Brennan, K.M.; Tayler, T.D.; Phelps, P.O.; Patapoutian, A.; Garrity, P.A. The Drosophila ortholog of vertebrate TRPA1 regulates thermotaxis. *Genes Dev.* **2005**, *19*, 419–424. [CrossRef] [PubMed]

155. Viswanath, V.; Story, G.M.; Peier, A.M.; Petrus, M.J.; Lee, V.M.; Hwang, S.W.; Patapoutian, A.; Jegla, T. Opposite thermosensor in fruitfly and mouse. *Nature* **2003**, *423*, 822–823. [CrossRef] [PubMed]

156. Gracheva, E.O.; Ingolia, N.T.; Kelly, Y.M.; Cordero-Morales, J.F.; Hollopeter, G.; Chesler, A.T.; Sanchez, E.E.; Perez, J.C.; Weissman, J.S.; Julius, D. Molecular basis of infrared detection by snakes. *Nature* **2010**, *464*, 1006–1011. [CrossRef] [PubMed]

157. Story, G.M.; Peier, A.M.; Reeve, A.J.; Eid, S.R.; Mosbacher, J.; Hricik, T.R.; Earley, T.J.; Hergarden, A.C.; Andersson, D.A.; Hwang, S.W.; et al. ANKTM1, a TRP-like channel expressed in nociceptive neurons, is activated by cold temperatures. *Cell* **2003**, *112*, 819–829. [CrossRef]

158. Moparthi, L.; Survery, S.; Kreir, M.; Simonsen, C.; Kjellbom, P.; Hogestatt, E.D.; Johanson, U.; Zygmunt, P.M. Human TRPA1 is intrinsically cold- and chemosensitive with and without its N-terminal ankyrin repeat domain. *Proc. Natl. Acad. Sci. USA* **2014**, *111*, 16901–16906. [CrossRef] [PubMed]

159. Wang, S.; Lee, J.; Ro, J.Y.; Chung, M.K. Warmth suppresses and desensitizes damage-sensing ion channel TRPA1. *Mol. Pain* **2012**, *8*, 22. [CrossRef] [PubMed]

160. Moparthi, L.; Kichko, T.I.; Eberhardt, M.; Hogestatt, E.D.; Kjellbom, P.; Johanson, U.; Reeh, P.W.; Leffler, A.; Filipovic, M.R.; Zygmunt, P.M. Human TRPA1 is a heat sensor displaying intrinsic u-shaped thermosensitivity. *Sci. Rep.* **2016**, *6*, 28763. [CrossRef] [PubMed]

161. Miyake, T.; Nakamura, S.; Zhao, M.; So, K.; Inoue, K.; Numata, T.; Takahashi, N.; Shirakawa, H.; Mori, Y.; Nakagawa, T.; et al. Cold sensitivity of TRPA1 is unveiled by the prolyl hydroxylation blockade-induced sensitization to ROS. *Nat. Commun.* **2016**, *7*, 12840. [CrossRef] [PubMed]

162. Meseguer, V.; Alpizar, Y.A.; Luis, E.; Tajada, S.; Denlinger, B.; Fajardo, O.; Manenschijn, J.A.; Fernandez-Pena, C.; Talavera, A.; Kichko, T.; et al. TRPA1 channels mediate acute neurogenic inflammation and pain produced by bacterial endotoxins. *Nat. Commun.* **2014**, *5*, 3125. [CrossRef] [PubMed]

163. Park, C.K.; Xu, Z.Z.; Berta, T.; Han, Q.; Chen, G.; Liu, X.J.; Ji, R.R. Extracellular micrornas activate nociceptor neurons to elicit pain via TLR7 and TRPA1. *Neuron* **2014**, *82*, 47–54. [CrossRef] [PubMed]

164. Kerstein, P.C.; del Camino, D.; Moran, M.M.; Stucky, C.L. Pharmacological blockade of TRPA1 inhibits mechanical firing in nociceptors. *Mol. Pain* **2009**, *5*, 19. [CrossRef] [PubMed]

165. Kwan, K.Y.; Glazer, J.M.; Corey, D.P.; Rice, F.L.; Stucky, C.L. TRPA1 modulates mechanotransduction in cutaneous sensory neurons. *J. Neurosci.* **2009**, *29*, 4808–4819. [CrossRef] [PubMed]

166. Lennertz, R.C.; Kossyreva, E.A.; Smith, A.K.; Stucky, C.L. TRPA1 mediates mechanical sensitization in nociceptors during inflammation. *PLoS ONE* **2012**, *7*, e43597. [CrossRef] [PubMed]

167. Zhang, X.F.; Chen, J.; Faltynek, C.R.; Moreland, R.B.; Neelands, T.R. Transient receptor potential A1 mediates an osmotically activated ion channel. *Eur. J. Neurosci.* **2008**, *27*, 605–611. [CrossRef] [PubMed]

168. Bautista, D.M.; Jordt, S.E.; Nikai, T.; Tsuruda, P.R.; Read, A.J.; Poblete, J.; Yamoah, E.N.; Basbaum, A.I.; Julius, D. TRPA1 mediates the inflammatory actions of environmental irritants and proalgesic agents. *Cell* **2006**, *124*, 1269–1282. [CrossRef] [PubMed]

169. McNamara, C.R.; Mandel-Brehm, J.; Bautista, D.M.; Siemens, J.; Deranian, K.L.; Zhao, M.; Hayward, N.J.; Chong, J.A.; Julius, D.; Moran, M.M.; et al. TRPA1 mediates formalin-induced pain. *Proc. Natl. Acad. Sci. USA* **2007**, *104*, 13525–13530. [CrossRef] [PubMed]

170. del Camino, D.; Murphy, S.; Heiry, M.; Barrett, L.B.; Earley, T.J.; Cook, C.A.; Petrus, M.J.; Zhao, M.; D'Amours, M.; Deering, N.; et al. TRPA1 contributes to cold hypersensitivity. *J. Neurosci.* **2010**, *30*, 15165–15174. [CrossRef] [PubMed]

171. Andersson, D.A.; Gentry, C.; Light, E.; Vastani, N.; Vallortigara, J.; Bierhaus, A.; Fleming, T.; Bevan, S. Methylglyoxal evokes pain by stimulating TRPA1. *PLoS ONE* **2013**, *8*, e77986. [CrossRef]

172. Nassini, R.; Gees, M.; Harrison, S.; De Siena, G.; Materazzi, S.; Moretto, N.; Failli, P.; Preti, D.; Marchetti, N.; Cavazzini, A.; et al. Oxaliplatin elicits mechanical and cold allodynia in rodents via TRPA1 receptor stimulation. *Pain* **2011**, *152*, 1621–1631. [CrossRef] [PubMed]

173. Andersson, D.A.; Filipovic, M.R.; Gentry, C.; Eberhardt, M.; Vastani, N.; Leffler, A.; Reeh, P.; Bevan, S. Streptozotocin stimulates the ion channel TRPA1 directly: Involvement of peroxynitrite. *J. Biol. Chem.* **2015**, *290*, 15185–15196. [CrossRef] [PubMed]

174. Koivisto, A.; Hukkanen, M.; Saarnilehto, M.; Chapman, H.; Kuokkanen, K.; Wei, H.; Viisanen, H.; Akerman, K.E.; Lindstedt, K.; Pertovaara, A. Inhibiting TRPA1 ion channel reduces loss of cutaneous nerve fiber function in diabetic animals: Sustained activation of the TRPA1 channel contributes to the pathogenesis of peripheral diabetic neuropathy. *Pharmacol. Res.* **2012**, *65*, 149–158. [CrossRef] [PubMed]

175. Kremeyer, B.; Lopera, F.; Cox, J.J.; Momin, A.; Rugiero, F.; Marsh, S.; Woods, C.G.; Jones, N.G.; Paterson, K.J.; Fricker, F.R.; et al. A gain-of-function mutation in TRPA1 causes familial episodic pain syndrome. *Neuron* **2010**, *66*, 671–680. [CrossRef] [PubMed]

176. Babes, A.; Sauer, S.K.; Moparthi, L.; Kichko, T.I.; Neacsu, C.; Namer, B.; Filipovic, M.; Zygmunt, P.M.; Reeh, P.W.; Fischer, M.J. Photosensitization in porphyrias and photodynamic therapy involves TRPA1 and TRPV1. *J. Neurosci.* **2016**, *36*, 5264–5278. [CrossRef] [PubMed]

177. Wilson, S.R.; Gerhold, K.A.; Bifolck-Fisher, A.; Liu, Q.; Patel, K.N.; Dong, X.; Bautista, D.M. TRPA1 is required for histamine-independent, Mas-related G protein-coupled receptor-mediated itch. *Nat. Neurosci.* **2011**, *14*, 595–602. [CrossRef] [PubMed]

178. Wilson, S.R.; The, L.; Batia, L.M.; Beattie, K.; Katibah, G.E.; McClain, S.P.; Pellegrino, M.; Estandian, D.M.; Bautista, D.M. The epithelial cell-derived atopic dermatitis cytokine TSLP activates neurons to induce itch. *Cell* **2013**, *155*, 285–295. [CrossRef] [PubMed]

179. Lieu, T.; Jayaweera, G.; Zhao, P.; Poole, D.P.; Jensen, D.; Grace, M.; McIntyre, P.; Bron, R.; Wilson, Y.M.; Krappitz, M.; et al. The bile acid receptor TGR5 activates the TRPA1 channel to induce itch in mice. *Gastroenterology* **2014**, *147*, 1417–1428. [CrossRef] [PubMed]

180. Wilson, S.R.; Nelson, A.M.; Batia, L.; Morita, T.; Estandian, D.; Owens, D.M.; Lumpkin, E.A.; Bautista, D.M. The ion channel TRPA1 is required for chronic itch. *J. Neurosci.* **2013**, *33*, 9283–9294. [CrossRef] [PubMed]

181. Oh, M.H.; Oh, S.Y.; Lu, J.; Lou, H.; Myers, A.C.; Zhu, Z.; Zheng, T. TRPA1-dependent pruritus in IL-13-induced chronic atopic dermatitis. *J. Immunol.* **2013**, *191*, 5371–5382. [CrossRef] [PubMed]

182. Liu, B.; Escalera, J.; Balakrishna, S.; Fan, L.; Caceres, A.I.; Robinson, E.; Sui, A.; McKay, M.C.; McAlexander, M.A.; Herrick, C.A.; et al. TRPA1 controls inflammation and pruritogen responses in allergic contact dermatitis. *FASEB J.* **2013**, *27*, 3549–3563. [CrossRef] [PubMed]

183. Saarnilehto, M.; Chapman, H.; Savinko, T.; Lindstedt, K.; Lauerma, A.I.; Koivisto, A. Contact sensitizer 2,4-dinitrochlorobenzene is a highly potent human TRPA1 agonist. *Allergy* **2014**, *69*, 1424–1427. [CrossRef] [PubMed]

184. Caceres, A.I.; Brackmann, M.; Elia, M.D.; Bessac, B.F.; del Camino, D.; D'Amours, M.; Witek, J.S.; Fanger, C.M.; Chong, J.A.; Hayward, N.J.; et al. A sensory neuronal ion channel essential for airway inflammation and hyperreactivity in asthma. *Proc. Natl. Acad. Sci. USA* **2009**, *106*, 9099–9104. [CrossRef] [PubMed]

185. Denda, M.; Tsutsumi, M.; Goto, M.; Ikeyama, K.; Denda, S. Topical application of TRPA1 agonists and brief cold exposure accelerate skin permeability barrier recovery. *J. Investig. Dermatol.* **2010**, *130*, 1942–1945. [CrossRef] [PubMed]

186. Uta, D.; Furue, H.; Pickering, A.E.; Rashid, M.H.; Mizuguchi-Takase, H.; Katafuchi, T.; Imoto, K.; Yoshimura, M. TRPA1-expressing primary afferents synapse with a morphologically identified subclass of substantia gelatinosa neurons in the adult rat spinal cord. *Eur. J. Neurosci.* **2010**, *31*, 1960–1973. [CrossRef] [PubMed]

187. Chiu, I.M.; Heesters, B.A.; Ghasemlou, N.; Von Hehn, C.A.; Zhao, F.; Tran, J.; Wainger, B.; Strominger, A.; Muralidharan, S.; Horswill, A.R.; et al. Bacteria activate sensory neurons that modulate pain and inflammation. *Nature* **2013**, *501*, 52–57. [CrossRef] [PubMed]

188. Pinter, E.; Helyes, Z.; Szolcsanyi, J. Inhibitory effect of somatostatin on inflammation and nociception. *Pharmacol. Ther.* **2006**, *112*, 440–456. [CrossRef] [PubMed]

189. Zappia, K.J.; Garrison, S.R.; Palygin, O.; Weyer, A.D.; Barabas, M.E.; Lawlor, M.W.; Staruschenko, A.; Stucky, C.L. Mechanosensory and atp release deficits following keratin14-cre-mediated TRPA1 deletion despite absence of TRPA1 in murine keratinocytes. *PLoS ONE* **2016**, *11*, e0151602. [CrossRef] [PubMed]

190. Bellono, N.W.; Kammel, L.G.; Zimmerman, A.L.; Oancea, E. Uv light phototransduction activates transient receptor potential a1 ion channels in human melanocytes. *Proc. Natl. Acad. Sci. USA* **2013**, *110*, 2383–2388. [CrossRef] [PubMed]

191. Oehler, B.; Scholze, A.; Schaefer, M.; Hill, K. TRPA1 is functionally expressed in melanoma cells but is not critical for impaired proliferation caused by allyl isothiocyanate or cinnamaldehyde. *Naunyn Schmiedebergs Arch. Pharmacol.* **2012**, *385*, 555–563. [CrossRef] [PubMed]

192. Oancea, E.; Wicks, N.L. TRPM1: New trends for an old TRP. *Adv. Exp. Med. Biol.* **2011**, *704*, 135–145. [PubMed]

193. Miller, A.J.; Du, J.; Rowan, S.; Hershey, C.L.; Widlund, H.R.; Fisher, D.E. Transcriptional regulation of the melanoma prognostic marker melastatin (TRPM1) by MITF in melanocytes and melanoma. *Cancer Res.* **2004**, *64*, 509–516. [CrossRef] [PubMed]

194. Guo, H.; Carlson, J.A.; Slominski, A. Role of TRPM in melanocytes and melanoma. *Exp. Dermatol.* **2012**, *21*, 650–654. [CrossRef] [PubMed]

195. Devi, S.; Markandeya, Y.; Maddodi, N.; Dhingra, A.; Vardi, N.; Balijepalli, R.C.; Setaluri, V. Metabotropic glutamate receptor 6 signaling enhances TRPM1 calcium channel function and increases melanin content in human melanocytes. *Pigment Cell Melanoma Res.* **2013**, *26*, 348–356. [CrossRef] [PubMed]

196. Mansuri, M.S.; Singh, M.; Begum, R. miRNA signatures and transcriptional regulation of their target genes in vitiligo. *J. Dermatol. Sci* **2016**, *84*, 50–58. [CrossRef] [PubMed]

197. Bellone, R.R.; Brooks, S.A.; Sandmeyer, L.; Murphy, B.A.; Forsyth, G.; Archer, S.; Bailey, E.; Grahn, B. Differential gene expression of TRPM1, the potential cause of congenital stationary night blindness and coat spotting patterns (LP) in the Appaloosa horse (Equus caballus). *Genetics* **2008**, *179*, 1861–1870. [CrossRef] [PubMed]

198. Oancea, E.; Vriens, J.; Brauchi, S.; Jun, J.; Splawski, I.; Clapham, D.E. TRPM1 forms ion channels associated with melanin content in melanocytes. *Sci. Signal.* **2009**, *2*, ra21. [CrossRef] [PubMed]

199. Kunisada, T.; Lu, S.Z.; Yoshida, H.; Nishikawa, S.; Nishikawa, S.; Mizoguchi, M.; Hayashi, S.; Tyrrell, L.; Williams, D.A.; Wang, X.; et al. Murine cutaneous mastocytosis and epidermal melanocytosis induced by keratinocyte expression of transgenic stem cell factor. *J. Exp. Med.* **1998**, *187*, 1565–1573. [CrossRef] [PubMed]

200. Levy, C.; Khaled, M.; Iliopoulos, D.; Janas, M.M.; Schubert, S.; Pinner, S.; Chen, P.H.; Li, S.; Fletcher, A.L.; Yokoyama, S.; et al. Intronic miR-211 assumes the tumor suppressive function of its host gene in melanoma. *Mol. Cell* **2010**, *40*, 841–849. [CrossRef] [PubMed]

201. Tan, C.H.; McNaughton, P.A. The TRPM2 ion channel is required for sensitivity to warmth. *Nature* **2016**, *536*, 460–463. [CrossRef] [PubMed]

202. Held, K.; Voets, T.; Vriens, J. TRPM3 in temperature sensing and beyond. *Temperature (Austin)* **2015**, *2*, 201–213. [CrossRef] [PubMed]

203. Vriens, J.; Held, K.; Janssens, A.; Toth, B.I.; Kerselaers, S.; Nilius, B.; Vennekens, R.; Voets, T. Opening of an alternative ion permeation pathway in a nociceptor TRP channel. *Nat. Chem. Biol.* **2014**, *10*, 188–195. [CrossRef] [PubMed]

204. McNeill, M.S.; Paulsen, J.; Bonde, G.; Burnight, E.; Hsu, M.Y.; Cornell, R.A. Cell death of melanophores in zebrafish TRPM7 mutant embryos depends on melanin synthesis. *J. Investig. Dermatol.* **2007**, *127*, 2020–2030. [CrossRef] [PubMed]

205. Bautista, D.M.; Siemens, J.; Glazer, J.M.; Tsuruda, P.R.; Basbaum, A.I.; Stucky, C.L.; Jordt, S.E.; Julius, D. The menthol receptor TRPM8 is the principal detector of environmental cold. *Nature* **2007**, *448*, 204–208. [CrossRef] [PubMed]

206. Colburn, R.W.; Lubin, M.L.; Stone, D.J., Jr.; Wang, Y.; Lawrence, D.; D'Andrea, M.R.; Brandt, M.R.; Liu, Y.; Flores, C.M.; Qin, N. Attenuated cold sensitivity in TRPM8 null mice. *Neuron* **2007**, *54*, 379–386. [CrossRef] [PubMed]

207. Dhaka, A.; Murray, A.N.; Mathur, J.; Earley, T.J.; Petrus, M.J.; Patapoutian, A. TRPM8 is required for cold sensation in mice. *Neuron* **2007**, *54*, 371–378. [CrossRef] [PubMed]

208. Chung, M.K.; Caterina, M.J. TRP channel knockout mice lose their cool. *Neuron* **2007**, *54*, 345–347. [CrossRef] [PubMed]

209. Bromm, B.; Scharein, E.; Darsow, U.; Ring, J. Effects of menthol and cold on histamine-induced itch and skin reactions in man. *Neurosci. Lett.* **1995**, *187*, 157–160. [CrossRef]

210. Shapovalov, G.; Gkika, D.; Devilliers, M.; Kondratskyi, A.; Gordienko, D.; Busserolles, J.; Bokhobza, A.; Eschalier, A.; Skryma, R.; Prevarskaya, N. Opiates modulate thermosensation by internalizing cold receptor TRPM8. *Cell Rep.* **2013**, *4*, 504–515. [CrossRef] [PubMed]

211. Asuthkar, S.; Demirkhanyan, L.; Sun, X.; Elustondo, P.A.; Krishnan, V.; Baskaran, P.; Velpula, K.K.; Thyagarajan, B.; Pavlov, E.V.; Zakharian, E. The TRPM8 protein is a testosterone receptor: II. Functional evidence for an ionotropic effect of testosterone on TRPM8. *J. Biol. Chem.* **2015**, *290*, 2670–2688. [CrossRef] [PubMed]

212. Asuthkar, S.; Elustondo, P.A.; Demirkhanyan, L.; Sun, X.; Baskaran, P.; Velpula, K.K.; Thyagarajan, B.; Pavlov, E.V.; Zakharian, E. The TRPM8 protein is a testosterone receptor: I. Biochemical evidence for direct TRPM8-testosterone interactions. *J. Biol. Chem.* **2015**, *290*, 2659–2669. [CrossRef] [PubMed]

213. Zhang, L.; Barritt, G.J. Evidence that TRPM8 is an androgen-dependent Ca^{2+} channel required for the survival of prostate cancer cells. *Cancer Res.* **2004**, *64*, 8365–8373. [CrossRef] [PubMed]

214. Bidaux, G.; Borowiec, A.S.; Gordienko, D.; Beck, B.; Shapovalov, G.G.; Lemonnier, L.; Flourakis, M.; Vandenberghe, M.; Slomianny, C.; Dewailly, E.; et al. Epidermal TRPM8 channel isoform controls the balance between keratinocyte proliferation and differentiation in a cold-dependent manner. *Proc. Natl. Acad. Sci. USA* **2015**, *112*, E3345–E3354. [CrossRef] [PubMed]

215. Denda, M.; Tsutsumi, M.; Denda, S. Topical application of TRPM8 agonists accelerates skin permeability barrier recovery and reduces epidermal proliferation induced by barrier insult: Role of cold-sensitive TRP receptors in epidermal permeability barrier homoeostasis. *Exp. Dermatol.* **2010**, *19*, 791–795. [CrossRef] [PubMed]

216. Park, N.H.; Na, Y.J.; Choi, H.T.; Cho, J.C.; Lee, H.K. Activation of transient receptor potential melastatin 8 reduces ultraviolet B-induced prostaglandin E2 production in keratinocytes. *J. Dermatol.* **2013**, *40*, 919–922. [CrossRef] [PubMed]

217. Mergler, S.; Derckx, R.; Reinach, P.S.; Garreis, F.; Bohm, A.; Schmelzer, L.; Skosyrski, S.; Ramesh, N.; Abdelmessih, S.; Polat, O.K.; et al. Calcium regulation by temperature-sensitive transient receptor potential channels in human uveal melanoma cells. *Cell Signal.* **2014**, *26*, 56–69. [CrossRef] [PubMed]

218. Yamamura, H.; Ugawa, S.; Ueda, T.; Morita, A.; Shimada, S. TRPM8 activation suppresses cellular viability in human melanoma. *Am. J. Physiol. Cell Physiol.* **2008**, *295*, C296–C301. [CrossRef] [PubMed]

219. Xu, H.; Delling, M.; Li, L.; Dong, X.; Clapham, D.E. Activating mutation in a mucolipin transient receptor potential channel leads to melanocyte loss in varitint-waddler mice. *Proc. Natl. Acad. Sci. USA* **2007**, *104*, 18321–18326. [CrossRef] [PubMed]

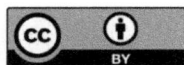

pharmaceuticals

MDPI

Review

Development of TRPM8 Antagonists to Treat Chronic Pain and Migraine

Andy D. Weyer [1] and Sonya G. Lehto [2],*

[1] Pacific University School of Physical Therapy, Hillsboro, OR 97123, USA; andy.weyer@pacificu.edu
[2] One Amgen Center Dr, Thousand Oaks, CA 91320, USA
*   Correspondence: slehto@amgen.com; Tel.: +1-850-313-5325

Academic Editors: Susan M. Huang, Arpad Szallasi and Jean Jacques Vanden Eynde
Received: 16 February 2017; Accepted: 23 March 2017; Published: 30 March 2017

Abstract: A review. Development of pharmaceutical antagonists of transient receptor potential melastatin 8 (TRPM8) have been pursued for the treatment of chronic pain and migraine. This review focuses on the current state of this progress.

Keywords: transient receptor potential melastatin 8 (TRPM*); pain; menthol; cold hyperalgesia; cold analgesia; mechanical hyperalgesia; migraine

1. Introduction

Transient receptor potential melastatin 8 (TRPM8) is a non-selective cation channel encoded by the *TRPM8* gene, first characterized as a detector of cold [1,2]. TRPM8 is found on both $A\delta$ and C fiber afferents, and in addition to activation by cold temperatures, TRPM8 is activated by a number of chemical agonists that are known to produce cool sensations such as menthol, icilin, and eucalyptol [3,4]. As a natural extension of these findings, much research over the past decade has been devoted to the role of TRPM8-expressing afferents in the complex interpretation of hot and cold temperatures. Furthermore, the role of TRPM8 in pain sensation has been debated; indeed, while a large body of research has supported a role for TRPM8 in reducing or limiting pain sensation under injury conditions, an equally large number of publications propose that TRPM8 actually exaggerates pain after injury. From a pharmaceutical perspective, this complicates whether specific agonists or antagonists of TRPM8 should be developed to treat different pain conditions. In this review, we summarize the literature concerning the contribution of TRPM8 to both analgesia and nociception, and provide an update on the current state of drug development involving this versatile protein.

2. The Role for TRPM8 in Mechanical and Heat Analgesia

Intimately tied to our understanding of a potential role for TRPM8 in promoting analgesia is the effect of one of its prime agonists, menthol. Menthol is a common component of topical creams that have long been used to reduce pain and provide a cooling sensation [5]. Although some data has indicated that menthol may activate a variety of other channels, including transient receptor potential Ankyrin 1 (TRPA1), gamma-aminobutyric acid (GABA), and voltage-gated calcium and sodium channels [6,7], more recent studies have demonstrated that the prime target of menthol is indeed TRPM8, as genetic deletion of this receptor in mice prevents responsiveness to menthol at both the behavioral and cellular levels [8].

In animal studies, menthol has been shown to block the mechanical and heat hyperalgesia caused by injection of inflammatory compounds such as Complete Freund's Adjuvant (CFA) or the transient receptor potential vanilloid 1 (TRPV1) agonist capsaicin [7,9,10]. Furthermore, injection of the TRPM8 agonist icilin significantly reduced the colonic damage observed in two different mouse models of inflammatory bowel disease [11]. In support of these inflammatory studies, it has been shown that components of the "inflammatory soup" that develops after an injury can inhibit TRPM8. Andersson and colleagues reported that low pH inactivates TRPM8, making it less responsive to the TRPM8 agonist icilin and cold temperatures (but interestingly not menthol) [12]. Similarly, another study found that bradykinin, a key potentiator of pain and component of the inflammatory soup, reduces TRPM8 activity through the action of protein kinase C in both the periphery and at the central synapse in the dorsal horn [10].

Adding to the view that TRPM8 promotes analgesia following injury are data from studies in which TRPM8 is either genetically deleted or experimentally knocked down. Proudfoot and colleagues first demonstrated this concept in a chronic constriction injury (CCI) model. Experimental rats in this study exhibited significantly reduced heat and mechanical pain behaviors when topical icilin was applied to the paw, but this effect was completely reversed when TRPM8 expression was knocked down via intrathecal injection of antisense oligonucleotides [13]. In similar experiments utilizing the CCI model, cooling or applying menthol to the affected paw resulted in reduced hypersensitivity in response to mechanical stimuli [14,15], but this effect was not seen when TRPM8 was knocked out or when TRPM8-expressing afferents were ablated [14]. Likewise, one of the first studies to utilize TRPM8 knockout mice demonstrated that TRPM8 was responsible for the analgesia provided by a cold plate during the first phase of the formalin test [16], and later studies using mice deficient in TRPM8 showed that menthol was unable to exert its analgesic effects in models of inflammatory pain using capsaicin or CFA [7].

A number of studies in humans also point toward a role for TRPM8 in mediating analgesia. In a recent study, injections of the TRPA1 agonist cinnamaldehyde into the forearm resulted in significant pain and neurogenic flare; however, simultaneous injection of menthol resulted in lower pain ratings, elevated mechanical pain thresholds, and reduced neurogenic flare as compared to cinnamaldehyde alone [17]. Two case studies also demonstrate the analgesic role of TRPM8 in patients suffering from chronic neuropathic pain. One individual developed neuropathic pain after long-term dosing with the chemotherapeutic Bortezomib, which causes neuropathy in up to 35% of patients. This individual suffered from a severe burning sensation in his lower limbs and "lightning-like" sensations in his hands. However, topical application of a 0.5% menthol cream to his lower extremities in a stocking distribution and the lumbosacral region overlying the affected nerve roots resulted in a significant improvement in response to suprathreshold mechanical stimuli and overall pain ratings [18]. Similarly, in another case where a patient suffered from severe allodynia following a case of post-herpetic neuralgia, application of menthol oil in concentrations of 2 or 10% resulted in a significant abatement of symptoms [19]. Further proof of the analgesic effects through TRPM8 can be observed in the ability of menthol or eucalyptol (another TRPM8 agonist) to prevent the irritant effects of acrolein and other cigarette smoke components [20].

3. The Role of TRPM8 in Cold Hyperalgesia

Much data also suggests that TRPM8 plays a role in amplifying pain sensation after injury, especially in models of neuropathic pain. Hypersensitivity to cold is a common complaint of individuals with neuropathies, with 20–30% of individuals diagnosed with different types of neuropathies complaining of cold hyperalgesia and elevated cold pain thresholds [21–23]. Likewise, other studies report significant elevations in cold pain thresholds in patients treated with the chemotherapeutic oxaliplatin, indicating that innocuous temperatures had become painful for these individuals [23,24]. In addition to alterations in cold thresholds, these individuals also rated specific cold temperatures as 3–4 times more painful than at baseline.

The cold hypersensitivity following neuropathic injury observed in human subjects has been consistently paralleled in animal models of nerve injury, and has been further extended to identify a definitive role for TRPM8 in mediating this pain. For instance, oxaliplatin-induced neuropathies in mice cause cold hypersensitivity on the behavioral level and also result in an increased percentage of isolated sensory neurons that respond to cold temperatures [25,26]. When TRPM8 knockout mice are utilized for these same experiments, this cold hyperalgesia is absent, implicating TRPM8 as a critical player in this phenomenon [25]. At this time it is unclear whether TRPM8 expression increases after installation of oxaliplatin-induced neuropathy, with one study reporting increased mRNA expression [27] and another reporting no change in mRNA expression levels [25].

Another popular neuropathic model is the CCI, in which ligatures are tied around the sciatic nerve. This model has consistently been shown to cause cold hypersensitivity, and multiple studies have reported that the increased responsiveness to the acetone evaporative cooling test following CCI was significantly reduced when TRPM8 was genetically deleted or when TRPM8-expressing afferents were chemically ablated [15,26]. Similarly, another study has reported that knockdown of TRPM8 with antisense oligonucleotides results in reduced responsiveness to cold as compared to animals injected with the missense oligonucleotide [14]. Additionally, this study and others have reported an increase in the number of neurons expressing TRPM8 [14,28,29] and an increase in total amount of TRPM8 protein in the DRG following CCI surgery [14]. Functionally, an increased number of isolated sensory neurons are responsive to cold and menthol after CCI, and these responses are potentiated as compared to controls [28].

4. The Role of TRPM8 in Bladder Pain

Interstitial cystitis/bladder pain syndrome is a condition characterized by pain in the bladder region and by urinary urgency and increased urination frequency [30]. Current therapeutics are often insufficient for treating this condition, so the identification of new drug targets is of particular interest. Much like in animal models of neuropathic pain, animal models of bladder pain reveal TRPM8 to be pro-nociceptive. For instance, the use of a novel TRPM8 antagonist, AMTB, increased intercontraction intervals in a rodent model of overactive bladder syndrome, and also decreased the visceromotor reflex [31]. A similar phenomenon was observed in guinea pigs, as a novel TRPM8 antagonist reversed the reduction in bladder voiding volume induced by cold saline and menthol infusion in to the bladder [32]. Whether these effects are mediated via inhibition of TRPM8 channels on bladder-projecting afferents or on TRPM8 located in the bladder itself is unclear, as TRPM8 expression at the mRNA and protein levels has been observed in both afferents innervating the bladder [31,33,34] and in the bladder itself [34,35]. A recent study may shed some light on this, as recordings from C-fiber afferents demonstrated reduced firing in response to bladder distention in the presence of menthol when a novel TRPM8 antagonist was infused into the bladder [36]. Interestingly, increased TRPM8 immunostaining was observed in bladder samples from individuals with bladder pain syndrome, and this was moderately correlated with increased pain scores in those patients [34].

5. The Role of TRPM8 in Migraine

In addition to its role in somatic pain sensation, recent genome-wide association studies have found a significant correlation between migraine incidence and single nucleotide polymorphisms (SNPs) located near the TRPM8 coding region (for a review see [37]). Interestingly, this connection seems to be present only for individuals of Northern European ancestry [38–42], as studies involving populations from Spain, India, and China found either no association or weak associations between migraine incidence and SNPs near the *TRPM8* locus [43–47].

These human studies have naturally sparked interest in exploring the contribution of TRPM8 to migraine through the use of rodent models. Unfortunately, these studies have found opposing results concerning TRPM8's involvement. Burgos-Vega and colleagues observed that application of icilin to the dura mater resulted in reduced paw and facial withdrawal thresholds in response to a mechanical stimulus, indicating that activation of TRPM8 caused migraine-like behaviors [48]. These behaviors were then subsequently blocked by dosing animals with a novel TRPM8 antagonist. Perhaps most interesting, however, was that sumatriptan, a drug commonly used to treat migraines, also prevented the migraine-like behaviors, which strongly implicates a role for TRPM8 in migraine generation. Conversely, a recent study by Ren and colleagues found opposing results, with application of menthol to the dura mater relieving migraine-like symptoms brought on by the application of inflammatory mediators to the dura. Symptom relief could then be subsequently blocked by injection of a TRPM8 antagonist. Finally, adding even more confusion to the matter is a study from Huang et al. that reported that TRPM8-expressing afferents were virtually absent from the dura [49]. However, further interest in strategies targeting TRP channels as migraine therapeutics is supported by clinical success of CGRP receptor antagonism since activation of TRP channels can elicit CGRP release [50].

6. Why is TRPM8 Analgesic in Some Cases and Nociceptive in Others?

An important point about TRPM8's roles in nociception and analgesia is that activation of TRPM8 seems to consistently cause cold pain following injury, while simultaneously reducing mechanical and heat pain. Therefore, whether to target TRPM8 with either an agonist or antagonist may depend on which symptom is most troublesome to the patient; individuals with a primary complaint of mechanical hyperalgesia may respond best to TRPM8 agonists, while those with cold hyperalgesia may respond best to TRPM8 antagonists. Importantly, this is not to suggest that TRPM8 itself is sensitive to both mechanical and cold stimuli; indeed, afferent recordings indicate that pharmacological blockade of TRPM8 has no effect on baseline mechanical responsiveness [51] and genetic deletion of TRPM8 or pharmacological ablation of TRPM8-expressing afferents does not impact behavioral responses to mechanical stimuli [15]. Rather, it seems that the effects of TRPM8 agonism/antagonism are due to effects at the spinal level, with TRPM8-expressing afferents either directly or indirectly inhibiting mechanonociceptive afferents. Indeed, Proudfoot et al. reported that the analgesic effects of TRPM8 activation may be due to axoaxonic synapses on mechanonociceptive and heat-nociceptive afferent terminals, which contain inhibitory mGluRII and mGluRIII receptors [13]. Thus, release of glutamate from TRPM8-expressing afferents may decrease the amount of excitatory neurotransmitters released onto nociceptive projection neurons in lamina I and II of the dorsal horn. There is also a suggestion that topical menthol-induced pain relief may occur through blockade of voltage gated sodium channels [52].

At the same time, cold hyperalgesia following injury may be due to activation of a separate population of TRPM8-expressing nociceptors that relay painful information to the central nervous system. These nociceptors may have reduced thresholds for activation under injury conditions, leading to the observed strong hyperalgesic responses to cold. Additionally, they may be triggered by especially strong stimuli that facilitate TRPM8 activation; indeed, studies in humans consistently report that application of high concentrations of menthol (30%–40%) induces pain, cold allodynia, and cold hyperalgesia [53–55], whereas the lower concentrations used in topical agents induce analgesia.

7. Development of TRPM8 Antagonists for Chronic Pain

Antagonists of TRPM8 as therapeutics for chronic pain, migraine or inflammation have been pursued over the recent decade by many pharmaceutical companies such as Hydra Biosciences, Glenmark, Janssen, Pfizer, Bayer, Grunenthal, Mitsubishi Tanabe, RaQualia, Dompe/Axxam, BASF, Dendreon and Amgen. These efforts have led to the publication of many patents (for a review see [56–58]).

Janssen has published several potent and selective small molecule antagonists that suppresses icilin-induced wet-dog shakes, cold pressor response, as well as cold-induced allodynia in a neuropathic pain model in rats with a similar resulting dose-response range of effect in either of the cold-induced endpoints [59–63]. Glenmark also similarly reported efficacy with their antagonist in both wet-dog shakes and oxaliplatin-induced cold allodynia at the same 30 mg/kg dose [64]. RaQualia published RQ-00203078 which is a single digit nM antagonist at human or rat TRPM8 that also potently blocks icilin-induced wet-dog shakes in rats and is now commercially available, though evaluation in analgesic models has not been published [65].

AMG2850 is a ~200 nM potent and selective antagonist from Amgen that blocks both TRPM8 agonist-induced behavioral responses (wet-dog shakes) and cold-induced increases in blood pressure (cold pressor test)—both considered pharmacodynamic models of TRPM8 antagonism in vivo. Although the effect in cold allodynia was not evaluated, the effective dose would presumably be similar to that in the reported cold endpoint, the cold pressor test. There was, however, no evidence of meaningful reversal of inflammatory nor neuropathic-induced mechanical hypersensitivities in rats. This lack of efficacy occurred even at unbound plasma concentrations in excess of 21-fold the IC_{90} pharmacodynamic model suggesting that TRPM8 does not play a role in these mechanical pain behaviors at what would be reasonably considered more than enough target coverage [51,66,67], thus casting doubt on the therapeutic potential of TRPM8 as an analgesic in non-cold related conditions.

Pfizer did advance to clinical trials with a ~100 nM molecule, PF-05105679, which successfully inhibited the cold pressor response in humans, but also produced hot sensations that were both unexpected and considered adverse. The lack of therapeutic index to this event coupled with the short half-life in humans limited further clinical progression as well as the ability to evaluate the analgesic effect [32,68]. It has been demonstrated that cutaneous TRPM8 controls autonomic and behavioral thermoeffectors involved in body temperature maintenance with antagonists decreasing body temperature in rodents [26,69–71]. While the Pfizer antagonist did not produce a significant alteration of body temperature in healthy volunteers, further understanding is needed to elucidate whether and how these hot sensations may be on-target side effects in humans.

Chemotherapeutic drug-induced cold allodynia can be dose limiting, resulting in the cessation of treatment, enduring years beyond treatment, and for which there are currently no proven therapies [72–74]. Since chemotherapy is associated with changes in TRPM8 expression [25,75], perhaps TRPM8 antagonists could be beneficial in the prevention and/or reversal of this chemotherapy-induced cold allodynia. Or, perhaps TRPM8 antagonists could still be useful therapeutics for any other cold-related painful allodynia or hyperalgesia associated with other neuropathic or inflammatory conditions or even migraine or bladder pain. Currently, there are no ongoing trials with TRPM8 antagonists [76].

Acknowledgments: Funding to publish this review was paid by Amgen Inc.

Conflicts of Interest: S.G.L. is employed by Amgen Inc.

References

1. Peier, A.M.; Moqrich, A.; Hergarden, A.C.; Reeve, A.J.; Andersson, D.A.; Story, G.M.; Earley, T.J.; Dragoni, I.; McIntyre, P.; Bevan, S.; et al. A TRP channel that senses cold stimuli and menthol. *Cell* **2002**, *108*, 705–715. [CrossRef]
2. McKemy, D.D.; Neuhausser, W.M.; Julius, D. Identification of a cold receptor reveals a general role for TRP channels in thermosensation. *Nature* **2002**, *416*, 52–58. [CrossRef] [PubMed]
3. Behrendt, H.J.; Germann, T.; Gillen, C.; Hatt, H.; Jostock, R. Characterization of the mouse cold-menthol receptor TRPM8 and vanilloid receptor type-1 VR1 using a fluorometric imaging plate reader (FLIPR) assay. *Br. J. Pharmacol.* **2004**, *141*, 737–745. [CrossRef] [PubMed]
4. Dai, Y. TRPs and pain. *Semin. Immunopathol.* **2016**, *38*, 277–291. [CrossRef] [PubMed]
5. Eccles, R. Menthol and related cooling compounds. *J. Pharm. Pharmacol.* **1994**, *46*, 618–630. [CrossRef] [PubMed]
6. Karashima, Y.; Damann, N.; Prenen, J.; Talavera, K.; Segal, A.; Voets, T.; Nilius, B. Bimodal action of menthol on the transient receptor potential channel TRPA1. *J. Neurosci.* **2007**, *27*, 9874–9884. [CrossRef] [PubMed]
7. Pan, R.; Tian, Y.; Gao, R.; Li, H.; Zhao, X.; Barrett, J.E.; Hu, H. Central mechanisms of menthol-induced analgesia. *J. Pharm. Exp. Ther.* **2012**, *343*, 661–672. [CrossRef] [PubMed]
8. Liu, B.; Fan, L.; Balakrishna, S.; Sui, A.; Morris, J.B.; Jordt, S.E. TRPM8 is the principal mediator of menthol-induced analgesia of acute and inflammatory pain. *Pain* **2013**, *154*, 2169–2177. [CrossRef] [PubMed]
9. Alpizar, Y.A.; Boonen, B.; Gees, M.; Sanchez, A.; Nilius, B.; Voets, T.; Talavera, K. Allyl isothiocyanate sensitizes TRPV1 to heat stimulation. *Pflugers Arch. EJP* **2014**, *466*, 507–515. [CrossRef] [PubMed]

10. Premkumar, L.S.; Raisinghani, M.; Pingle, S.C.; Long, C.; Pimentel, F. Downregulation of transient receptor potential melastatin 8 by protein kinase C-mediated dephosphorylation. *J. Neurosci.* **2005**, *25*, 11322–11329. [CrossRef] [PubMed]

11. Ramachandran, R.; Hyun, E.; Zhao, L.; Lapointe, T.K.; Chapman, K.; Hirota, C.L.; Ghosh, S.; McKemy, D.D.; Vergnolle, N.; Beck, P.L.; et al. TRPM8 activation attenuates inflammatory responses in mouse models of colitis. *Proc. Natl. Acad. Sci. USA* **2013**, *110*, 7476–7481. [CrossRef] [PubMed]

12. Andersson, D.A.; Chase, H.W.; Bevan, S. TRPM8 activation by menthol, icilin, and cold is differentially modulated by intracellular pH. *J. Neurosci.* **2004**, *24*, 5364–5369. [CrossRef] [PubMed]

13. Proudfoot, C.J.; Garry, E.M.; Cottrell, D.F.; Rosie, R.; Anderson, H.; Robertson, D.C.; Fleetwood-Walker, S.M.; Mitchell, R. Analgesia mediated by the TRPM8 cold receptor in chronic neuropathic pain. *Curr. Boil.* **2006**, *16*, 1591–1605. [CrossRef] [PubMed]

14. Su, L.; Wang, C.; Yu, Y.-H.; Ren, Y.-Y.; Xie, K.-L.; Wang, G.-L. Role of TRPM8 in dorsal root ganglion in nerve injury-induced chronic pain. *BMC Neurosci.* **2011**, *12*, 120. [CrossRef] [PubMed]

15. Knowlton, W.M.; Palkar, R.; Lippoldt, E.K.; McCoy, D.D.; Baluch, F.; Chen, J.; McKemy, D.D. A sensory-labeled line for cold: TRPM8-expressing sensory neurons define the cellular basis for cold, cold pain, and cooling-mediated analgesia. *J. Neurosci.* **2013**, *33*, 2837–2848. [CrossRef] [PubMed]

16. Dhaka, A.; Murray, A.N.; Mathur, J.; Earley, T.J.; Petrus, M.J.; Patapoutian, A. TRPM8 is required for cold sensation in mice. *Neuron* **2007**, *54*, 371–378. [CrossRef] [PubMed]

17. Andersen, H.H.; Gazerani, P.; Arendt-Nielsen, L. High-Concentration L-Menthol Exhibits Counter-Irritancy to Neurogenic Inflammation, Thermal and Mechanical Hyperalgesia Caused by Trans-cinnamaldehyde. *J. Pain* **2016**, *17*, 919–929. [CrossRef] [PubMed]

18. Colvin, L.A.; Johnson, P.R.; Mitchell, R.; Fleetwood-Walker, S.M.; Fallon, M. From bench to bedside: A case of rapid reversal of bortezomib-induced neuropathic pain by the TRPM8 activator, menthol. *J. Clin. Oncol.* **2008**, *26*, 4519–4520. [CrossRef] [PubMed]

19. Davies, S.J.; Harding, L.M.; Baranowski, A.P. A novel treatment of postherpetic neuralgia using peppermint oil. *Clin. J. Pain* **2002**, *18*, 200–202. [CrossRef] [PubMed]

20. Willis, D.N.; Liu, B.; Ha, M.A.; Jordt, S.E.; Morris, J.B. Menthol attenuates respiratory irritation responses to multiple cigarette smoke irritants. *FASEB J.* **2011**, *25*, 4434–4444. [CrossRef] [PubMed]

21. Eberle, T.; Doganci, B.; Kramer, H.H.; Geber, C.; Fechir, M.; Magerl, W.; Birklein, F. Warm and cold complex regional pain syndromes: Differences beyond skin temperature? *Neurology* **2009**, *72*, 505–512. [CrossRef] [PubMed]

22. Maier, C.; Baron, R.; Tolle, T.R.; Binder, A.; Birbaumer, N.; Birklein, F.; Gierthmuhlen, J.; Flor, H.; Geber, C.; Huge, V.; et al. Quantitative sensory testing in the German Research Network on Neuropathic Pain (DFNS): Somatosensory abnormalities in 1236 patients with different neuropathic pain syndromes. *Pain* **2010**, *150*, 439–450. [CrossRef] [PubMed]

23. Attal, N.; Bouhassira, D.; Gautron, M.; Vaillant, J.N.; Mitry, E.; Lepere, C.; Rougier, P.; Guirimand, F. Thermal hyperalgesia as a marker of oxaliplatin neurotoxicity: A prospective quantified sensory assessment study. *Pain* **2009**, *144*, 245–252. [CrossRef] [PubMed]

24. Binder, A.; Stengel, M.; Maag, R.; Wasner, G.; Schoch, R.; Moosig, F.; Schommer, B.; Baron, R. Pain in oxaliplatin-induced neuropathy—sensitisation in the peripheral and central nociceptive system. *Eur. J. Cancer* **2007**, *43*, 2658–2663. [CrossRef] [PubMed]

25. Descoeur, J.; Pereira, V.; Pizzoccaro, A.; Francois, A.; Ling, B.; Maffre, V.; Couette, B.; Busserolles, J.; Courteix, C.; Noel, J.; et al. Oxaliplatin-induced cold hypersensitivity is due to remodelling of ion channel expression in nociceptors. *EMBO Mol. Med.* **2011**, *3*, 266–278. [CrossRef] [PubMed]

26. Knowlton, W.M.; Daniels, R.L.; Palkar, R.; McCoy, D.D.; McKemy, D.D. Pharmacological blockade of TRPM8 ion channels alters cold and cold pain responses in mice. *PLoS ONE* **2011**, *6*, e25894. [CrossRef] [PubMed]

27. Gauchan, P.; Andoh, T.; Kato, A.; Kuraishi, Y. Involvement of increased expression of transient receptor potential melastatin 8 in oxaliplatin-induced cold allodynia in mice. *Neurosci. Lett.* **2009**, *458*, 93–95. [CrossRef] [PubMed]

28. Xing, H.; Chen, M.; Ling, J.; Tan, W.; Gu, J.G. TRPM8 mechanism of cold allodynia after chronic nerve injury. *J. Neurosci.* **2007**, *27*, 13680–13690. [CrossRef] [PubMed]

29. Frederick, J.; Buck, M.E.; Matson, D.J.; Cortright, D.N. Increased TRPA1, TRPM8, and TRPV2 expression in dorsal root ganglia by nerve injury. *Biochem. Biophys. Res. Commun.* **2007**, *358*, 1058–1064. [CrossRef] [PubMed]

30. Berry, S.H.; Elliott, M.N.; Suttorp, M.; Bogart, L.M.; Stoto, M.A.; Eggers, P.; Nyberg, L.; Clemens, J.Q. Prevalence of symptoms of bladder pain syndrome/interstitial cystitis among adult females in the United States. *J. Urol.* **2011**, *186*, 540–544. [CrossRef] [PubMed]

31. Lashinger, E.S.; Steiginga, M.S.; Hieble, J.P.; Leon, L.A.; Gardner, S.D.; Nagilla, R.; Davenport, E.A.; Hoffman, B.E.; Laping, N.J.; Su, X. AMTB, a TRPM8 channel blocker: Evidence in rats for activity in overactive bladder and painful bladder syndrome. *Am. J. Physiol. Renal Physiol.* **2008**, *295*, F803–F810. [CrossRef] [PubMed]

32. Winchester, W.J.; Gore, K.; Glatt, S.; Petit, W.; Gardiner, J.C.; Conlon, K.; Postlethwaite, M.; Saintot, P.P.; Roberts, S.; Gosset, J.R.; et al. Inhibition of TRPM8 channels reduces pain in the cold pressor test in humans. *J. Pharm. Exp. Ther.* **2014**, *351*, 259–269. [CrossRef] [PubMed]

33. Hayashi, T.; Kondo, T.; Ishimatsu, M.; Yamada, S.; Nakamura, K.; Matsuoka, K.; Akasu, T. Expression of the TRPM8-immunoreactivity in dorsal root ganglion neurons innervating the rat urinary bladder. *J. Neurosci. Res.* **2009**, *65*, 245–251. [CrossRef] [PubMed]

34. Mukerji, G.; Yiangou, Y.; Corcoran, S.L.; Selmer, I.S.; Smith, G.D.; Benham, C.D.; Bountra, C.; Agarwal, S.K.; Anand, P. Cool and menthol receptor TRPM8 in human urinary bladder disorders and clinical correlations. *BMC Urol.* **2006**, *6*, 6. [CrossRef] [PubMed]

35. Kobayashi, H.; Yoshiyama, M.; Zakoji, H.; Takeda, M.; Araki, I. Sex differences in the expression profile of acid-sensing ion channels in the mouse urinary bladder: A possible involvement in irritative bladder symptoms. *BJU Int.* **2009**, *104*, 1746–1751. [CrossRef] [PubMed]

36. Ito, H.; Aizawa, N.; Sugiyama, R.; Watanabe, S.; Takahashi, N.; Tajimi, M.; Fukuhara, H.; Homma, Y.; Kubota, Y.; Andersson, K.E.; et al. Functional role of the transient receptor potential melastatin 8 (TRPM8) ion channel in the urinary bladder assessed by conscious cystometry and ex vivo measurements of single-unit mechanosensitive bladder afferent activities in the rat. *BJU Int.* **2016**, *117*, 484–494. [CrossRef] [PubMed]

37. Dussor, G.; Cao, Y.Q. TRPM8 and Migraine. *Headache* **2016**, *56*, 1406–1417. [CrossRef] [PubMed]

38. Chasman, D.I.; Anttila, V.; Buring, J.E.; Ridker, P.M.; Schurks, M.; Kurth, T. Selectivity in genetic association with sub-classified migraine in women. *PLoS Genet.* **2014**, *10*, e1004366. [CrossRef] [PubMed]

39. Chasman, D.I.; Schurks, M.; Anttila, V.; de Vries, B.; Schminke, U.; Launer, L.J.; Terwindt, G.M.; van den Maagdenberg, A.M.; Fendrich, K.; Volzke, H.; et al. Genome-wide association study reveals three susceptibility loci for common migraine in the general population. *Nat. Genet.* **2011**, *43*, 695–698. [CrossRef] [PubMed]

40. Freilinger, T.; Anttila, V.; de Vries, B.; Malik, R.; Kallela, M.; Terwindt, G.M.; Pozo-Rosich, P.; Winsvold, B.; Nyholt, D.R.; van Oosterhout, W.P.; et al. Genome-wide association analysis identifies susceptibility loci for migraine without aura. *Nat. Genet.* **2012**, *44*, 777–782. [CrossRef] [PubMed]

41. Esserlind, A.L.; Christensen, A.F.; Le, H.; Kirchmann, M.; Hauge, A.W.; Toyserkani, N.M.; Hansen, T.; Grarup, N.; Werge, T.; Steinberg, S.; et al. Replication and meta-analysis of common variants identifies a genome-wide significant locus in migraine. *Eur. J. Neurol.* **2013**, *20*, 765–772. [CrossRef] [PubMed]

42. Zhao, H.; Eising, E.; de Vries, B.; Vijfhuizen, L.S.; International Headache Genetics Consortium; Anttila, V.; Winsvold, B.S.; Kurth, T.; Stefansson, H.; Kallela, M.; et al. Gene-based pleiotropy across migraine with aura and migraine without aura patient groups. *Cephalalgia* **2016**, *36*, 648–657. [CrossRef] [PubMed]

43. Carreno, O.; Corominas, R.; Fernandez-Morales, J.; Camina, M.; Sobrido, M.J.; Fernandez-Fernandez, J.M.; Pozo-Rosich, P.; Cormand, B.; Macaya, A. SNP variants within the vanilloid TRPV1 and TRPV3 receptor genes are associated with migraine in the Spanish population. *Am. J. Med. Genet. B Neuropsychiatr. Genet.* **2012**, *159B*, 94–103. [CrossRef] [PubMed]

44. An, X.K.; Ma, Q.L.; Lin, Q.; Zhang, X.R.; Lu, C.X.; Qu, H.L. PRDM16 rs2651899 variant is a risk factor for Chinese common migraine patients. *Headache* **2013**, *53*, 1595–1601. [CrossRef] [PubMed]

45. Ghosh, J.; Pradhan, S.; Mittal, B. Genome-wide-associated variants in migraine susceptibility: A replication study from North India. *Headache* **2013**, *53*, 1583–1594. [CrossRef] [PubMed]

46. Sintas, C.; Fernandez-Morales, J.; Vila-Pueyo, M.; Narberhaus, B.; Arenas, C.; Pozo-Rosich, P.; Macaya, A.; Cormand, B. Replication study of previous migraine genome-wide association study findings in a Spanish sample of migraine with aura. *Cephalalgia* **2015**, *35*, 776–782. [CrossRef] [PubMed]

47. Fan, X.; Wang, J.; Fan, W.; Chen, L.; Gui, B.; Tan, G.; Zhou, J. Replication of migraine GWAS susceptibility loci in Chinese Han population. *Headache* **2014**, *54*, 709–715. [CrossRef] [PubMed]

48. Burgos-Vega, C.C.; Ahn, D.D.; Bischoff, C.; Wang, W.; Horne, D.; Wang, J.; Gavva, N.; Dussor, G. Meningeal transient receptor potential channel M8 activation causes cutaneous facial and hindpaw allodynia in a preclinical rodent model of headache. *Cephalalgia* **2016**, *36*, 185–193. [CrossRef] [PubMed]

49. Huang, D.; Li, S.; Dhaka, A.; Story, G.M.; Cao, Y.Q. Expression of the transient receptor potential channels TRPV1, TRPA1 and TRPM8 in mouse trigeminal primary afferent neurons innervating the dura. *Mol. Pain* **2012**, *8*, 66. [CrossRef] [PubMed]

50. Dussor, G.; Yan, J.; Xie, J.Y.; Ossipov, M.H.; Dodick, D.W.; Porreca, F. Targeting TRP channels for novel migraine therapeutics. *ACS Chem. Neurosci.* **2014**, *5*, 1085–1096. [CrossRef] [PubMed]

51. Lehto, S.G.; Weyer, A.D.; Zhang, M.; Youngblood, B.D.; Wang, J.; Wang, W.; Kerstein, P.C.; Davis, C.; Wild, K.D.; Stucky, C.L.; et al. AMG2850, a potent and selective TRPM8 antagonist, is not effective in rat models of inflammatory mechanical hypersensitivity and neuropathic tactile allodynia. *Naunyn Schmiedebergs Arch. Pharmacol.* **2015**, *388*, 465–476. [CrossRef] [PubMed]

52. Gaudioso, C.; Hao, J.; Martin-Eauclaire, M.F.; Gabriac, M.; Delmas, P. Menthol pain relief through cumulative inactivation of voltage-gated sodium channels. *Pain* **2012**, *153*, 473–484. [CrossRef] [PubMed]

53. Namer, B.; Seifert, F.; Handwerker, H.O.; Maihofner, C. TRPA1 and TRPM8 activation in humans: Effects of cinnamaldehyde and menthol. *Neuroreport* **2005**, *16*, 955–959. [CrossRef] [PubMed]

54. Wasner, G.; Schattschneider, J.; Binder, A.; Baron, R. Topical menthol–a human model for cold pain by activation and sensitization of C nociceptors. *Brain* **2004**, *127*, 1159–1171. [CrossRef] [PubMed]

55. Hatem, S.; Attal, N.; Willer, J.C.; Bouhassira, D. Psychophysical study of the effects of topical application of menthol in healthy volunteers. *Pain* **2006**, *122*, 190–196. [CrossRef] [PubMed]

56. DeFalco, J.; Duncton, M.A.; Emerling, D. TRPM8 biology and medicinal chemistry. *Curr. Top. Med. Chem.* **2011**, *11*, 2237–2252. [CrossRef] [PubMed]

57. Eid, S.R. Therapeutic targeting of TRP channels–the TR(i)P to pain relief. *Curr. Top. Med. Chem.* **2011**, *11*, 2118–2130. [CrossRef] [PubMed]

58. Premkumar, L.S.; Abooj, M. TRP channels and analgesia. *Life Sci.* **2013**, *92*, 415–424. [CrossRef] [PubMed]

59. Feketa, V.V.; Zhang, Y.; Cao, Z.; Balasubramanian, A.; Flores, C.M.; Player, M.R.; Marrelli, S.P. Transient receptor potential melastatin 8 channel inhibition potentiates the hypothermic response to transient receptor potential vanilloid 1 activation in the conscious mouse. *Crit. Care Med.* **2014**, *42*, e355–e363. [CrossRef] [PubMed]

60. Zhu, B.; Xia, M.; Xu, X.; Ludovici, D.W.; Tennakoon, M.; Youngman, M.A.; Matthews, J.M.; Dax, S.L.; Colburn, R.W.; Qin, N.; et al. Arylglycine derivatives as potent transient receptor potential melastatin 8 (TRPM8) antagonists. *Bioorg. Med. Chem. Lett.* **2013**, *23*, 2234–2237. [CrossRef] [PubMed]

61. Matthews, J.M.; Qin, N.; Colburn, R.W.; Dax, S.L.; Hawkins, M.; McNally, J.J.; Reany, L.; Youngman, M.A.; Baker, J.; Hutchinson, T.; et al. The design and synthesis of novel, phosphonate-containing transient receptor potential melastatin 8 (TRPM8) antagonists. *Bioorg. Med. Chem. Lett.* **2012**, *22*, 2922–2926. [CrossRef] [PubMed]

62. Calvo, R.R.; Meegalla, S.K.; Parks, D.J.; Parsons, W.H.; Ballentine, S.K.; Lubin, M.L.; Schneider, C.; Colburn, R.W.; Flores, C.M.; Player, M.R. Discovery of vinylcycloalkyl-substituted benzimidazole TRPM8 antagonists effective in the treatment of cold allodynia. *Bioorg. Med. Chem. Lett.* **2012**, *22*, 1903–1907. [CrossRef] [PubMed]

63. Parks, D.J.; Parsons, W.H.; Colburn, R.W.; Meegalla, S.K.; Ballentine, S.K.; Illig, C.R.; Qin, N.; Liu, Y.; Hutchinson, T.L.; Lubin, M.L.; et al. Design and optimization of benzimidazole-containing transient receptor potential melastatin 8 (TRPM8) antagonists. *J. Med. Chem.* **2011**, *54*, 233–247. [CrossRef] [PubMed]

64. Chaudhari, S.S.; Kadam, A.B.; Khairatkar-Joshi, N.; Mukhopadhyay, I.; Karnik, P.V.; Raghuram, A.; Rao, S.S.; Vaiyapuri, T.S.; Wale, D.P.; Bhosale, V.M.; et al. Synthesis and pharmacological evaluation of novel N-aryl-3,4-dihydro-1'H-spiro[chromene-2,4'-piperidine]-1'-carboxamides as TRPM8 antagonists. *Bioorg. Med. Chem. Lett.* **2013**, *21*, 6542–6553. [CrossRef] [PubMed]

65. Ohmi, M.; Shishido, Y.; Inoue, T.; Ando, K.; Fujiuchi, A.; Yamada, A.; Watanabe, S.; Kawamura, K. Identification of a novel 2-pyridyl-benzensulfonamide derivative, RQ-00203078, as a selective and orally active TRPM8 antagonist. *Bioorg. Med. Chem. Lett.* **2014**, *24*, 5364–5368. [CrossRef] [PubMed]

66. Tamayo, N.A.; Bo, Y.; Gore, V.; Ma, V.; Nishimura, N.; Tang, P.; Deng, H.; Klionsky, L.; Lehto, S.G.; Wang, W.; et al. Fused piperidines as a novel class of potent and orally available transient receptor potential melastatin type 8 (TRPM8) antagonists. *J. Med. Chem.* **2012**, *55*, 1593–1611. [CrossRef] [PubMed]

67. Horne, D.B.; Tamayo, N.A.; Bartberger, M.D.; Bo, Y.; Clarine, J.; Davis, C.D.; Gore, V.K.; Kaller, M.R.; Lehto, S.G.; Ma, V.V.; et al. Optimization of Potency and Pharmacokinetic Properties of Tetrahydroisoquinoline Transient Receptor Potential Melastatin 8 (TRPM8) Antagonists. *J. Med. Chem.* **2014**, *57*, 2989–3004. [CrossRef] [PubMed]

68. Andrews, M.D.; Af Forselles, K.; Beaumont, K.; Galan, S.R.; Glossop, P.A.; Grenie, M.; Jessiman, A.; Kenyon, A.S.; Lunn, G.; Maw, G.; et al. Discovery of a Selective TRPM8 Antagonist with Clinical Efficacy in Cold-Related Pain. *ACS Med. Chem. Lett.* **2015**, *6*, 419–424. [CrossRef] [PubMed]

69. Almeida, M.C.; Hew-Butler, T.; Soriano, R.N.; Rao, S.; Wang, W.; Wang, J.; Tamayo, N.; Oliveira, D.L.; Nucci, T.B.; Aryal, P.; et al. Pharmacological blockade of the cold receptor TRPM8 attenuates autonomic and behavioral cold defenses and decreases deep body temperature. *J. Neurosci.* **2012**, *32*, 2086–2099. [CrossRef] [PubMed]

70. Miller, S.; Rao, S.; Wang, W.; Liu, H.; Wang, J.; Gavva, N.R. Antibodies to the extracellular pore loop of TRPM8 act as antagonists of channel activation. *PLoS ONE* **2014**, *9*, e107151. [CrossRef] [PubMed]

71. Gavva, N.R.; Davis, C.; Lehto, S.G.; Rao, S.; Wang, W.; Zhu, D.X. Transient receptor potential melastatin 8 (TRPM8) channels are involved in body temperature regulation. *Mol. Pain* **2012**, *8*, 36. [CrossRef] [PubMed]

72. Grisold, W.; Cavaletti, G.; Windebank, A.J. Peripheral neuropathies from chemotherapeutics and targeted agents: Diagnosis, treatment, and prevention. *Neuro-Oncology* **2012**. [CrossRef] [PubMed]

73. Windebank, A.J.; Grisold, W. Chemotherapy-induced neuropathy. *J. Peripher. Nerv. Syst.* **2008**, *13*, 27–46. [CrossRef] [PubMed]

74. Pachman, D.R.; Barton, D.L.; Watson, J.C.; Loprinzi, C.L. Chemotherapy-induced peripheral neuropathy: Prevention and treatment. *Clin. Pharmacol. Ther.* **2011**, *90*, 377–387. [CrossRef] [PubMed]

75. Basso, L.; Altier, C. Transient Receptor Potential Channels in neuropathic pain. *Curr. Opin. Pharmacol.* **2016**, *32*, 9–15. [CrossRef] [PubMed]

76. Clinical Trials.gov. Available online: https://clinicaltrials.gov/ (accessed on 24 March 2017).

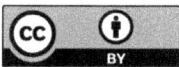

pharmaceuticals

MDPI

Review

Blocking TRPA1 in Respiratory Disorders: Does It Hold a Promise?

Indranil Mukhopadhyay, Abhay Kulkarni and Neelima Khairatkar-Joshi *

Biological Research, Glenmark Research Centre, Glenmark Pharmaceuticals Ltd. Navi Mumbai, Maharashtra 400709, India; Indranil.Mukhopadhyay@glenmarkpharma.com (I.M.); Abhay.Kulkarni@glenmarkpharma.com (A.K.)
* Correspondence: Neelima.Joshi@glenmarkpharma.com; Tel.: +91-22-6772-0000 (Ext. 3252)

Academic Editors: Arpad Szallasi and Jean Jacques Vanden Eynde
Received: 14 July 2016; Accepted: 28 September 2016; Published: 5 November 2016

Abstract: Transient Receptor Potential Ankyrin 1 (TRPA1) ion channel is expressed abundantly on the C fibers that innervate almost entire respiratory tract starting from oral cavity and oropharynx, conducting airways in the trachea, bronchi, terminal bronchioles, respiratory bronchioles and upto alveolar ducts and alveoli. Functional presence of TRPA1 on non-neuronal cells got recognized recently. TRPA1 plays a well-recognized role of "chemosensor", detecting presence of exogenous irritants and endogenous pro-inflammatory mediators that are implicated in airway inflammation and sensory symptoms like chronic cough, asthma, chronic obstructive pulmonary disease (COPD), allergic rhinitis and cystic fibrosis. TRPA1 can remain activated chronically due to elevated levels and continued presence of such endogenous ligands and pro-inflammatory mediators. Several selective TRPA1 antagonists have been tested in animal models of respiratory disease and their performance is very promising. Although there is no TRPA1 antagonist in advanced clinical trials or approved on market yet to treat respiratory diseases, however, limited but promising evidences available so far indicate likelihood that targeting TRPA1 may present a new therapy in treatment of respiratory diseases in near future. This review will focus on in vitro, animal and human evidences that strengthen the proposed role of TRPA1 in modulation of specific airway sensory responses and also on preclinical and clinical progress of selected TRPA1 antagonists.

Keywords: TRPA1; airway inflammation; airway sensory responses; asthma; COPD; cough

1. TRPA1 Receptor

TRPA1 ion channel and its biology is known for more than a decade now. It has attracted academic scientists due to its interesting tissue distribution and functions. TRPA1 is abundantly expressed in peripheral nervous system and has demonstrated a chemosensory function. Hence, it has been assigned a role of "warning system" against external as well as internal assaults. Industrial researchers are interested in TRPA1 as a target for therapeutic intervention due to its implicated role in miscellaneous diseases. Evidence for potential role of TRPA1 in pain signaling based on TRPA1 knockout (TRPA1 KO) mice and siRNA studies emerged much earlier compared to its involvement in airway diseases—which is relatively recent and still emerging. TRPA1 is highly expressed on pulmonary innervation—an anatomically relevant region for respiratory diseases, and could be one of the major players in orchestration of airway inflammatory response. A large number of recent studies have implicated TRPA1 in the pathogenesis of several respiratory diseases including chronic cough, asthma, COPD, allergic rhinitis and cystic fibrosis. Blockade of TRPA1 is perceived as a novel strategy for its therapeutic intervention.

2. TRPA1—Expression and Activation in Airways

TRPA1 was first identified in cultured human lung fibroblasts [1]. Later on, TRPA1 expression on mouse lung was reported, albeit to a lesser extent compared to other tissues [2]. TRPA1 is abundantly expressed on the innervations of almost entire respiratory tract including the C-fibers of the trigeminal and vagal ganglia, which innervate upper regions of oral cavity and oropharynx and on conducting airways in the trachea, bronchi, terminal bronchioles, respiratory bronchioles, alveolar ducts and alveoli. C-fibers largely "sense" the presence of potentially toxic inhaled irritants and toxicants. TRPA1 was initially recognized as an irritant sensing ion channel on majority of vagal nociceptive C-fibers in the bronchopulmonary region [3]. It is well known now that unlike traditional chemoreceptors, TRPA1 is activated by a wide variety of structurally different molecules with high chemical reactivity spanning from exogenous irritants to endogenously produced reactive reagents [4–11]. Functional presence of TRPA1 on non-neuronal cells got recognized recently. TRPA1 is shown to be expressed on lung fibroblasts, epithelial and smooth muscle cells [12–15].

The role of TRPA1 in airway pathologies has been corroborated by studies using the TRPA1 KO mice and TRPA1 antagonists. In wild-type mice, airway exposure to hypochlorite or Hydrogen peroxide (H_2O_2) evoke respiratory depression as manifested by a reduction in breathing frequency and increase in end expiratory pause, both of which were attenuated in TRPA1 KO mice [6]. A host of chemicals are known to be specifically associated with respiratory diseases and airway reflex responses such as coughing, sneezing and bronchoconstriction. Acrolein and crotonaldehyde induce strong tussive response in animals as well as in man. H_2O_2, 4-Hydroxynonenal (4-HNE), photochemical smog, zinc, toluene diisocyanate are associated with allergic asthma in humans. All the above listed chemicals are direct and potent activators of TRPA1. α,β-unsaturated aldehydes are earliest recognized TRPA1 activators, and are detected in air spaces, breath, sputum, lungs, and blood from patients with asthma as well as COPD. Fragrance chemicals like menthol, 1,8-Cineole, borneol, fenchyl alcohol etc. are associated with TRPA1 activation and play a key role in allergic reactions [16]. Cigarette smoke, wood smoke, diesel exhaust, and other combustion-derived particles activate TRPA1, causing irritation and inflammation in the respiratory tract [17,18]. TRPA1 is a molecular sensor for wood smoke particulate and several chemical constituents such as 3,5-ditert-butylphenol, coniferaldehyde, formaldehyde, perinaphthenone, agathic acid, and isocupressic acid are TRPA1 agonists [18]. Nassini R et al. [14] demonstrated that TRPA1 is expressed in non-neuronal cells in human and murine airways, and promote a non-neurogenic inflammatory response. This raises an alternate possibility that airway inflammation may also be promoted by non-neuronal mediators. Thus, TRPA1 ion channel with its wide range of expression in neuronal and non-neuronal cells and its activation by several exogenous and endogenous stimuli relevant to airway sensory responses may be a major regulator in driving several respiratory diseases.

3. TRPA1 in Chronic Cough

Cough is a vagally mediated defensive mechanism to protect the airway to clear respiratory tract from continuously exposed airborne environmental irritants. Despite wide prevalence of chronic cough, therapy options are very inadequate and often symptomatic. Currently available treatments such as dextromethorphan, hydrocodone and codeine are inadequate due to limited efficacy, central nervous system (CNS) side effects or abuse liability, respiratory depression and gastrointestinal disturbances. The paucity, if not absence of effective medicine to treat cough is mainly because the molecular mechanisms that orchestrate chronic cough are not clearly understood in experimental animal models as well as in man. Scientists are attempting to shed some light on the possible mechanism behind the occurrence of chronic cough. A number of TRP channels (TRPA1, TRPV1 and TRPV4) have been linked to sensory perception relevant to cough response [19]. A large number of in vitro and in vivo studies have recently indicated important role of TRPA1 activation in driving cough reflex. Acrolein and crotonaldehyde are contained in cigarette smoke and polluted air which are well recognized cough inducers. TRPA1 agonists are shown to induce activation of recombinant human TRPA1 channels in vitro in human embryonic kidney cells (HEK293), depolarization of murine, guinea pig and human vagal sensory nerves and produce cough in healthy human volunteers [20]. Allyl isothiocyanate (AITC), acrolein, crotonaldehyde and cinnamaldehyde—all are potent TRPA1 agonists and shown to induce dose dependent and robust tussive response in guinea pigs which was attenuated by non-selective TRP channel blockers (camphor, gentamicin) as well as by selective TRPA1 antagonist from Hydra Biosciences—HC-030031 (Figure 1) [9]. The cough response however remained unchanged upon administration of capsazepine which is a TRPV1 antagonist as well as desensitizing TRPA1 agonist [21]. We demonstrated direct in vitro activation of TRPA1 receptor by citric acid which is routinely used to evoke cough in preclinical and clinical studies [22]. Citric acid induced tussive response in guinea pigs was inhibited by a potent and selective TRPA1 antagonist from our laboratory, GRC 17536 (structure not disclosed). Anti-tussive effect of other TRPA1 antagonists is also demonstrated in animal cough model. Recently, a poster from Almirall at European Respiratory Society Conference (2015) reported a potent oral TRPA1 antagonist-Compound A, that showed inhibition of isolated guinea pig vagus nerve depolarization with EC_{50} of 80 nM. Furthermore, in the in vivo model of AITC induced cough, Compound-A showed dose dependent inhibition of cough response with ED_{50} of 0.17 mg/kg dose [23].

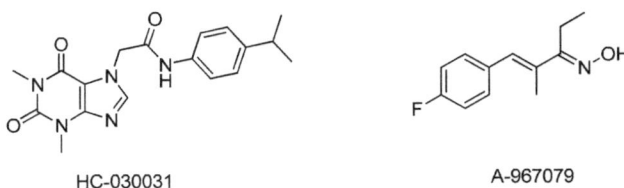

HC-030031   A-967079

Figure 1. Chemical structure of Hydra Biosciences (HC-030031) and Abbott (A-967079).

Importantly, TRPA1 mediated tussive response is associated with both exogenous TRPA1 agonists as well as endogenous biochemicals that are produced during diseases associated with cough. For example, prostaglandin E2 (PGE_2) and bradykinin are produced during tissue inflammation. Mucoid secretions containing similar pro-tussive inflammatory mediators are produced in patients with post nasal drip syndrome (PNDS). 4-HNE, reactive oxygen species (ROS), reactive nitrogen species (RNS), 15-deoxy-delta-12,14-prostaglandin J2 ($15d$-PGJ_2) are produced in the airways during asthma, COPD and in the esophagus during gastroesophageal reflux disease (GERD) [24] and lastly, toll like receptors (TLRs) that are produced during post viral cough condition. [25–27]. Thus, TRPA1 could have a central role in producing chronic cough associated with diverse pathologies but via a common mechanism of vagal nerve activation due to its activators prevailing during specific diseases as described above [9,20,28,29]. Hence TRPA1 has emerged as one of the most promising targets for the development of medicines to treat chronic cough.

4. TRPA1 and Asthma

Asthma is an inflammatory disease of the lungs characterized by bronchoconstriction and airway hyperreactivity, leading to shortness of breath, wheezing, and coughing. It is triggered by exposure to allergen or irritant and manifested as episodes or attacks of airway narrowing that are mediated by airway nerves and muscles. Studies focusing on airway smooth muscle and epithelial function strongly indicate involvement of immunogenic and neurogenic mechanisms in airway inflammation. TRPA1 could be a key integrator of immune and neuronal signaling in the airways [30].

Various noxious chemicals and environmental/industrial irritants that activate TRPA1 happen to be triggers for asthma or reactive airways dysfunction syndrome (RADS) and are known to worsen asthma attacks [31]. Toluene diisocyanate is a potent TRPA1 activator and exposure to this chemical is the leading cause of occupational asthma. Exposure to cigarette smoke strongly correlates with asthma severity. Cigarette smoke ingredients-acrolein and crotonaldehyde activate native and recombinant TRPA1 and produce tracheal extravasation in wild type animals in TRPA1 dependent manner. Asthmatics are sensitive to photochemical smog that contains acrolein and other oxidant species which are also known to activate TRPA1. Several TRPA1 activators or sensitizers are endogenously produced in lungs of patients which are also efficient triggers of asthma e.g., H_2O_2, 4-HNE, cyclic prostaglandin PGJ_2 and bradykinin. Elevated levels of bradykinin and nerve growth factor (NGF) are found in bronchoalveolar lavage of asthma and rhinitis patients while elevated 4-HNE and acrolein are detected in lungs, air spaces, breath, sputum and blood of asthma and COPD patients. Experiments with TRPA1 KO mice revealed reduced airway infiltration by inflammatory leukocytes accompanied by decreased production of pro-inflammatory cytokines and neuropeptide release in the airways in the ovalbumin (OVA) asthma model [30]. In the wild type mice that developed asthma upon OVA challenge, pharmacological blockade of TRPA1 receptor with HC-030031 reiterated the above observation. HC-030031 also inhibited OVA-induced late asthmatic response in dose dependent manner in B/N rats [32]. During late asthmatic response, allergen challenge is implicated to trigger airway sensory nerves via TRPA1 activation to further initiate a central reflex event. A couple of recent posters presented in conferences have reported similar findings as above using TRPA1 selective antagonists [33,34]. GRC 17536 showed significant inhibition of lung eosinophilia, mucus production and airway hyperresponsiveness in mouse asthma model, and, inhibition of eosinophils and early airway reactivity in guinea pig allergic asthma model [33]. Another TRPA1 antagonist from Cubist Pharmaceuticals, CB-625 (structure not disclosed), was effective in reducing the late asthmatic response and antigen induced airway hyperresponsiveness upon oral dosing in sheep model of asthma [34]. Epidemiological evidence has linked therapeutic acetaminophen doses with risk of COPD and asthma [35]. Recent studies by Nassini et al. [36] demonstrated that N-acetyl-p-benzoquinoneimine (NAPQ1), a metabolite of acetaminophen, evoked pro-inflammatory responses in the lung. They further demonstrated that NAPQ1 selectively activates TRPA1, and selective inhibition of TRPA1 abated the pro-inflammatory effect of acetaminophen. It remains to be seen if TRPA1 antagonists attenuate asthma in clinics.

5. Role of TRPA1 in COPD

COPD is a disease characterized by increased infiltration of inflammatory cells in the lung, increased oxidative and nitrosative burden in the lung and parenchymal destruction, associated with progressive decline in lung function. COPD is strongly associated with smoking status of an individual but other environmental factors such as bio mass fuel exposure are also implicated in the etiology of COPD [37].

TRPA1 is shown to be a major neuronal sensor for oxidants in the airways [6]. Various pollutants, oxidants, cigarette smoke extract (CSE) and cigarette smoke (CS) ingredients such as acrolein, crotonaldehyde, 4-HNE that are associated with the pathobiology of COPD, are potent agonists of TRPA1. Some of these are associated with interleukin 8 (IL8) release in the human macrophagic cell lines [7,38]. Our TRPA1 antagonist GRC 17536 was effective in inhibiting CSE, crotonaldehyde and acrolein induced Ca^{2+} influx in vitro and AITC induced Ca^{2+} influx and IL8 production in human lung fibroblast cells (CCD19-Lu) and human pulmonary alveolar epithelial cell line (A549) [22]. CSE induced increase in TRPA1 expression and IL8 release in human bronchial epithelial cells (HBEC) was attenuated by HC-030031 [39].

Further corroborating evidence to support the role of TRPA1 in COPD came from the studies in animal models of COPD. CS and acrolein induced release of keratinocyte chemoattractant (KC) (CXCL1/GRO alpha; mouse homolog of human IL-8) in bronchoalveolar lavage fluid (BALf) of mice was significantly reduced in TRPA1 KO mice [14]. Pretreatment of animals with HC-030031 showed protection from CS induced plasma protein extravasation whereas capsazepine was not effective suggesting selective involvement of TRPA1 in inducing CS associated inflammation. When C57BL/6 mice was exposed to CS for 4 weeks, significant increase in TRPA1 mRNA was observed in trigeminal and nodose/jugular ganglia of CS-exposed mice with a positive correlation to cellular infiltration. An increase in leukocytes, macrophages and neutrophils was observed in BALf of mice [40]. Increased immunostaining for TRPA1 was observed in wild type mice chronically exposed to CS whereas TRPA1 KO mice revealed reduced inflammation and structural changes [39]. All these observations suggest strong involvement of TRPA1 in mediating CS induced inflammation in the animal models.

Although COPD is directly linked to the smoking history, recently it was shown that other factors like biomass fuels and biomass smoke exposure is also a risk factor for COPD development [41]. Wood smoke and its chemical constituents are activators of TRPA1 and are known for their damaging effects on respiratory system. Wood smoke particulate matter (WSPM) at low concentration, which is relevant in terms of potential human exposure levels are known to activate TRPA1 [18]. There is ample evidence to show involvement of TRPA1 in COPD and TRPA1 antagonists seem promising treatment options in clinical management of COPD.

6. Role of TRPA1 in Allergic Rhinitis

Allergic rhinitis and asthma are chronic inflammatory atopic disorders characterized by overlapping symptoms and pathophysiology. Toluene diisocyanate (TDI) is a highly reactive chemical associated with respiratory symptoms resembling allergic rhinitis and a most prevalent cause of occupational asthma [42,43]. Exposure of mice to TDI showed decreased breathing rates, increased cytokines accompanied by increased eosinophils and allergic inflammation in nasal cavity [44]. It is an effective TRPA1 activator with in vitro EC_{50} of 10 µM which is a physiologically relevant concentration known to cause decreased breathing rate and sensory irritation in mice. Interestingly, these symptoms were absent in TRPA1 KO mice [45] suggesting an important role of TRPA1 in allergic or occupational asthma and rhinitis. A recent study showed increased level of TRPA1 mRNA in subjects with rhinitis compared to normal controls ($p = 0.03$) suggesting potential involvement of TRPA1 in allergic rhinitis [46].

7. Role of TRPA1 in Cystic Fibrosis

Cystic fibrosis (CF) is a disease associated with mutation in the gene for cystic fibrosis transmembrane conductance regulator (CFTR) and can affect many organs. When upper and lower airways are involved, it causes impaired mucociliary clearance leading to mucus plugging in the airways, failure in effective clearing of inhaled bacteria and lung neutrophilia. Respiratory failure is a major cause of mortality associated with CF. Recently TRPA1 expression was reported on different epithelial cells obtained from lung tissues of CF patients [47]. IL8 expression was observed in the bronchial epithelial cells co-expressing TRPA1. Furthermore TRPA1 specific inhibitors from Hydra Biosciences (HC-030031) and Abbott (A-967079) (Figure 1) [48] inhibited *P. aeruginosa* induced transcription of IL8, IL1b, IL6 and tumor necrosis factor α (TNFα) in A549 and human cystic fibrosis cell line (CuFi-1). *P. aeruginosa* is a gram negative bacteria and releases lipopolysaccharide (LPS) which is a direct TRPA1 agonist and sensitizer [49]. Silencing TRPA1 significantly reduced the release of IL-8, IL-1β and TNF-α from HBECs from CF patients. This is the first study which revealed the potential of TRPA1 antagonists in controlling inflammation associated with CF.

8. TRPA1 Antagonists: What's the Status?

Till date, there is limited published literature showing efficacy of TRPA1 antagonists in respiratory diseases. The accumulating evidence supporting TRPA1 as an attractive target in respiratory disease has resulted in large number of small molecules patents (Table 1). Some of the compounds have been evaluated in animal models of respiratory diseases as summarized in earlier sections and the data is very encouraging. However it remains to be seen if such promising results in animal will eventually translate to efficacy in humans. Until then, translational studies to assess their pharmacological effects on patient derived lung tissues ex vivo could strengthen the claim of their potential utility to treat human respiratory diseases. Such study tools are established for assessing translatability of TRPA1 antagonist pharmacology in pain where in calcitonin gene-related peptide (CGRP) release from human dental pulp is assayed as a biomarker. Recently, TRPA1 antagonist—GRC 17536 from our laboratory has shown positive proof of concept in reducing peripheral diabetic neuropathic pain in patients with intact nerves [50]. The clinical features of chronic pain and refractory chronic cough seem overlapping. Clinical presentation of chronic pain typically includes paraesthesia (abnormal sensation in the absence of a stimulus), hyperalgesia (pain triggered by a low exposure to a known painful stimulus), and allodynia (pain triggered by a non-painful stimulus) and shows similarities with the clinical features of refractory chronic cough, such as an abnormal throat sensation or tickle (laryngeal paraesthesia), increased cough sensitivity in response to known tussigens (hypertussia), and cough triggered in response to non-tussive stimuli such as talking or cold air (allotussia). Gabapentin, which is used to treat neuropathic pain, is also reported to show antitussive effect in human chronic cough patients recently [51]. Hence there is optimism to believe that TRPA1 antagonists could work in treatment of chronic cough.

Table 1. TRPA1 in Respiratory Diseases: A Patent Update.

Patent Number	Owner Companies	Indications
WO2013084153; WO2013014597; WO2012176143; WO2012172475; WO2012176105; WO2011132017; WO2014203210; WO2010125469; WO2010004390; WO2010109287; WO2013183035; WO2009118596; WO2012085662; WO2009144548; WO2011114184	Glenmark Pharmaceuticals SA	Asthma; COPD; Bronchitis, COPD, Cough, Respiratory disorder
WO2009140517; WO2010132838; WO2007073505; WO2010039289; WO2015164643; WO2016044792; WO2010036821	Hydra Biosciences Inc.	Asthma, Cough; Respiratory disease; Asthma; COPD; Lung injury
WO2009071631; WO2010141805	Janssen Pharmaceutica NV	COPD; Lung disease; Cough
WO2015052264; WO2014060341; WO2014056958; WO2014049047; WO2014072325	F Hoffmann-La Roche AG; Hoffmann-La Roche Inc.; Roche Holding AG Genentech Inc.	Asthma; COPD; Cough; Allergic rhinitis; Respiratory disease; Bronchospasm
WO2015144976; WO2012152983; WO2014053694; WO2015144977	Orion Corp	Asthma; COPD; Cough
WO2013023102; WO2014113671	Cubist Pharmaceuticals Inc.; Hydra Biosciences Inc.	Asthma; COPD; Respiratory disease
WO2015115507; WO2014098098; WO2013108857	Ajinomoto Co Inc.	Asthma; COPD; Cough; Lung disease
JP2014024810	Kao Corp	Respiratory failure
WO2009089082	AbbVie Deutschland GmbH & Co KG; Abbott Laboratories	Lung disease
WO2016028325	Duke University; University of California	Fibrosis
WO2015155306	Almirall Prodesfarma SA	Respiratory disease
WO2014135617	Ario Pharma Ltd; PharmEste SRL	Asthma; COPD; Cough

As far as COPD is concerned, cigarette smoke and wood smoke have a close and proven involvement in COPD pathobiology. Constituents of cigarette smoke and wood smoke are potent activators of TRPA1. Hence, TRPA1 antagonists such as GRC 17536, which have started to show promising clinical benefits in human pain proof of concept trials, could also be effective in treating respiratory diseases. Several pharmaceutical companies have active drug discovery programs targeting TRPA1 receptor for potential treatment of miscellaneous respiratory disorders (Table 1).

9. TRPA1 Antagonists: Any Safety Concerns?

TRPA1 KO mice are viable, normal in appearance and fertile with no auditory dysfunction [4,52]. Unlike TRPV1 or TRPM8, TRPA1 is not involved in body temperature regulation at basal level or under cold challenge [53,54]. Hence TRPA1 antagonists are expected to be devoid of adverse effects on body temperature unlike the TRPV1 antagonists (hyperthermia) or TRPM8 antagonists (hypothermia). Human healthy volunteers administered with CB-625 show normal body temperature and also unimpaired thermosensation in heat and cold tests [55]. This is in line with TRPA1 KO mice data that exhibits unimpaired heat and cold sensitivity [4]. Also, wild type (WT) animals in spinal nerve ligation (SNL) nerve injury model when treated with antisense TRPA1 were protected against cold hyperalgesia while showing no effect on normal cold sensitivity [56]. Animals treated with TRPA1 antagonist have normal performance in hot and cold plate tests and no paradoxical sensation [53].

Although TRPA1 is predominantly expressed in sensory neurons, it is also expressed in other non-neuronal tissues, albeit at a much lower level. This raises a question if targeting TRPA1 could have unintended/unrecognized adverse effects on physiological functions or on known protective functions such as sensing environmental irritants. TRPA1 KO mice are recently reported to show physical hyperactivity [57]. Since several TRPA1 antagonists are at different stages of evaluation including chemical synthesis, preclinical studies and clinical trials, their long term safety in patients is likely to be addressed soon.

10. Summary

The role of TRPA1 in the respiratory system has been summarized in Figure 2. TRPA1 is expressed on pulmonary innervation - an anatomically relevant region for respiratory diseases and implicated in the orchestration of inflammatory response in animal models of airway diseases, including chronic cough, asthma, COPD, allergic rhinitis and cystic fibrosis. TRPA1 can remain activated chronically due to elevated levels and continued presence of endogenous ligands and pro-inflammatory mediators. Phenotype of TRPA1 KO mice in allergen-induced asthma model and CS model is in line with this since these animals show reduced leukocyte infiltration in the airways, reduction of cytokine and mucus production.

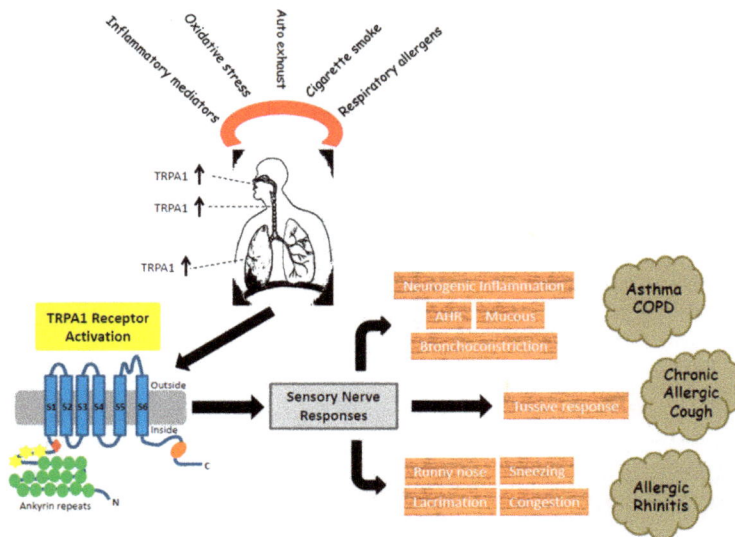

Figure 2. TRPA1 in respiratory diseases.

Preclinical performance of TRPA1 antagonists in respiratory disease models is promising. There is no TRPA1 antagonist in advanced clinical trials or approved on market yet to treat respiratory diseases. We are in the wait to see if they can attenuate undesirable airway sensory responses in man and additionally if they are capable of reversing disease progression and outperform current standard of care such as anti-inflammatory drugs. Available evidences and underlying science indicate likelihood that they may live up to the expectations and help clinicians in treatment of chronic airway diseases with unmet medical need in near future.

Conflicts of Interest: The authors declare no conflict of interest.

Abbreviations

TRPA1	Transient Receptor Potential Ankyrin 1
COPD	Chronic obstructive pulmonary disease
TRPA1 KO	TRPA1 knockout
H_2O_2	Hydrogen peroxide
4-HNE	4-Hydroxynonenal
CNS	Central nervous system
HEK293	Human embryonic kidney cells
AITC	Allyl isothiocyanate
PGE_2	Prostaglandin E2
PNDS	Post nasal drip syndrome
ROS	Reactive oxygen species
RNS	Reactive nitrogen species
15d-PGJ_2	15-deoxy-delta-12,14-prostaglandin J2
GERD	Gastroesophageal reflux disease
TLRs	Toll like receptors
RADS	Reactive airways dysfunction syndrome
NGF	Nerve growth factor
OVA	Ovalbumin
NAPQ1	*N*-acetyl-p-benzoquinoneimine
CSE	Cigarette smoke extract
CS	Cigarette smoke
IL8	Interleukin 8
CCD19-Lu	Human lung fibroblast cells
A549	Human pulmonary alveolar epithelial cell line
HBEC	Human bronchial epithelial cells
KC	Keratinocyte chemoattractant
BALf	Bronchoalveolar lavage fluid
WSPM	Wood smoke particulate matter
TDI	Toluene diisocyanate
CF	Cystic fibrosis
CFTR	Cystic fibrosis transmembrane conductance regulator
$TNF\alpha$	Tumor necrosis factor α
CuFi-1	Human cystic fibrosis cell line
LPS	Lipopolysaccharide
CGRP	Calcitonin gene-related peptide
WT	Wild type
SNL	Spinal nerve ligation

References

1. Jaquemar, D.; Schenker, T.; Trueb, B. An ankyrin-like protein with transmembrane domains is specifically lost after oncogenic transformation of human fibroblasts. *J. Biol. Chem.* **1999**, *274*, 7325–7333. [CrossRef]
2. Kunert-Keil, C.; Bisping, F.; Krüger, J.; Brinkmeier, H. Tissue-specific expression of TRP channel genes in the mouse and its variation in three different mouse strains. *BMC Genom.* **2006**, *7*, 159. [CrossRef]
3. Nassenstein, C.; Kwong, K.; Taylor-Clark, T.; Kollarik, M.; Macglashan, D.M.; Braun, A.; Undem, B.J. Expression and function of the ion channel TRPA1 in vagal afferent nerves innervating mouse lungs. *J. Physiol.* **2008**, *586*, 1595–1604. [CrossRef]
4. Bautista, D.M.; Jordt, S.E.; Nikai, T.; Tsuruda, P.R.; Read, A.J.; Poblete, J.; Yamoah, E.N.; Basbaum, A.I.; Julius, D. TRPA1 mediates the inflammatory actions of environmental irritants and proalgesic agents. *Cell* **2006**, *124*, 1269–1282. [CrossRef]
5. Trevisani, M.; Siemens, J.; Materazzi, S.; Bautista, D.M.; Nassini, R.; Campi, B.; Imamachi, N.; Andrè, E.; Patacchini, R.; Cottrell, G.S.; et al. 4-Hydroxynonenal, an endogenous aldehyde, causes pain and neurogenic inflammation through activation of the irritant receptor TRPA1. *Proc. Natl. Acad. Sci. USA* **2007**, *104*, 13519–13524. [CrossRef]
6. Bessac, B.F.; Sivula, M.; von Hehn, C.A.; Escalera, J.; Cohn, L.; Jordt, S.E. TRPA1 is a major oxidant sensor in murine airway sensory neurons. *J. Clin. Invest.* **2008**, *118*, 1899–1910. [CrossRef]
7. Andrè, E.; Campi, B.; Materazzi, S.; Trevisani, M.; Amadesi, S.; Massi, D.; Creminon, C.; Vaksman, N.; Nassini, R.; Civelli, M.; et al. Cigarette smoke-induced neurogenic inflammation is mediated by α,β-unsaturated aldehydes and the TRPA1 receptor in rodents. *J. Clin. Invest.* **2008**, *118*, 2574–2582. [CrossRef]
8. Matta, J.A.; Cornett, P.M.; Miyares, R.L.; Abe, K.; Sahibzada, N.; Ahern, G.P. General anesthetics activate a nociceptive ion channel to enhance pain and inflammation. *Proc. Natl. Acad. Sci. USA* **2008**, *105*, 8784–8789. [CrossRef]
9. Andrè, E.; Gatti, R.; Trevisani, M.; Preti, D.; Baraldi, P.G.; Patacchini, R.; Geppetti, P. Transient receptor potential ankyrin receptor 1 is a novel target for pro-tussive agents. *Br. J. Pharmacol.* **2009**, *158*, 1621–1628. [CrossRef]
10. Hu, H.; Bandell, M.; Petrus, M.J.; Zhu, M.X.; Patapoutian, A. Zinc activates damage-sensing TRPA1 ion channels. *Nat. Chem. Biol.* **2009**, *5*, 183–190. [CrossRef]
11. Taylor-Clark, T.E.; Ghatta, S.; Bettner, W.; Undem, B.J. Nitrooleic acid, an endogenous product of nitrative stress, activates nociceptive sensory nerves via the direct activation of TRPA1. *Mol. Pharmacol.* **2009**, *75*, 820–829. [CrossRef]
12. Nagata, K.; Duggan, A.; Kumar, G.; García-Añoveros, J. Nociceptor and hair cell transducer properties of TRPA1, a channel for pain and hearing. *J. Neurosci.* **2005**, *25*, 4052–4061. [CrossRef]
13. Mukhopadhyay, I.; Gomes, P.; Aranake, S.; Shetty, M.; Karnik, P.; Damle, M.; Kuruganti, S.; Thorat, S.; Khairatkar-Joshi, N. Expression of functional TRPA1 receptor on human lung fibroblast and epithelial cells. *J. Recept. Signal Transduct.* **2011**, *31*, 350–358. [CrossRef]
14. Nassini, R.; Pedretti, P.; Moretto, N.; Fusi, C.; Carnini, C.; Facchinetti, F.; Viscomi, A.R.; Pisano, A.R.; Stokesberry, S.; Brunmark, C.; et al. Transient receptor potential ankyrin 1 channel localized to non-neuronal airway cells promotes non-neurogenic inflammation. *PLoS ONE* **2012**, *7*, e42454. [CrossRef]
15. Büch, T.R.; Schäfer, E.A.; Demmel, M.T.; Boekhoff, I.; Thiermann, H.; Gudermann, T.; Steinritz, D.; Schmidt, A. Functional expression of the transient receptor potential channel TRPA1, a sensor for toxic lung inhalants, in pulmonary epithelial cells. *Chem. Biol. Interact.* **2013**, *206*, 462–471. [CrossRef]
16. Mihara, S.; Shibamoto, T. The role of flavor and fragrance chemicals in TRPA1 (transient receptor potential cation channel, member A1) activity associated with allergies. *Allergy Asthma Clin. Immunol.* **2015**, *11*. [CrossRef]
17. Kichko, T.I.; Kobal, G.; Reeh, P.W. Cigarette smoke has sensory effects through nicotinic and TRPA1 but not TRPV1 receptors on the isolated mouse trachea and larynx. *Am. J. Physiol. Lung Cell. Mol. Physiol.* **2015**, *309*, L812–L820. [CrossRef]

18. Shapiro, D.; Deering-Rice, C.E.; Romero, E.G.; Hughen, R.W.; Light, A.R.; Veranth, J.M.; Reilly, C.A. Activation of transient receptor potential ankyrin-1 (TRPA1) in lung cells by wood smoke particulate material. *Chem. Res. Toxicol.* **2013**, *26*, 750–758. [CrossRef]
19. Grace, M.S.; Dubuis, E.; Birrell, M.A.; Belvisi, M.G. Pre-clinical studies in cough research: Role of Transient Receptor Potential (TRP) channels. *Pulm. Pharmacol. Ther.* **2013**, *26*, 498–507. [CrossRef]
20. Birrell, M.A.; Belvisi, M.G.; Grace, M.; Sadofsky, L.; Faruqi, S.; Hele, D.J.; Maher, S.A.; Freund-Michel, V.; Morice, A.H. TRPA1 agonists evoke coughing in guinea pig and human volunteers. *Am. J. Respir. Crit. Care Med.* **2009**, *180*, 1042–1047. [CrossRef]
21. Kistner, K.; Siklosi, N.; Babes, A.; Khalil, M.; Selescu, T.; Zimmermann, K.; Wirtz, S.; Becker, C.; Neurath, M.F.; Reeh, P.W.; et al. Systemic desensitization through TRPA1 channels by capsazepine and mustard oil—A novel strategy against inflammation and pain. *Sci. Rep.* **2016**, *6*, 28621. [CrossRef]
22. Mukhopadhyay, I.; Kulkarni, A.; Aranake, S.; Karnik, P.; Shetty, M.; Thorat, S.; Ghosh, I.; Wale, D.; Bhosale, V.; Khairatkar-Joshi, N. Transient receptor potential ankyrin 1 receptor activation in vitro and in vivo by pro-tussive agents: GRC 17536 as a promising anti-tussive therapeutic. *PLoS ONE* **2014**, *9*, e97005. [CrossRef]
23. Aparici, M.; Tarrasón, G.; Jover, I.; Carcasona, C.; Fernández-Blanco, J.; Eichhorn, P.; Gavaldà, A.; De Alba, J.; Roberts, R.; Miralpeix, M. Pharmacological profile of a novel, potent and oral TRPA1 antagonist. Characterization in a preclinical model of induced cough. *Eur. Respir. J.* **2015**, *46*, PA3948. [CrossRef]
24. Canning, B.J. Afferent nerves regulating the cough reflex: Mechanisms and mediators of cough in disease. *Otolaryngol. Clin. North Am.* **2010**, *43*, 15–25. [CrossRef]
25. Bezemer, G.F.G.; Sagar, S.; van Bergenhenegouwen, J.; Georgiou, N.A.; Garssen, J.; Kraneveld, A.D.; Folkerts, G. Dual Role of Toll-Like Receptors in Asthma and Chronic Obstructive Pulmonary Disease. *Pharmacol. Rev.* **2012**, *64*, 337–358. [CrossRef]
26. Zhang, L.; Liu, J.; Bai, J.; Wang, X.; Li, Y.; Jiang, P. Comparative expression of Toll-like receptors and inflammatory cytokines in pigs infected with different virulent porcine reproductive and respiratory syndrome virus isolates. *J. Virol.* **2013**, *10*, 135. [CrossRef]
27. Qi, J.; Buzas, K.; Fan, H.; Cohen, J.I.; Wang, K.; Mont, E.; Klinman, D.; Oppenheim, J.J.; Howard, O.M. Painful pathways induced by TLR stimulation of dorsal root ganglion neurons. *J. Immunol.* **2011**, *186*, 6417–6426. [CrossRef]
28. Belvisi, M.G.; Dubuis, E.; Birrell, M.A. Transient receptor potential A1 channels: Insights into cough and airway inflammatory disease. *Chest* **2011**, *140*, 1040–1047. [CrossRef]
29. Lavinka, P.C.; Dong, X. Molecular signaling and targets from itch: Lessons for cough. *Cough* **2013**, *9*, 8. [CrossRef]
30. Caceres, A.I.; Brackmann, M.; Elia, M.D.; Bessac, B.F.; del Camino, D.; D'Amours, M.; Witek, J.S.; Fanger, C.M.; Chong, J.A.; Hayward, N.J.; et al. A sensory neuronal ion channel essential for airway inflammation and hyperreactivity in asthma. *Proc Natl Acad Sci USA* **2009**, *106*, 9099–9104. [CrossRef]
31. Facchinetti, F.; Patacchini, R. The rising role of TRPA1 in asthma. *Open Drug Discov. J.* **2010**, *2*, 71–80. [CrossRef]
32. Raemdonck, K.; de Alba, J.; Birrell, M.A.; Grace, M.; Maher, S.A.; Irvin, C.G.; Fozard, J.R.; O'Byrne, P.M.; Belvisi, M.G. A role for sensory nerves in the late asthmatic response. *Thorax* **2012**, *67*, 19–25. [CrossRef]
33. Anupindi, R.; Mukhopadhyay, I.; Thomas, A.; Kumar, S.; Chaudhari, S.S.; Kulkarni, A.; Gudi, G.; Khairatkar-Joshi, N. GRC 17536, a novel, selective TRPA1 antagonist for potential treatment of respiratory disorders. *Eur. Respir. J.* **2010**, *36*, E5645.
34. Camino, D.; Chong, J.A.; Hayward, N.J.; Monsen, J.; Moran, M.M.; Curtis, R.; Murphy, C.; Mortin, L.I.; Abraham, W.M. Effects of blocking TRPA1 in a sheep model of asthma. In Proceedings of the International Workshop on Transient Receptor Potential Channels, a TRiP to Spain, Valencia, Spain, 12–14 September 2012; p. 68.
35. Beasley, R.; Clayton, T.; Crane, J.; von Mutius, E.; Lai, C.K.; Montefort, S.; Stewart, A. Association between paracetamol use in infancy and childhood, and risk of asthma, rhinoconjunctivitis, and eczema in children aged 6–7 years: Analysis from phase three of the ISAAC programme. *Lancet* **2008**, *372*, 1039–1048. [CrossRef]
36. Nassini, R.; Materazzi, S.; Andre', E.; Sartiani, L.; Aldini, G.; Trevisani, M.; Carnini, C.; Massi, D.; Pedretti, P.; Carini, M.; et al. Acetaminophen, *via* its reactive metabolite N-acetyl-pbenzo-quinoneimine and transient receptor potential ankyrin-1 stimulation, causes neurogenic inflammation in the airways and other tissues in rodents. *FASEB J.* **2010**, *24*, 4904–4916. [CrossRef]

37. Liu, S.; Zhou, Y.; Wang, X.; Wang, D.; Lu, J.; Zheng, J.; Zhong, N.; Ran, P. Biomass fuels are the probable risk factor for chronic obstructive pulmonary disease in rural South China. *Thorax* **2007**, *62*, 889–897. [CrossRef]

38. Facchinetti, F.; Amadei, F.; Geppetti, P.; Tarantini, F.; Serio, C.; Dragotto, A.; Gigli, P.M.; Catinella, S.; Civelli, M.; Patacchini, R. α,β-Unsaturated aldehydes in cigarette smoke release inflammatory mediators from human macrophages. *Am. J. Respir. Cell Mol. Biol.* **2007**, *37*, 617–623. [CrossRef]

39. Lin, A.H.; Liu, M.H.; Ko, H.K.; Perng, D.W.; Lee, T.S.; Kou, Y.R. Lung epithelial TRPA1 transduces the extracellular ROS into transcriptional regulation of lung inflammation induced by cigarette smoke: The role of influxed Ca^{2+}. *Mediat. Inflamm.* **2015**, *2015*, 148367. [CrossRef]

40. Dupont, L.L.; Alpizar, Y.A.; Brusselle, G.G.; Bracke, K.R.; Talavera, K.; Joos, G.F.; Maes, T. Expression of transient receptor potential (TRP) channels in a murine model of cigarette smoke exposure. In Proceedings of the C34. Insights into COPD Pathogenesis from Pre-Clinical Studies, San Diego, CA, USA, 16–21 May 2014; Volume 189, p. A4286.

41. Hu, G.; Zhou, Y.; Tian, J.; Yao, W.; Li, J.; Li, B.; Ran, P. Risk of COPD from exposure to biomass smoke: A metaanalysis. *Chest* **2010**, *1381*, 20–31. [CrossRef]

42. Hur, G.Y.; Kohw, D.H.; Choi, G.S.; Park, H.J.; Choi, S.J.; Ye, Y.M.; Kimw, K.S.; Park, H.S. Clinical and immunologic findings of methylene Diphenyl diisocyanate-induced occupational asthma in a car upholstery factory. *Clin. Exp. Allergy* **2008**, *38*, 586–593. [CrossRef]

43. Fisseler-Eckhoff, A.; Bartsch, H.; Zinsky, R.; Schirren, J. Environmental isocyanate-induced asthma: Morphologic and pathogenetic aspects of an increasing occupational disease. *Int. J. Environ. Res. Public Health* **2011**, *8*, 3672–3687. [CrossRef]

44. Johnson, V.J.; Yucesoy, B.; Reynolds, J.S.; Fluharty, K.; Wang, W.; Richardson, D.; Luster, M.I. Inhalation of toluene diisocyanate vapor induces allergic rhinitis in mice. *J. Immunol.* **2007**, *179*, 1864–1871. [CrossRef]

45. Taylor-Clark, T.E.; Kiros, F.; Carr, M.J.; McAlexander, M.A. Transient receptor potential ankyrin 1 mediates toluene diisocyanate–evoked respiratory irritation. *Am. J. Respir. Cell Mol. Biol.* **2009**, *40*, 756–762. [CrossRef]

46. Tourangeau, L.M.; Christiansen, S.C.; Herschbach, J.; Brooks, S.M.; Eddleston, J.; Zuraw, B. Nasal mucosal TRPA1 and TRPV1 levels in human rhinitis. *J. Allergy Clin. Immunol.* **2011**, *127*, AB52. [CrossRef]

47. Prandini, P.; De Logu, F.; Fusi, C.; Provezza, L.; Nassini, R.; Montagner, G.; Materazzi, S.; Munari, S.; Gilioli, E.; Bezzerri, V.; et al. TRPA1 channels modulate inflammatory response in respiratory cells from cystic fibrosis patients. *Am. J. Respir. Cell. Mol. Biol.* **2016**, *55*. [CrossRef]

48. Chen, J.; Hackos, D.H. TRPA1 as drug target-Promise and challenges. *Naunyn-Schmiedeberg's Arch. Pharmacol.* **2015**, *388*, 451–463. [CrossRef]

49. Meseguer, V.; Alpizar, Y.A.; Luis, E.; Tajada, S.; Denlinger, B.; Fajardo, O.; Manenschijn, J.A.; Fernández-Peña, C.; Talavera, A.; Kichko, T.; et al. TRPA1 channels mediate acute neurogenic inflammation and pain produced by bacterial endotoxins. *Nat. Commun.* **2014**, *5*, 3125. [CrossRef]

50. Tandon, M.; Jain, S.M.; Balamurugan, R.; Koslowski, M.; Keohane, P. Treatment of pain associated with diabetic peripheral neuropathy with the novel TRPA1 antagonist GRC 17536 in patients with intact peripheral nerve function. In Proceedings of the Fifth International Meeting of The Special Interest Group on Neuropathic Pain (NeuPSIG), Nice, France, 14–17 May 2015.

51. Ryan, N.M.; Birring, S.S.; Gibson, P.G. Gabapentin for refractory chronic cough: A randomised, double-blind, placebo-controlled trial. *Lancet* **2012**, *380*, 1583–1589. [CrossRef]

52. Kwan, K.Y.; Allchorne, A.J.; Vollrath, M.A.; Christensen, A.P.; Zhang, D.S.; Woolf, C.J.; Corey, D.P. TRPA1 contributes to cold, mechanical, and chemical nociception but is not essential for hair-cell transduction. *Neuron* **2006**, *50*, 277–289. [CrossRef]

53. Chen, J.; Joshi, S.K.; DiDomenico, S.; Perner, R.J.; Mikusa, J.P.; Gauvin, D.M.; Segreti, J.A.; Han, P.; Zhang, X.F.; Niforatos, W.; et al. Selective blockade of TRPA1 channel attenuates pathological pain without altering noxious cold sensation or body temperature regulation. *Pain* **2011**, *152*, 1165–1172. [CrossRef]

54. de Oliveira, C.; Garami, A.; Lehto, S.G.; Pakai, E.; Tekus, V.; Pohoczky, K.; Youngblood, B.D.; Wang, W.; Kort, M.E.; Kym, P.R.; et al. Transient receptor potential channel ankyrin-1 is not a cold sensor for autonomic thermoregulation in rodents. *J. Neurosci.* **2014**, *34*, 4445–4452. [CrossRef]

55. Curtis, R.; Coleman, S.; Camino, D.D.; Hayward, N.J.; Moran, M.M.; Bokesch, P. Transient Receptor Potential A1 (TRPA1) is not involved in thermoregulation in dogs and humans. In Proceedings of the A Trip to Spain: International workshop on transient receptor potential channels, Valencia, Spain, 12–14 September 2012; p. 65.

56. Obata, K.; Katsura, H.; Mizushima, T.; Yamanaka, H.; Kobayashi, K.; Dai, Y.; Fukuoka, T.; Tokunaga, A.; Tominaga, M.; Noguchi, K. TRPA1 induced in sensory neurons contributes to cold hyperalgesia after inflammation and nerve injury. *J. Clin. Invest.* **2005**, *115*, 2393–2401. [CrossRef]

57. Bodkin, J.V.; Thakore, P.; Aubdool, A.A.; Liang, L.; Fernandes, E.S.; Nandi, M.; Spina, D.; Clark, J.E.; Aaronson, P.I.; Shattock, M.J.; et al. Investigating the potential role of TRPA1 in locomotion and cardiovascular control during hypertension. *Pharmacol. Res. Perspect.* **2014**, *2*, e00052. [CrossRef]

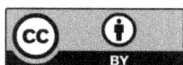

pharmaceuticals

MDPI

Review
TRPV1 and TRPM8 in Treatment of Chronic Cough

Eva Millqvist

Department of Allergology, Institution of Internal Medicine,
The Sahlgrenska Academy at University of Gothenburg, 413 45 Gothenburg, Sweden;
eva.millqvist@medfak.gu.se; Tel.: +46-708-43-3819; Fax: +46-500-43-3819

Academic Editors: Arpad Szallasi and Susan M. Huang
Received: 1 June 2016; Accepted: 22 July 2016; Published: 28 July 2016

Abstract: Chronic cough is common in the population, and among some there is no evident medical explanation for the symptoms. Such a refractory or idiopathic cough is now often regarded as a neuropathic disease due to dysfunctional airway ion channels, though the knowledge in this field is still limited. Persistent coughing and a cough reflex easily triggered by irritating stimuli, often in combination with perceived dyspnea, are characteristics of this disease. The patients have impaired quality of life and often reduced work capacity, followed by social and economic consequences. Despite the large number of individuals suffering from such a persisting cough, there is an unmet clinical need for effective cough medicines. The cough treatment available today often has little or no effect. Adverse effects mostly follow centrally acting cough drugs comprised of morphine and codeine, which demands the physician's awareness. The possibilities of modulating airway transient receptor potential (TRP) ion channels may indicate new ways to treat the persistent cough "without a reason". The TRP ion channel vanilloid 1 (TRPV1) and the TRP melastin 8 (TRPM8) appear as two candidates in the search for cough therapy, both as single targets and in reciprocal interaction.

Keywords: chronic cough; TRPV1; TRPM8; TRP antagonists; desensitization

1. Introduction

1.1. Chronic Cough

Coughing by humans is a necessary protective mechanism to prohibit food and foreign substances from reaching and harming the lower airways. However, coughing is also a symptom that signals attention in the diagnosis of several diseases.

Coughing is one of the most common symptoms for which patients consult a doctor in the western world, and the most usual cause is a common cold with associated cough [1–3]. However, when coughing is not effective enough to "clear" the airways from phlegm and mucus, it can lead to a variety of pathological conditions like atelectasis, bronchiectasis, pneumonia, lung abscesses, and pulmonary scarring [4].

The definition of coughing varies in literature, but daily coughing, when it lasts for more than two months, is, in general, regarded as chronic [5]. In addition, epidemiologic information on the prevalence of chronic cough varies, and it is reported that up to 20% of the adult population suffers from long lasting cough [2,6] with the condition related to a negative influence on quality of life and social activities [7–9].

When clinical tests do not give any indication of well-known causes for coughing like airway infection, asthma, post-nasal drip, chronic obstructive pulmonary disease (COPD), gastroesophageal reflux disease, cancer, alveolitis, heart failure or medication with angiotensin-converting enzyme (ACE) inhibitors, there is still a group of patients left over with chronic cough without a specific diagnosis having an ongoing cough, often refractory to available cough medications. In the present review, such patients will be referred to as having chronic idiopathic cough (CIC). How common this condition is has, however, been debated [5,10]. A similar group of patients with airway symptoms induced by environmental irritants, reporting problems with chronic coughing, chest discomfort, dyspnea, rhinitis, and eye irritation, has been identified [11,12]. The symptoms mimic asthma, but asthma-specific tests are negative. These patients have an increased cough reaction to inhaled capsaicin (the active compound of chili peppers), a tasteless and odorless substance that stimulates sensory nerves, and the provoked cough reflects sensory nerve reactivity [13]. Such airway symptoms are interpreted as airway sensory hyperreactivity (SHR). Cigarette smoke, car exhaust, perfumed products, and cold air are some of the triggers for SHR symptoms [11]. SHR affects more than 6% of the adult population in Sweden, mainly women, according to a population-based epidemiologic study [12]. In most cases, the patients could also be diagnosed with CIC [14] or the recently established cough hypersensitivity syndrome (CHS) [15]. This syndrome includes several airway conditions characterized by easily evoked cough reflex and increased cough sensitivity to inhaled capsaicin [15–18]. There was a high degree of agreement in a recent article reporting how opinion leaders in cough research regarded the suggestion of CHS as a cause underlying the cough etiology in CIC [19], and it is today, together with some forms of itch and pain [20], regarded as a possible neuropathic disease following neural injuries from various inflammatory, infective, and irritative influences [21–23].

1.2. The Medical Problem of Treating CIC

Patients with pronounced CIC have, with little success in most cases, frequently tried a variety of asthma, COPD, and cough medications. The international market for over the counter cough medication is huge, reaching several billion euros [24], though there are few scientific data supporting the effects of these products [25]. Whereas centrally acting medications like codeine and morphine can decrease coughing temporarily, they are connected with well-known adverse effects like drowsiness, difficulty concentrating, symptoms of the gall bladder, and constipation. In addition, there is a risk of habituation or abuse. Recent research indicates that pregabalin and gabapentin may have a role in treating severe CIC [23,26], though it is necessary to be aware of potential adverse reactions. There is an unmet clinical need for new, safe, and effective cough therapies with few adverse effects [10].

2. TRP Ion Channels in the Airways

The TRP ion channels can be found abundantly in the airways, as in most of the human organ systems and have during the last decades been important for studying multiple organ systems and their interaction with the environment [13,27]. Many of these ion channels are present in primary airway sensory neurons, some of which transmit nociceptive information to the brain. Furthermore, TRPV1 channels are expressed not only in sensory neurons but also in airway smooth muscle and epithelial cells [28,29], and some evidence suggests that TRPV1 has functional roles in the immune system [30,31].

The TRPV1 ion channel together with the later identified transient ion channel ankyrin 1 (TRPA1) have important functions in airway chemo-sensation and reflex control regarding temperature, osmolarity and oxidant stress [30,32,33]. These ion channels are believed to play an important role in asthma as well as in COPD [34–36]. Asthma is an inflammatory disease and many hopes have been attached to TRP antagonists as potential asthma relievers, though the research in this field is not unison [37]. However, a recent study, in a mice model of allergic asthma, also showed that a TRPV1 inhibitor decreased airway inflammation, immunoglobulin E (IgE) levels and airway hyperreactivity [38].

In addition, non-neuronal TRPV1 channels may be involved in airway disorders, and epithelial cells play a significant role in both asthma and COPD. McGarvey et al. recently found increased epithelial TRPV1 expression in severe asthma, indicating that the TRPV1 channels could represent a possibility to treat severe asthma where available medications have not been successful [29].

3. TRP Ion Channels in Chronic Cough

There is increasing evidence of the role of TRP ion channels, expressed by C and Aδ fibers in the cough mechanism. The cough reflex is induced by activation of airway sensory nerves and TRP ion channels related to the vanilloid (TRPV) and the ankyrin (TRPA) families [33,39–41]. In thermal nociception and in inflammatory hyperalgesia, the TRPV1 is an integrator of triggering stimuli and plays a role in protective reflexes like coughing and sneezing. In CIC, increased expression of TRPV1 was found and also a correlation between cough sensitivity to inhaled capsaicin and the quantity of TRPV1-positive nerves [42,43]. Several studies have pointed to heightened capsaicin cough sensitivity in CIC [14,44]. Capsaicin is the main, often used agonist for TRPV1; as an inhalant, it has for decades been used in cough provocation, regarded as a safe and reproducible procedure [2,11,45–50]. The results from such cough provocation studies suggest that the pathophysiology of CIC is related to airway mucosal TRP receptors in sensory nerves, reacting to noxious stimuli [33], and today there is a common opinion that the "cough without explanation" could be regarded as a neuropathic disorder [21,23]. Whether the main mechanisms in CIC are generally peripherally or centrally controlled is, however, debated [51–53], though both peripheral and central mechanisms may be involved.

3.1. TRP Ion Channels as Therapeutic Targets for CIC

In recent years, there has been an emerging interest in the family of TRP ion channels as possible therapeutic targets for a number of airway diseases, among them CIC [31,37,54]. The focus has been not only on TRPV1 but also on TRPA1 and TRPM8 [55]. Modulation of these TRP ion channels may be followed by disease improvement in a variety of airway disorders including CIC [34,54].

3.1.1. TRPV1 as a Therapeutic Target for CIC

TRPV1 is, in addition to being involved in cough and rhinitis, a major actor in pain and pain sensitivity, subsequently followed by increasing interest in the development of TRPV1 antagonists, both for cough treatment and for neuropathic pain disorders [37,56,57]. For the treatment of pain, there have long been several products available (creams and patches) targeting the TRPV1, using topical capsaicin to desensitize the sensory C fibers, probably by "exhausting" signal substances of the sensory nerves [57]. A recent study showed that higher concentration of capsaicin in patches provided better relief of neuropathic and chronic pain [58]. Topical treatment with capsaicin solution may also reduce symptoms in non-allergic chronic rhinitis [59]. A current study found, in such patients, increased levels of substance P in nasal lavage and overexpression of TRPV1 in nasal mucosa and treatment with topical capsaicin decreased symptoms and lowered nasal hyperreactivity [60]. The authors hypothesized that, in the nasal mucosa, capsaicin ablated the TRPV1–substance P nociceptive signaling pathway.

The TRPV1 ion channel was initially also called the "capsaicin receptor", due to capsaicin's close relation to this receptor [61]. The noxious effect of capsaicin in chili fruits is well known and is used in spices and pepper spray [62].

In light of the current lack of effective cough medications, it is natural that a number of commercial pharmaceutical companies are developing drugs acting as antagonists on TRP ion channels [37]. Resolvin D2 is a potent endogenous antagonists for TRPV1 [63], and there have been many exogenous TRPV1 antagonists identified, some of them synthetic analogs of capsaicin, such as capsazepine [55]. There have been hopeful findings in animal testing [64], but some of these projects seem to have problems when the medication is finally tested in humans beings, having adverse effects including hyperthermia and impaired noxious heat sensation, which has been extensively reviewed earlier [31,37,65,66]. A recent study on the TRPV1 antagonist SB-705498 did reduce the capsaicin cough sensitivity in patients with chronic cough, but not the cough frequency [65]. Up to now, there has been no oral TRPV1 antagonist available on the market for either cough or pain.

Desensitization is a complex, not exactly defined process, but it has a therapeutic potential and when inhaled, capsaicin in humans is known to cause a short period of desensitization in terms of less cough sensitivity [67,68].

Capsaicin, the major trigger of TRPV1, is found naturally in a great variety of food dishes comprising different kinds of chili products, giving a "hot" taste and further inducing a number of physiological reactions of which some seem to be health promoting [69]. The use of chili in food varies between different countries and cultures. Most western countries have no long tradition of the use of chili in cooking. A dish with a lot of hot chili can result in undesired symptoms like irritation in the mouth and throat, sneezing, eye irritation, and sometimes coughing. It is "common knowledge" that it is possible to get used to spicy food by gradually increasing the intake. The TRPV1 receptors use neuropeptides to evoke brain signals, and if these receptors are regularly stimulated, neuropeptides are depleted, and few or no symptoms are awakened by spicy food [37,70]. Previously, it was thought that capsaicin desensitization is only possible when capsaicin is applied locally on skin or inhaled. For ingested capsaicin to have an effect on coughing, it must act systemically after transport in the circulatory system. Little is known about the absorption and distribution of capsaicin in humans, and only one study has looked at capsaicin human pharmacokinetics—after a large meal of Thai capsicums [71]. This study found a low bioavailability of capsaicin, though this is likely explained by conversion of capsaicin in the intestine to dihydrocapsaicin, an intestinal metabolite of capsaicin, which was not measured but probably induced reactions similar to those from capsaicin. Given the interest in capsaicin, both for the purpose of cough and pain suppression and also as an emerging therapy for obesity and cancer [31,69,72], this is a major knowledge gap. A method developed to analyze capsaicin in human sera with high performance liquid cromatography (HPLC) gives new possibilities of reducing this gap and studying any dose-response relation [73].

In the clinic, we have encountered patients who claim to have "treated" their cough by eating very spicy food equivalent to several fresh chili pepper fruits per day. However, the same dietary recommendations have not been feasible because of the experience of the strong flavor. In a recent pilot study, 21 patients with chronic cough had fewer symptoms and reduced cough reflex sensitivity if they regularly consumed capsules containing concentrated capsaicin from chili peppers [74]. There were no adverse effects and the daily intake of capsaicin corresponded to what it is common to eat regularly in countries such as Mexico and Thailand. Epidemiological research found the incidence of chronic cough in countries with regular intake of spicy food to be around 2%, compared to up to 20% in western countries [75], supporting the observation that first led to this work in Sweden. Since the current pilot study [74] has showed convincing results, orally given capsaicin has been identified as a possible treatment of cough, offering a good option for those people not used to spicy foods.

3.1.2. TRPM8 as a Therapeutic Target for CIC

Patients with CIC and SHR often complain that exercising in cold air is an inducing factor for cough [47,48,76,77], and exercise in a cold air chamber was followed both by both coughing and increased capsaicin sensitivity [78]. It seems likely that TRPM8 and TRPA1, known to react to low temperatures, are involved in airway symptoms induced by cold air. The sensation of cold evoked by menthol was explained by the discovery of the TRPM8 ion channel reacting to cool temperatures and menthol [79–81]. Menthol ($C_{10}H_{20}O$), synthetically produced or extracted from mint oils, is a covalent organic compound that is present in a number of over the counter (OTC) products for ameliorating symptoms in rhinitis, common cold and throat irritation. Eccles et al. found no significant effect on nasal patency [82]. Whereas OTC products comprising menthol for relief of airway symptoms have been available for decades, only a few scientific studies support the cough-relieving effects from menthol products, though the interest in a potential effect in cough treatment seems to be increasing.

Menthol is also used in the tobacco industry as a cigarette brand to improve flavor and disguise the airway irritation evoked by smoking [83,84]. Already in 1994, Morice et al. published results from a study proving that, in humans, cough induced by inhaling citric acid could be prevented from *pre* inhalation of menthol [85]. A year later, the concordant results were shown in guinea pigs [85]. However, in children, Kenia et al. found no difference in cough count compared to placebo when a provocation with citric acid was preceded by inhalation of menthol, whereas the perception of nasal patency increased [86]. Another study showed that premedication of menthol inhalation before bronchoscopy did not improve coughing during the process, but late symptoms of cough and dyspnea improved as did peak expiratory flow [87]. Later reports indicated the possibility of reducing cough sensitivity with inhaled or intranasal menthol given before a provocation with cough-inducing agents [88–91]. In summary, menthol seems to have a capacity to reduce the sensitivity of an important airway defense mechanism that could be used for good (in cough medications) or for bad (in cigarette brands) [84].

Also regarding TRPM8 and menthol, there is a parallel between the airways and the skin regarding the treatment of itch and pain, with some studies reporting a beneficial effect from topical menthol preparations [92–94]. However, in healthy humans, topical cutaneous menthol provoked cold allodynia, suggested as being the results from a sensitization of nociceptors reacting on cold stimuli [95,96], indicating complex innervation mechanisms where menthol in some situations may be hyperalgesic but may be analgesic in some patients with peripheral and central neuropathic pain. Also illustrating the confusing role of menthol and the TRP channels are the findings that the TRPA1 ion channel, known to evoke cough from noxious stimuli and cold, is a highly sensitive receptor for menthol, probably involved in a variety of menthol induced physiological reactions [36,97]. Takaishi et al. elucidated these questions, demonstrating a reciprocal effect of capsaicin and menthol wherein menthol proved to have an anti-nociceptive effect on TRPV1, and capsaicin inhibited TRPM8-mediated currents [98]. Furthermore, there was a mutual inhibition of temperature activation in human TRPV1 or TRPM8 and a binding site of menthol was identified in TRPV1.

Although it is better understood today, the theoretical explanation as to why menthol has an ameliorating effect on cough reflex sensitivity remains in part obscure, but acting via TRPM8, menthol may interfere with TRPV1 and the cough outcome from capsaicin and environmental irritants [34,35].

4. Conclusions

During the last decade, a new paradigm has been developed of CIC as a possible neuropathic disease that could be linked to the TRP ion channels, with persisting cough as an unmistakable symptom. The lack of effective medical treatment in CIC is obvious and frustrating, though neuromodulators and new receptor antagonists indicate different novel options to ameliorate cough and cough sensitivity, as does the possibility of TRPV1 desensitization [23,74,99]. The TRPV1 antagonist SB-705498 revealed no negative properties but a somewhat surprising effect only on the capsaicin cough sensitivity, not on the cough symptoms [65]. However, this is in concordance with other reports studying rhinitis and pruritus [100–103] showing no improvement from treatment with SB-705498. The results could suggest that TRPV1 may not be of such great importance in chronic cough as earlier believed, but the evident relation between chronic cough, TRPV1 expression and cough sensitivity to inhaled capsaicin contradicts such a paradigm change. The SB-705498 is a highly selective molecule and the blocking of TRPV1 in terms of both lowering capsaicin sensitivity and improving cough symptoms may demand a more complex structure interacting on different binding sites. It would, however, be interesting to carry out a clinical study with SB-705498 in patients with severe, refractory asthma, since the mechanisms in such asthma is quite different from those in chronic cough and recent findings showed increased epithelial TRPV1 expression in this difficult to treat condition [29]. One major problem is the lack of tools to study how TRP channels appear and change in CIC and other airway disorders.

There is a rich "flora" of OTC medications based on a diversity of substances, though few scientific studies can confirm measurable effects. Future research in cough medication should focus on proving reliable effects with few adverse events.

Acknowledgments: The author's work was supported by grants from the Swedish Heart and Lung Foundation, the Swedish Asthma and Allergy Association's Research Fund, and the Swedish Cancer and Allergy Fund.

Conflicts of Interest: Millqvist filed an international patent application (PCT application) for the use of capsaicin as a cough-reducing product on 3 January 2014. The author declares no other conflict of interest, financial or otherwise, related to this study.

References

1. Irwin, R.S.; Curley, F.J.; French, C.L. Chronic cough. The spectrum and frequency of causes, key components of the diagnostic evaluation, and outcome of specific therapy. *Am. Rev. Respir. Dis.* **1990**, *141*, 640–647. [CrossRef] [PubMed]

2. Chung, K.F.; Pavord, I.D. Prevalence, pathogenesis, and causes of chronic cough. *Lancet* **2008**, *371*, 1364–1374. [CrossRef]

3. Schappert, S.M.; Rechtsteiner, E.A. Ambulatory medical care utilization estimates for 2007. *Vital Health Stat. Ser. 13 Data Natl. Health Surv.* **2011**, *169*, 1–38.

4. Madison, J.M.; Irwin, R.S. Cough: A worldwide problem. *Otolaryngol. Clin. North Am.* **2010**, *43*, 1–13. [CrossRef] [PubMed]

5. Morice, A.H.; Fontana, G.A.; Sovijarvi, A.R.; Pistolesi, M.; Chung, K.F.; Widdicombe, J.; O'Connell, F.; Geppetti, P.; Gronke, L.; De Jongste, J.; et al. The diagnosis and management of chronic cough. *Eur. Respir. J.* **2004**, *24*, 481–492. [CrossRef] [PubMed]

6. Song, W.J.; Chang, Y.S.; Faruqi, S.; Kim, J.Y.; Kang, M.G.; Kim, S.; Jo, E.J.; Kim, M.H.; Plevkova, J.; Park, H.W.; et al. The global epidemiology of chronic cough in adults: A systematic review and meta-analysis. *Eur. Respir. J.* **2015**, *45*, 1479–1481. [CrossRef] [PubMed]

7. French, C.L.; Irwin, R.S.; Curley, F.J.; Krikorian, C.J. Impact of chronic cough on quality of life. *Arch. Intern. Med.* **1998**, *158*, 1657–1661. [CrossRef] [PubMed]

8. Young, E.C.; Smith, J.A. Quality of life in patients with chronic cough. *Ther. Adv. Respir. Dis.* **2010**, *4*, 49–55. [CrossRef] [PubMed]

9. Ternesten-Hasseus, E.; Larsson, S.; Millqvist, E. Symptoms induced by environmental irritants and health-related quality of life in patients with chronic cough—A cross-sectional study. *Cough* **2011**, *7*, 6. [CrossRef] [PubMed]

10. Dicpinigaitis, P.V. Cough: An unmet clinical need. *Br. J. Pharmacol.* **2011**, *163*, 116–124. [CrossRef] [PubMed]

11. Millqvist, E.; Bende, M.; Löwhagen, O. Sensory hyperreactivity—A possible mechanism underlying cough and asthma-like symptoms. *Allergy* **1998**, *53*, 1208–1212. [CrossRef] [PubMed]

12. Johansson, A.; Millqvist, E.; Nordin, S.; Bende, M. Relationship between self-reported odor intolerance and sensitivity to inhaled capsaicin: Proposed definition of airway sensory hyperreactivity and estimation of its prevalence. *Chest* **2006**, *129*, 1623–1628. [CrossRef] [PubMed]

13. Clapham, D.E. TRP channels as cellular sensors. *Nature* **2003**, *426*, 517–524. [CrossRef] [PubMed]

14. Ternesten-Hasseus, E.; Larsson, C.; Larsson, S.; Millqvist, E. Capsaicin sensitivity in patients with chronic cough—Results from a cross-sectional study. *Cough* **2013**, *9*, 5. [CrossRef] [PubMed]

15. Morice, A.H.; Faruqi, S.; Wright, C.E.; Thompson, R.; Bland, J.M. Cough hypersensitivity syndrome: A distinct clinical entity. *Lung* **2011**, *189*, 73–79. [CrossRef] [PubMed]

16. Morice, A.H. The cough hypersensitivity syndrome: A novel paradigm for understanding cough. *Lung* **2009**, *188*, 87–90. [CrossRef] [PubMed]

17. Chung, K.F. Chronic 'cough hypersensitivity syndrome': A more precise label for chronic cough. *Pulm. Pharmacol. Ther.* **2011**, *24*, 267–271. [CrossRef] [PubMed]

18. Morice, A.H.; Millqvist, E.; Belvisi, M.G.; Bieksiene, K.; Birring, S.S.; Chung, K.F.; Dal Negro, R.W.; Dicpinigaitis, P.; Kantar, A.; McGarvey, L.P.; et al. Cough hypersensitivity syndrome: Clinical measurement is the key to progress. *Eur. Respir. J.* **2015**, *45*, 1509–1510. [CrossRef] [PubMed]

19. Morice, A.H.; Millqvist, E.; Belvisi, M.G.; Bieksiene, K.; Birring, S.S.; Chung, K.F.; Dal Negro, R.W.; Dicpinigaitis, P.; Kantar, A.; McGarvey, L.P.; et al. Expert opinion on the cough hypersensitivity syndrome in respiratory medicine. *Eur. Respir. J.* **2014**, *44*, 1132–1148. [CrossRef] [PubMed]

20. Ji, R.R. Neuroimmune interactions in itch: Do chronic itch, chronic pain, and chronic cough share similar mechanisms? *Pulm. Pharmacol. Ther.* **2015**, *35*, 81–86. [CrossRef] [PubMed]

21. Chung, K.; McGarvey, L.; Mazzone, S. Chronic cough as a neuropathic disorder. *Lancet Respir. Med.* **2013**, *1*, 412–422. [CrossRef]

22. Vertigan, A.E.; Gibson, P.G. Chronic refractory cough as a sensory neuropathy: Evidence from a reinterpretation of cough triggers. *J. Voice* **2011**, *25*, 596–601. [CrossRef] [PubMed]

23. Gibson, P.; Wang, G.; McGarvey, L.; Vertigan, A.E.; Altman, K.W.; Birring, S.S.; Panel, C.E.C. Treatment of unexplained chronic cough: Chest guideline and expert panel report. *Chest* **2016**, *149*, 27–44. [CrossRef] [PubMed]

24. Morice, A.H. Over-the-counter cough medicines: New approaches. *Pulm. Pharmacol. Ther.* **2015**, *35*, 149–151. [CrossRef] [PubMed]

25. Morice, A.H.; McGarvey, L. Clinical cough II: Therapeutic treatments and management of chronic cough. *Handb. Exp. Pharmacol.* **2009**, *187*, 277–295. [PubMed]

26. Vertigan, A.E.; Kapela, S.L.; Ryan, N.M.; Birring, S.S.; McElduff, P.; Gibson, P.G. Pregabalin and speech pathology combination therapy for refractory chronic cough: A randomized controlled trial. *Chest* **2016**, *149*, 639–648. [CrossRef] [PubMed]

27. Lehmann, R.; Schobel, N.; Hatt, H.; van Thriel, C. The involvement of trp channels in sensory irritation: A mechanistic approach toward a better understanding of the biological effects of local irritants. *Arch. Toxicol.* **2016**, *90*, 1399–1413. [CrossRef] [PubMed]

28. Guibert, C.; Ducret, T.; Savineau, J.P. Expression and physiological roles of trp channels in smooth muscle cells. *Adv. Exp. Med. Biol.* **2011**, *704*, 687–706. [PubMed]

29. McGarvey, L.P.; Butler, C.A.; Stokesberry, S.; Polley, L.; McQuaid, S.; Abdullah, H.; Ashraf, S.; McGahon, M.K.; Curtis, T.M.; Arron, J.; et al. Increased expression of bronchial epithelial transient receptor potential vanilloid 1 channels in patients with severe asthma. *J. Allergy Clin. Immunol.* **2014**, *133*, 704–712.e4. [CrossRef] [PubMed]

30. Fernandes, E.S.; Fernandes, M.A.; Keeble, J.E. The functions of trpa1 and trpv1: Moving away from sensory nerves. *Br. J. Pharmacol.* **2012**, *166*, 510–521. [CrossRef] [PubMed]

31. Kaneko, Y.; Szallasi, A. Transient receptor potential (TRP) channels: A clinical perspective. *Br. J. Pharmacol.* **2014**, *171*, 2474–2507. [CrossRef] [PubMed]

32. Macpherson, L.J.; Dubin, A.E.; Evans, M.J.; Marr, F.; Schultz, P.G.; Cravatt, B.F.; Patapoutian, A. Noxious compounds activate trpa1 ion channels through covalent modification of cysteines. *Nature* **2007**, *445*, 541–545. [CrossRef] [PubMed]

33. Bessac, B.F.; Jordt, S.E. Breathtaking trp channels: Trpa1 and trpv1 in airway chemosensation and reflex control. *Physiology (Bethesda)* **2008**, *23*, 360–370. [CrossRef] [PubMed]

34. Banner, K.H.; Igney, F.; Poll, C. Trp channels: Emerging targets for respiratory disease. *Pharmacol. Ther.* **2011**, *130*, 371–384. [CrossRef] [PubMed]

35. Abbott-Banner, K.; Poll, C.; Verkuyl, J.M. Targeting trp channels in airway disorders. *Curr. Top. Med. Chem.* **2013**, *13*, 310–321. [CrossRef] [PubMed]

36. Grace, M.S.; Baxter, M.; Dubuis, E.; Birrell, M.A.; Belvisi, M.G. Transient receptor potential (TRP) channels in the airway: Role in airway disease. *Br. J. Pharmacol.* **2014**, *171*, 2593–2607. [CrossRef] [PubMed]

37. Preti, D.; Szallasi, A.; Patacchini, R. TRP channels as therapeutic targets in airway disorders: A patent review. *Expert Opin. Ther. Pat.* **2012**, *22*, 663–695. [CrossRef] [PubMed]

38. Baker, K.; Raemdonck, K.; Dekkak, B.; Snelgrove, R.J.; Ford, J.; Shala, F.; Belvisi, M.G.; Birrell, M.A. Role of the ion channel, transient receptor potential cation channel subfamily v member 1 (TRPV1), in allergic asthma. *Respir. Res.* **2016**, *17*, 67. [CrossRef] [PubMed]

39. Nilius, B. Trp channels in disease. *Biochim. Biophys. Acta* **2007**, *1772*, 805–812. [CrossRef] [PubMed]

40. Venkatachalam, K.; Montell, C. Trp channels. *Annu. Rev. Biochem.* **2007**, *76*, 387–417. [CrossRef] [PubMed]

41. Birrell, M.A.; Belvisi, M.G.; Grace, M.; Sadofsky, L.; Faruqi, S.; Hele, D.J.; Maher, S.A.; Freund-Michel, V.; Morice, A.H. Trpa1 agonists evoke coughing in guinea pig and human volunteers. *Am. J. Respir. Crit. Care Med.* **2009**, *180*, 1042–1047. [CrossRef] [PubMed]

42. Groneberg, D.A.; Niimi, A.; Dinh, Q.T.; Cosio, B.; Hew, M.; Fischer, A.; Chung, K.F. Increased expression of transient receptor potential vanilloid-1 in airway nerves of chronic cough. *Am. J. Respir. Crit. Care Med.* **2004**, *170*, 1276–1280. [CrossRef] [PubMed]

43. Mitchell, J.E.; Campbell, A.P.; New, N.E.; Sadofsky, L.R.; Kastelik, J.A.; Mulrennan, S.A.; Compton, S.J.; Morice, A.H. Expression and characterization of the intracellular vanilloid receptor (trpv1) in bronchi from patients with chronic cough. *Exp. Lung Res.* **2005**, *31*, 295–306. [CrossRef] [PubMed]

44. Nieto, L.; de Diego, A.; Perpina, M.; Compte, L.; Garrigues, V.; Martinez, E.; Ponce, J. Cough reflex testing with inhaled capsaicin in the study of chronic cough. *Respir. Med.* **2003**, *97*, 393–400. [CrossRef] [PubMed]

45. Dicpinigaitis, P.V. Short- and long-term reproducibility of capsaicin cough challenge testing. *Pulm. Pharmacol. Ther.* **2003**, *16*, 61–65. [CrossRef]

46. Dicpinigaitis, P.V.; Alva, R.V. Safety of capsaicin cough challenge testing. *Chest* **2005**, *128*, 196–202. [CrossRef] [PubMed]

47. Ternesten-Hasseus, E.; Johansson, Å.; Lowhagen, O.; Millqvist, E. Inhalation method determines outcome of capsaicin inhalation in patients with chronic cough due to sensory hyperreactivity. *Pulm. Pharmacol. Ther.* **2006**, *19*, 172–178. [CrossRef] [PubMed]

48. Ternesten-Hasseus, E.; Lowhagen, O.; Millqvist, E. Quality of life and capsaicin sensitivity in patients with airway symptoms induced by chemicals and scents: A longitudinal study. *Environ. Health Perspect.* **2007**, *115*, 425–429. [CrossRef] [PubMed]

49. Nejla, S.; Fujimura, M.; Kamio, Y. Comparison between tidal breathing and dosimeter methods in assessing cough receptor sensitivity to capsaicin. *Respirology* **2000**, *5*, 337–342. [CrossRef] [PubMed]

50. Couto, M.; de Diego, A.; Perpini, M.; Delgado, L.; Moreira, A. Cough reflex testing with inhaled capsaicin and trpv1 activation in asthma and comorbid conditions. *J. Investig. Allergol. Clin. Immunol.* **2013**, *23*, 289–301. [PubMed]

51. Millqvist, E. The problem of treating unexplained chronic cough. *Chest* **2016**, *149*, 613–614. [CrossRef] [PubMed]

52. Faruqi, S.; Morice, A.H. Cough reduction using capsaicin: An alternative mechanistic hypothesis. *Respir. Med.* **2015**, *109*, 926. [CrossRef] [PubMed]

53. Gibson, P.G.; Simpson, J.L.; Ryan, N.M.; Vertigan, A.E. Mechanisms of cough. *Curr. Opin. Allergy Clin. Immunol.* **2014**, *14*, 55–61. [CrossRef] [PubMed]

54. Planells-Cases, R.; Valente, P.; Ferrer-Montiel, A.; Qin, F.; Szallasi, A. Complex regulation of trpv1 and related thermo-trps: Implications for therapeutic intervention. *Adv. Exp. Med. Biol.* **2011**, *704*, 491–515. [PubMed]

55. Bonvini, S.J.; Birrell, M.A.; Smith, J.A.; Belvisi, M.G. Targeting trp channels for chronic cough: From bench to bedside. *Naunyn-Schmiedeb. Arch. Pharmacol.* **2015**, *388*, 401–420. [CrossRef] [PubMed]

56. Petrocellis, L.; Moriello, A. Modulation of the trpv1 channel: Current clinical trials and recent patents with focus on neurological conditions. *Recent Pat. CNS Drug Discov.* **2013**, *8*, 180–204. [CrossRef] [PubMed]

57. Szallasi, A.; Sheta, M. Targeting TRPV1 for pain relief: Limits, losers and laurels. *Expert Opin. Investig. Drugs* **2012**, *21*, 1351–1369. [CrossRef] [PubMed]

58. Peppin, J.F.; Pappagallo, M. Capsaicinoids in the treatment of neuropathic pain: A review. *Ther. Adv. Neurol. Disord.* **2014**, *7*, 22–32. [CrossRef] [PubMed]

59. Singh, U.; Bernstein, J.A. Intranasal capsaicin in management of nonallergic (vasomotor) rhinitis. In *Capsaicin as a Therapeutic Molecule*; Springer: Basel, Switzerland, 2014; Volume 68, pp. 147–170.

60. Van Gerven, L.; Alpizar, Y.A.; Wouters, M.M.; Hox, V.; Hauben, E.; Jorissen, M.; Boeckxstaens, G.; Talavera, K.; Hellings, P.W. Capsaicin treatment reduces nasal hyperreactivity and transient receptor potential cation channel subfamily v, receptor 1 (TRPV1) overexpression in patients with idiopathic rhinitis. *J. Allergy Clin. Immunol.* **2014**, *133*, 1332–1339. [CrossRef] [PubMed]

61. Caterina, M.J.; Schumacher, M.A.; Tominaga, M.; Rosen, T.A.; Levine, J.D.; Julius, D. The capsaicin receptor: A heat-activated ion channel in the pain pathway. *Nature* **1997**, *389*, 816–824. [PubMed]

62. Busker, R.W.; van Helden, H.P. Toxicologic evaluation of pepper spray as a possible weapon for the dutch police force: Risk assessment and efficacy. *Am. J. Forensic Med. Pathol.* **1998**, *19*, 309–316. [CrossRef] [PubMed]

63. Park, C.K.; Xu, Z.Z.; Liu, T.; Lu, N.; Serhan, C.N.; Ji, R.R. Resolvin D2 is a potent endogenous inhibitor for transient receptor potential subtype V1/A1, inflammatory pain, and spinal cord synaptic plasticity in mice: Distinct roles of resolvin D1, D2, and E1. *J. Neurosci. Off. J. Soc. Neurosci.* **2011**, *31*, 18433–18438. [CrossRef] [PubMed]

64. Grace, M.S.; Dubuis, E.; Birrell, M.A.; Belvisi, M.G. Pre-clinical studies in cough research: Role of transient receptor potential (TRP) channels. *Pulm. Pharmacol. Ther.* **2013**, *26*, 498–507. [CrossRef] [PubMed]

65. Khalid, S.; Murdoch, R.; Newlands, A.; Smart, K.; Kelsall, A.; Holt, K.; Dockry, R.; Woodcock, A.; Smith, J.A. Transient receptor potential vanilloid 1 (TRPV1) antagonism in patients with refractory chronic cough: A double-blind randomized controlled trial. *J. Allergy Clin. Immunol.* **2014**, *134*, 56–62. [CrossRef] [PubMed]

66. Brederson, J.D.; Kym, P.R.; Szallasi, A. Targeting trp channels for pain relief. *Eur. J. Pharmacol.* **2013**, *716*, 61–76. [CrossRef] [PubMed]

67. Collier, J.G.; Fuller, R.W. Capsaicin inhalation in man and the effects of sodium cromoglycate. *Br. J. Pharmacol.* **1984**, *81*, 113–117. [CrossRef] [PubMed]

68. Fuller, R.W. Pharmacology of inhaled capsaicin in humans. *Respir. Med.* **1991**, *85*, 31–34. [CrossRef]

69. Nilius, B.; Appendino, G. Spices: The savory and beneficial science of pungency. *Rev. Physiol. Biochem. Pharmacol.* **2013**, *164*, 1–76. [PubMed]

70. Szallasi, A.; Blumberg, P.M. Vanilloid (capsaicin) receptors and mechanisms. *Pharmacol. Rev.* **1999**, *51*, 159–212. [PubMed]

71. Chaiyasit, K.; Khovidhunkit, W.; Wittayalertpanya, S. Pharmacokinetic and the effect of capsaicin in capsicum frutescens on decreasing plasma glucose level. *J. Med. Assoc. Thail.* **2009**, *92*, 108–113.

72. Rollyson, W.D.; Stover, C.A.; Brown, K.C.; Perry, H.E.; Stevenson, C.D.; McNees, C.A.; Ball, J.G.; Valentovic, M.A.; Dasgupta, P. Bioavailability of capsaicin and its implications for drug delivery. *J. Controll. Release* **2014**, *196*, 96–105. [CrossRef] [PubMed]

73. Hartley, T.; Stevens, B.; Ahuja, K.D.; Ball, M.J. Development and experimental application of an hplc procedure for the determination of capsaicin and dihydrocapsaicin in serum samples from human subjects. *Indian J. Clin. Biochem.* **2013**, *28*, 329–335. [CrossRef] [PubMed]

74. Ternesten-Hasseus, E.; Johansson, E.L.; Millqvist, E. Cough reduction using capsaicin. *Respir. Med.* **2015**, *109*, 27–37. [CrossRef] [PubMed]

75. Mahesh, P.A.; Jayaraj, B.S.; Prabhakar, A.K.; Chaya, S.K.; Vijayasimha, R. Prevalence of chronic cough, chronic phlegm & associated factors in mysore, karnataka, india. *Indian J. Med. Res.* **2011**, *134*, 91–100. [PubMed]

76. Johansson, A.; Löwhagen, O.; Millqvist, E.; Bende, M. Capsaicin inhalation test for identification of sensory hyperreactivity. *Respir. Med.* **2002**, *96*, 731–735. [CrossRef] [PubMed]

77. Ternesten-Hasseus, E.; Farbrot, A.; Löwhagen, O.; Millqvist, E. Sensitivity to methacholine and capsaicin in patients with unclear respiratory symptoms. *Allergy* **2002**, *57*, 501–507. [CrossRef] [PubMed]

78. Ternesten-Hasseus, E.; Johansson, E.L.; Bende, M.; Millqvist, E. Dyspnea from exercise in cold air is not always asthma. *J. Asthma: Off. J. Assoc. Care Asthma* **2008**, *45*, 705–709. [CrossRef] [PubMed]

79. Bautista, D.M.; Siemens, J.; Glazer, J.M.; Tsuruda, P.R.; Basbaum, A.I.; Stucky, C.L.; Jordt, S.E.; Julius, D. The menthol receptor trpm8 is the principal detector of environmental cold. *Nature* **2007**, *448*, 204–208. [CrossRef] [PubMed]

80. McCoy, D.D.; Knowlton, W.M.; McKemy, D.D. Scraping through the ice: Uncovering the role of trpm8 in cold transduction. *Am. J. Physiol. Regul. Integr. Comp. Physiol.* **2011**, *300*, R1278–R1287. [CrossRef] [PubMed]

81. McKemy, D.D.; Neuhausser, W.M.; Julius, D. Identification of a cold receptor reveals a general role for trp channels in thermosensation. *Nature* **2002**, *416*, 52–58. [CrossRef] [PubMed]

82. Eccles, R. Menthol: Effects on nasal sensation of airflow and the drive to breathe. *Curr. Allergy Asthma Rep.* **2003**, *3*, 210–214. [CrossRef] [PubMed]

83. Anderson, S.J. Menthol cigarettes and smoking cessation behaviour: A review of tobacco industry documents. *Tob. Control* **2011**, *20* (Suppl. 2), ii49–ii56. [CrossRef] [PubMed]

84. Willis, D.N.; Liu, B.; Ha, M.A.; Jordt, S.E.; Morris, J.B. Menthol attenuates respiratory irritation responses to multiple cigarette smoke irritants. *FASEB J.* **2011**, *25*, 4434–4444. [CrossRef] [PubMed]

85. Morice, A.H.; Marshall, A.E.; Higgins, K.S.; Grattan, T.J. Effect of inhaled menthol on citric acid induced cough in normal subjects. *Thorax* **1994**, *49*, 1024–1026. [CrossRef] [PubMed]

86. Kenia, P.; Houghton, T.; Beardsmore, C. Does inhaling menthol affect nasal patency or cough? *Pediatr. Pulmonol.* **2008**, *43*, 532–537. [PubMed]

87. Haidl, P.; Kemper, P.; Butnarasu, S.J.; Klauke, M.; Wehde, H.; Kohler, D. Does the inhalation of a 1% l-menthol solution in the premedication of fiberoptic bronchoscopy affect coughing and the sensation of dyspnea? *Pneumologie* **2001**, *55*, 115–119. [CrossRef] [PubMed]

88. Plevkova, J.; Kollarik, M.; Poliacek, I.; Brozmanova, M.; Surdenikova, L.; Tatar, M.; Mori, N.; Canning, B.J. The role of trigeminal nasal trpm8-expressing afferent neurons in the antitussive effects of menthol. *J. Appl. Physiol.* **2013**, *115*, 268–274. [CrossRef] [PubMed]

89. Buday, T.; Brozmanova, M.; Biringerova, Z.; Gavliakova, S.; Poliacek, I.; Calkovsky, V.; Shetthalli, M.V.; Plevkova, J. Modulation of cough response by sensory inputs from the nose—Role of trigeminal TRPA1 versus trpm8 channels. *Cough* **2012**, *8*, 11. [CrossRef] [PubMed]

90. Millqvist, E.; Ternesten-Hasseus, E.; Bende, M. Inhalation of menthol reduces capsaicin cough sensitivity and influences inspiratory flows in chronic cough. *Respir. Med.* **2013**, *107*, 433–438. [CrossRef] [PubMed]

91. Wise, P.M.; Breslin, P.A.; Dalton, P. Sweet taste and menthol increase cough reflex thresholds. *Pulm. Pharmacol. Ther.* **2012**, *25*, 236–241. [CrossRef] [PubMed]

92. Roberts, K.; Shenoy, R.; Anand, P. A novel human volunteer pain model using contact heat evoked potentials (chep) following topical skin application of transient receptor potential agonists capsaicin, menthol and cinnamaldehyde. *J. Clin. Neurosci. Off. J. Neurosurg. Soc. Australas.* **2011**, *18*, 926–932. [CrossRef] [PubMed]

93. Gaudioso, C.; Hao, J.; Martin-Eauclaire, M.F.; Gabriac, M.; Delmas, P. Menthol pain relief through cumulative inactivation of voltage-gated sodium channels. *Pain* **2012**, *153*, 473–484. [CrossRef] [PubMed]

94. Yosipovitch, G.; Szolar, C.; Hui, X.Y.; Maibach, H. Effect of topically applied menthol on thermal, pain and itch sensations and biophysical properties of the skin. *Arch. Dermatol. Res.* **1996**, *288*, 245–248. [CrossRef] [PubMed]

95. Wasner, G.; Naleschinski, D.; Binder, A.; Schattschneider, J.; McLachlan, E.M.; Baron, R. The effect of menthol on cold allodynia in patients with neuropathic pain. *Pain Med.* **2008**, *9*, 354–358. [CrossRef] [PubMed]

96. Wasner, G.; Schattschneider, J.; Binder, A.; Baron, R. Topical menthol—A human model for cold pain by activation and sensitization of C nociceptors. *Brain* **2004**, *127*, 1159–1171. [CrossRef] [PubMed]

97. Karashima, Y.; Damann, N.; Prenen, J.; Talavera, K.; Segal, A.; Voets, T.; Nilius, B. Bimodal action of menthol on the transient receptor potential channel trpa1. *J. Neurosci. Off. J. Soc. Neurosci.* **2007**, *27*, 9874–9884. [CrossRef] [PubMed]

98. Takaishi, M.; Uchida, K.; Suzuki, Y.; Matsui, H.; Shimada, T.; Fujita, F.; Tominaga, M. Reciprocal effects of capsaicin and menthol on thermosensation through regulated activities of trpv1 and trpm8. *J. Physiol. Sci.* **2016**, *66*, 143–155. [CrossRef] [PubMed]

99. Abdulqawi, R.; Dockry, R.; Holt, K.; Layton, G.; McCarthy, B.G.; Ford, A.P.; Smith, J.A. P2x3 receptor antagonist (af-219) in refractory chronic cough: A randomised, double-blind, placebo-controlled phase 2 study. *Lancet* **2015**, *385*, 1198–1205. [CrossRef]

100. Gibson, R.A.; Robertson, J.; Mistry, H.; McCallum, S.; Fernando, D.; Wyres, M.; Yosipovitch, G. A randomised trial evaluating the effects of the trpv1 antagonist sb705498 on pruritus induced by histamine, and cowhage challenge in healthy volunteers. *PLoS ONE* **2014**, *9*, e100610. [CrossRef] [PubMed]

101. Bareille, P.; Murdoch, R.D.; Denyer, J.; Bentley, J.; Smart, K.; Yarnall, K.; Zieglmayer, P.; Zieglmayer, R.; Lemell, P.; Horak, F. The effects of a trpv1 antagonist, sb-705498, in the treatment of seasonal allergic rhinitis. *Int. J. Clin. Pharmacol. Ther.* **2013**, *51*, 576–584. [CrossRef] [PubMed]

102. Changani, K.; Hotee, S.; Campbell, S.; Pindoria, K.; Dinnewell, L.; Saklatvala, P.; Thompson, S.A.; Coe, D.; Biggadike, K.; Vitulli, G.; et al. Effect of the trpv1 antagonist sb-705498 on the nasal parasympathetic reflex response in the ovalbumin sensitized guinea pig. *Br. J. Pharmacol.* **2013**, *169*, 580–589. [CrossRef] [PubMed]

103. Murdoch, R.D.; Bareille, P.; Denyer, J.; Newlands, A.; Bentley, J.; Smart, K.; Yarnall, K.; Patel, D. Trpv1 inhibition does not prevent cold dry air-elicited symptoms in non-allergic rhinitis. *Int. J. Clin. Pharmacol. Ther.* **2014**, *52*, 267–276. [CrossRef] [PubMed]

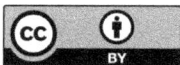

pharmaceuticals

MDPI

Review

TRPM8 Puts the Chill on Prostate Cancer

Guillaume P. Grolez and Dimitra Gkika *

Laboratoire de Physiologie cellulaire, Inserm U1003, Laboratory of Excellence,
Ion Channels Science and Therapeutics, Université de Lille, 59655 Villeneuve d'Ascq Cedex, France;
guillaume.grolez@etudiant.univ-lille1.fr
* Correspondence: dimitra.gkika@univ-lille1.fr; Tel.: +33-03-20-43-68-38

Academic Editors: Arpad Szallasi and Susan M. Huang
Received: 26 May 2016; Accepted: 4 July 2016; Published: 9 July 2016

Abstract: Prostate cancer (PCa) is one of the most frequently diagnosed cancers in developed countries. Several studies suggest that variations in calcium homeostasis are involved in carcinogenesis. Interestingly, (Transient Receptor Potential Melastatin member 8) TRPM8 calcium permeable channel expression is differentially regulated during prostate carcinogenesis, thereby suggesting a potential functional role for this channel in those cell processes, which are important for PCa evolution. Indeed, several studies have shown that TRPM8 plays a key role in processes such as the proliferation, viability and cell migration of PCa cells. Where cell migration is concerned, TRPM8 seems to have a protective anti-invasive effect and could be a particularly promising therapeutic target. The goal of this review is to inventory advances in understanding of the role of TRPM8 in the installation and progression of PCa.

Keywords: TRPM8; prostate cancer; migration

---

1. Introduction

In developed countries, prostate cancer is the second most frequently diagnosed cancer and the third most common cause of death by cancer in men [1]. Prostate cancer (PCa) development starts from epithelial cells in the peripheral zone of the prostate and is androgen-controlled [2]. In its first stages, the cancer develops slowly and remains localized, while in later stages the prostate capsule barrier can be crossed, and PCa becomes invasive, often leading to metastasis in lymph nodes and later mainly in the bone, liver and lung [3]. Metastasis development in the late PCa stages is the main cause of mortality due to PCa. To prevent PCa development, the main treatment is tumor ablation followed by hormone-therapy and more precisely androgen suppression. This treatment is the leading treatment in the case of metastasis, and currently the most successful since it leads to tumor regression. However, PCa cells can become androgen-independent for their survival and proliferation and therefore escape this treatment, leading to more aggressive forms of cancer [4]. This androgen insensitivity is a significantly increases PCa mortality rates and suggests that various androgen-related factors are involved in PCa progression.

Several studies suggest that variations or modifications to Ca^{2+} homeostasis are involved in PCa carcinogenesis and in metastasis development of since this affects the key cellular processes of carcinogenesis [5–8]. Indeed, malignant cell-transformation is the result of enhanced proliferation, aberrant differentiation, and an impaired ability to die [9]. These result in abnormal tissue growth, which can eventually turn into the uncontrolled expansion and invasion that is characteristic of cancer. Such transformation is often accompanied by changes in ion channel expression and, consequently, by the abnormal progression of the cellular responses with which they are involved. Members of TRP (Transient Receptor Potential) ion channel superfamily are implicated in all the hallmarks of cancer, while their expression levels are correlated with the emergence and/or progression of numerous epithelial cancers [10–14]. In addition, it should be noted that besides their transcriptional and translational regulation, ion channel trafficking to the cell surface as well as plasma membrane stabilization define channel activity. Therefore, modulation of TRP expression/activity on one of these levels affects intracellular Ca^{2+} concentrations and, consequently, those processes involved in carcinogenesis, such as proliferation, apoptosis, and migration [12].

2. TRPM8: An Androgen Target in Prostate Cancer

TRPM8 is one of the TRP channels involved in PCa and it seems to be one of the most promising clinical targets. Its androgen-dependent expression increases in both benign prostate hyperplasia and in prostate carcinoma cells, which both presented high androgen levels [15], while anti-androgen therapy greatly reduces the expression of TRPM8 [16]. It appears that the androgen dependency of TRPM8 expression is related to the differentiation degree of prostate epithelial cells [17,18]. Recent studies suggest that androgens could act in a non-genomic way on TRPM8 channel [19].

Furthermore, androgens have been shown to define the subcellular localization of TRPM8 toward different healthy and cancerous prostate cells [18]. Several studies have demonstrated both plasma membrane and endoplasmic reticulum (ER) membrane TRPM8 expression, in prostate cancer cell lines that are androgen-sensitive, such as LNCaP cells (Lymph Node Carcinoma of the Prostate) [20,21]. TRPM8 expression at the plasma membrane seems to increase in correlation with the increase of functional AR expression, while the ER isoform is less sensitive to androgens. At the functional level, the ER isoform has been shown to be involved in the activation of store-operated channels [20]. Thus, dual localization of TRPM8 in the two membranes significantly increases the spectrum of physiological and pathological processes the channel may be involved in. Indeed, plasma membrane or ER ion channels localization induce different calcium signaling patterns, which are responsible for the inception of various cellular processes. For example, when TRPM8 channel localizes at the plasma membrane, it is mainly involved in cancer proliferation and migration by activation of various calcium dependent pathways [22,23], whereas ER ion channel localization has been shown to be involved in the balance between apoptosis and proliferation [8,24]. These processes have been defined as being hallmarks of cancer and TRPM8 plays a role in all of these. Among these hallmarks, cell migration is the most involved in the evolution of cancer towards metastatic stages.

3. Roles of TRPM8 in PCa Progression

Malignant transformation of cells is the result of enhanced proliferation, aberrant differentiation, and an impaired ability to die, which results in tumor growth and potential invasion of the surrounding tissues and eventually metastasis [9]. This transformation is characterized by changes in the ion channel expression profile, which in turn modifies the cellular responses they are involved in. Different studies have shown an involvement of the TRPM8 channel in these processes in PCa cells and more particularly, TRPM8 has been shown to play a major role in migration.

3.1. Role of TRPM8 in Proliferation

The role of TRPM8 in the proliferation of PCa cells was shown using in vitro assays measuring cell viability, in cell cycle assays and with in vivo studies. Firstly, an anti-proliferative effect of TRPM8 on PCa cell lines was demonstrated using in vitro assays. Indeed, in androgen insensitive PCa cells (DU-145), endogenous TRPM8 activation by menthol treatment induces a decrease in proliferation [25]. Moreover, over-expression of TRPM8 in PC3 androgen insensitive cells that do not express TRPM8 at endogenous level induces a decrease in proliferation. To mediate this anti-proliferation effect, TRPM8 over-expression induces an arrest in the cell cycle from the G1 to S phase transition. This arrest is due to a down-regulation of Cdk4 and Cdk6 proteins after TRPM8 overexpression [26]. An in vivo study also showed an anti-proliferative effect of TRPM8 over-expression in PCa cells. Indeed, tumors monitored by xenograft in mice with PC3 cells overexpressing TRPM8, were less voluminous than tumors in PC3 cells, which were not [27].

On the other hand, a pro-proliferative role was shown in vitro for TRPM8 by using blockers and siRNA against TRPM8 [28]. In this study, the authors tested the effects of TRPM8 inhibition on various PCa cell lines. TRPM8 blockers and siRNA were shown to reduce the proliferation of LNCap cells and DU-145 cells, but not in PC3 cells and PNTA1 cells. The different effects of TRPM8 siRNA on PCa cell proliferation could not be explained by the difference in TRPM8 expression because TRPM8 was be shown to expressed at the same level in both PC3 and LNCaP cells [29].

The discrepancy in the TRPM8 effect on proliferation mentioned above could be explained by the distinct androgen sensitivity of the cell lines used. In fact, TRPM8 seems to play an anti-proliferative role in PCa androgen insensitive cells (PC3 and DU-145), yet a pro-proliferative role in PCa androgen sensitive cells (LNCaP). This result suggests that TRPM8 channels could be useful PCa proliferation arrest targets in the first stage of cancer, when pharmacological blockers could be used.

3.2. Role of TRPM8 in Cell Death or Survival

During cancer progression, cell survival balance is disturbed, thereby causing a resistance to cell death and a resistance to apoptosis in particular. Various studies have shown an interest in the TRPM8 role in cell viability in the PCa. Indeed, by its ER localization, TRPM8 was shown to be involved in the activation of store-operated channels [20], inducing an increase in cytosolic calcium concentration. Moreover, in LNCaP cell lines, ER store depletion has been shown to be sufficient to induce the apoptosis process [30] suggesting a possible role for TRPM8 in the apoptosis balance. Different studies seem to show a pro-apoptotic role of TRPM8 in PCa cells. In vitro assays using flow cytometry on PC3 cells show that TRPM8 overexpression increases apoptosis rates in starved conditions (1% FBS for 48 h). Moreover, as previously mentioned, TRPM8 overexpression in these cells induces arrest of the cell cycle in the G0/G1 stages [26] TRPM8 has also been shown to have a pro-apoptotic role in DU-145 cells after activation by menthol [25]. Finally, sustained activation of TRPM8 by menthol induces an increase in apoptosis in LNCaP cells due to the increase in the cytosolic calcium concentration [21].

On the other hand, one study using TRPM8 siRNA and blockers showed the opposite effects. Indeed, in LNCaP cells, siRNA-mediated knockdown of TRPM8, or a capsazepine treatment induced an apoptotic process shown by the increased numbers of cells with apoptotic nuclei [21]. By this study, authors show that TRPM8 are necessary for the survival and the anti-apoptotic role of TRPM8 in LNCaP cells. Another interesting study shows an anti-apoptotic role of a short isoform of TRPM8 expressed in PCa cells [31]. Overexpression of the short TRPM8 isoform, sM8a, reduces the apoptosis induced by starvation in LNCaP cells. This sM8a isoform is a 19 kDa protein, which was previously shown to negatively regulate the full length of TRPM8 by interaction [32].

Overall, these studies show that TRPM8 plays a role in cell viability, which seems to be regulated by androgens as well as the differential expression of TRPM8 isoforms expressed in PCa cells.

3.3. Role of TRPM8 in Migration

As mentioned above, metastasis development is the main cause of cancer-related mortality, and depends on two key processes: cell migration of cancer cells that invade adjacent tissues, followed by intravasation into blood/lymphatic vessels and tumor vascularization, which give access to the bloodstream. During the metastatic process, cell migration of both epithelial and endothelial cells is an essential step leading to the spread of the primary tumor and to the invasion of neighboring connective tissue, the lymphatic system and blood vessels. The role of TRPM8 channel in the PCa migration process in has been studied recently. Indeed, we as well as others suggest a putative protective role for TRPM8 in prostate metastatic cancer progression [33], since enhancement in channel expression and/or an activation, blocks prostate cancer cell migration [22,26,27]. In this context, we have shown that PCa cell treated with icilin, a TRPM8 agonist, results in a decrease in the cell mobility of PC3 cells overexpressing TRPM8 [22]. In line with these results, two other studies demonstrate that TRPM8 overexpression significantly inhibits PC3 cell migration and they show that this inhibition occurred through the inactivation of focal adhesion kinase (FAK) [26,27]. FAK is the non-receptor protein, tyrosine kinase, the phosphorylation of which is critical during focal adhesion formation and consequently in cellular processes such as migration and invasion [34]. These studies showed that TRPM8 activation by different agonists or overexpression of TRPM8 channels induces an inhibition of PCa migration. Nevertheless, it has to be noted that contrasting results concerning the role of TRPM8 in cell migration have been shown using pharmacological agents inhibiting TRPM8, which have led to a reduction in the speed of prostate cancer cells [28,35].

Further, TRPM8-mediated cancer cell migration has been seen to be regulated by the newly identified partner proteins of the channel. Firstly, Prostate Specific Antigen (PSA), shown to be an endogenous agonist of TRPM8 increasing the channel activity while supporting its plasma membrane expression, was shown to induce a decrease in cell mobility in PC3 cells overexpressing TRPM8 [22]. Moreover, the channel-associated protein TCAF1, which is also strongly expressed in the prostate [36], was shown to facilitate the opening state of TRPM8 and plasma membrane expression by direct interaction. This protein, by activating TRPM8 regulation, was shown to decrease the migration of PCa cells by reducing both cell speed and velocity [36]. In line with these results, the short TRPM8 isoform sM8a, acts as a partner protein to the channel inhibiting full length TRPM8 and promoting cell mobility and invasion when overexpressed in LNCaP cells [31].

In summary, taking into account the aforementioned studies using endogenous and exogenous agonists of the TRPM8 channel, as well as the overexpression of this protein in PCa cells, one can conclude that there is an anti-migratory role of this channel in PCa cells. Since migration is one of the key processes of metastatic development, these results suggest a protective role for TRPM8 in prostate metastatic cancer progression. To further confirm this hypothesis, Zhu et al. were interested in the role of TRPM8 on angiogenesis, which is also a key process for metastasis development. An in vivo study in nude mice showed that TRPM8 expression had a negative effect on angiogenesis [27]. Indeed, mice transplanted with prostate cancer cells over-expressing TRPM8 develop tumors that are less vascularized than control cases. The lower micro-vascular density of the TRPM8 xenografts can be explained by their lower expression of FAK and VEGF, which is one of the most potent angiogenic factors [27]. Taken together, these results reinforce the hypothesis that TRPM8 could play a protective role in prostate cancer progression by reducing both cell migration and angiogenesis.

4. Discussion

Several lines of evidence have been discovered over recent decades showing the importance of TRPM8 in prostate cancer. Firstly, it has been demonstrated that expression of TRPM8 varies during cancer progression and the androgen-dependence of TRPM8 expression has been demonstrated. A loss of TRPM8 expression is positively correlated with the aggressive androgen-independent state of PCa. Indeed, TRPM8 is strongly expressed in the first PCa stages and its expression disappears in the late and more aggressive states of the PCa. By this variation in its expression, TRPM8 may be considered and used as a diagnostic/prognostic marker as it is already used as a clinical marker in some countries [37,38].

Several studies cited in this review have shown by the use of agonists and blockers of TRPM8 that this channel has mainly anti-proliferative, pro-apoptotic and anti-migratory roles in PCa cells. As proliferation and cell viability data are contradictory, further experiments are needed and particularly in vivo data in order to confirm an anti-cancer role for this channel. However, there is less controversy concerning the TRPM8 anti-migratory role, consequently suggesting a protective role for this channel against metastasis in PCa. This is why several regulatory agents (listed in Table 1) could be used to prevent the metastatic evolution of PCa when the cancer is diagnosed.

Table 1. TRPM8 modulators can be used in research therapies against PCa.

Molecule	Agonist/Antagonist	PCa-Related Cellular Effect
Capsazepine [21]	Antagonist	Increased apoptosis in LnCaP cells
AMTB [28,39]	Antagonist	Decreased proliferation in LnCaP cells
JNJ-39267631 [40]	Antagonist	Not defined
BCTC [28]	Antagonist	Decreased cell proliferation
M8-B [41]	Antagonist	Not defined
Cannabigerol [42]	Antagonist	Pro-apoptotic effects in Pca cells
PBMC [43]	Antagonist	Not defined
PSA [22]	Agonist	Decreased cell mobility in PC3-TRPM8 cells
Icilin [22]	Agonist	Decreased cell mobility in PC3-TRPM8 cells
Menthol [21,25]	Agonist	Decreased proliferaion, increased apoptosis
WS12 [44]	Agonist	Not defined
D-3263 [45]	Agonist	Decrease mice prostate hyperplasia

Another way to prevent the metastatic evolution of PCa is to reinforce the activation of TRPM8 endogenous regulator proteins (listed on Table 2) and to target the channel's activity. These different endogenous or pharmacological modulators of TRPM8 are very promising for the prevention of the metastatic evolution of PCa and should therefore be validated in animal models.

Table 2. TRPM8 regulatory proteins can be used in research therapies against PCa.

Partners Protein	Agonist/Antagonist	PCa-Related Cellular Effect
G alpha protein [46]	Antagonist	Inhibition of TRPM8
sM8a protein [32]	Antagonist	Negative regulation of full length TRPM8
Pirt [47]	Agonist	Enhances TRPM8 channel properties
TCAF1 [36]	Agonist	Facilitates the opening state of TRPM8 and plasma membrane expression
PYR-41 [48]	Agonist	Facilitates TRPM8 plasma membrane expression

5. Conclusions

In conclusion, TRPM8 variation in expression during the evolution of PCa makes this channel an appealing clinical marker in order to separate the different stages of the disease. Concerning the therapeutic targeting of the channel, at first sight the evolution of TRPM8 expression during carcinogenesis might seem not in full accordance with the anti-cancer effect of the channel activation. In order to make sense of TRPM8's role in prostate carcinogenesis, the different hallmarks of cancer should be studied separately; at the beginning, by taking into account the androgen dependency of the PCa cells in the various stages of advancement. However, the results till now support the hypothesis that TRPM8 increase in the first androgen-dependent stages of PCa has a protective role regarding the invasive character of prostate cancer cells. Indeed, to support this hypothesis, a preclinical assay with a TRPM8 agonist (D-3263) show that TRPM8 activation decrease mice prostate hyperplasia [45]. Finally, for these early stages, how the high expression of the channel is functionally related to the growth of the tumor volume remains to be elucidated.

Acknowledgments: This study was supported by grants from the Ministère de l'Education Nationale, the Institut National de la Santé et de la Recherche Medicale (INSERM) and by the Lille I University. The research of DG was supported by the Fondation ARC pour la recherche sur le cancer (PJA 20141202010) and the Association pour la Recherche sur les Tumeurs de la Prostate (ARTP).

Conflicts of Interest: Authors declare no conflicts of interest.

References

1. Ferlay, J.; Soerjomataram, I.; Dikshit, R.; Eser, S.; Mathers, C.; Rebelo, M.; Parkin, D.M.; Forman, D.; Bray, F. Cancer incidence and mortality worldwide: Sources, methods and major patterns in GLOBOCAN 2012. *Int. J. Cancer* **2015**, *136*, E359–E386. [CrossRef] [PubMed]
2. Cunha, G.R.; Donjacour, A.A.; Cooke, P.S.; Mee, H.; Bigsby, R.M.; Higgins, S.J.; Sugilura, Y. The Endocrinology and Developmental Biology of the Prostate. *Endocr. Rev.* **1987**, *8*, 338–362. [CrossRef] [PubMed]
3. Bubendorf, L.; Schöpfer, A.; Wagner, U.; Sauter, G.; Moch, H.; Willi, N.; Gasser, T.C.; Mihatsch, M.J. Metastatic patterns of prostate cancer: An autopsy study of 1589 patients. *Hum. Pathol.* **2000**, *31*, 578–583. [CrossRef] [PubMed]
4. Feldman, B.J.; Feldman, D. The development of androgen-independent prostate cancer. *Nat. Rev. Cancer* **2001**, *1*, 34–45. [CrossRef] [PubMed]
5. Thebault, S.; Flourakis, M.; Vanoverberghe, K.; Vandermoere, F.; Roudbaraki, M.; Lehen'kyi, V.; Slomianny, C.; Beck, B.; Mariot, P.; Bonnal, J.L.; et al. Differential Role of Transient Receptor Potential Channels in Ca^{2+} Entry and Proliferation of Prostate Cancer Epithelial Cells. *Cancer Res.* **2006**, *66*, 2038–2047. [CrossRef] [PubMed]
6. Monteith, G.R.; McAndrew, D.; Faddy, H.M.; Roberts-Thomson, S.J. Calcium and cancer: Targeting Ca^{2+} transport. *Nat. Rev. Cancer* **2007**, *7*, 519–530. [CrossRef] [PubMed]
7. Roderick, H.L.; Cook, S.J. Ca^{2+} signalling checkpoints in cancer: Remodelling Ca^{2+} for cancer cell proliferation and survival. *Nat. Rev. Cancer* **2008**, *8*, 361–375. [CrossRef] [PubMed]
8. Flourakis, M.; Prevarskaya, N. Insights into Ca^{2+} homeostasis of advanced prostate cancer cells. *Biochim. Biophys. Acta Mol. Cell Res.* **2009**, *1793*, 1105–1109. [CrossRef] [PubMed]
9. Hanahan, D.; Weinberg, R.A. Hallmarks of Cancer: The Next Generation. *Cell* **2011**, *144*, 646–674. [CrossRef] [PubMed]
10. Prevarskaya, N.; Zhang, L.; Barritt, G. TRP channels in cancer. *Biochim. Biophys. Acta Mol. Basis Dis.* **2007**, *1772*, 937–946. [CrossRef] [PubMed]
11. Santoni, G.; Farfariello, V. TRP Channels and Cancer: New Targets for Diagnosis and Chemotherapy. *Endocr. Metab. Immune Disord. Drug Targets* **2011**, *11*, 54–67. [CrossRef] [PubMed]
12. Gkika, D.; Prevarskaya, N. Molecular mechanisms of TRP regulation in tumor growth and metastasis. *Biochim. Biophys. Acta Mol. Cell Res.* **2009**, *1793*, 953–958. [CrossRef] [PubMed]
13. Fioro Pla, A.; Gkika, D. Emerging role of TRP channels in cell migration: From tumor vascularization to metastasis. *Front. Physiol.* **2013**, *4*, 311. [CrossRef] [PubMed]
14. Bernardini, M.; Fiorio Pla, A.; Prevarskaya, N.; Gkika, D. Human transient receptor potential (TRP) channel expression profiling in carcinogenesis. *Int. J. Dev. Biol.* **2015**, *59*, 399–406. [CrossRef] [PubMed]
15. Tsavaler, L.; Shapero, M.H.; Morkowski, S.; Laus, R. Trp-p8, a Novel Prostate-specific Gene, Is Up-Regulated in Prostate Cancer and Other Malignancies and Shares High Homology with Transient Receptor Potential Calcium Channel Proteins. *Cancer Res.* **2001**, *61*, 3760–3769. [PubMed]
16. Henshall, S.M.; Afar, D.E.H.; Hiller, J.; Horvath, L.G.; Quinn, D.I.; Rasiah, K.K.; Gish, K.; Willhite, D.; Kench, J.G.; Gardiner-Garden, M.; et al. Survival Analysis of Genome-Wide Gene Expression Profiles of Prostate Cancers Identifies New Prognostic Targets of Disease Relapse. *Cancer Res.* **2003**, *63*, 4196–4203. [PubMed]
17. Bidaux, G.; Roudbaraki, M.; Merle, C.; Crépin, A.; Delcourt, P.; Slomianny, C.; Thebault, S.; Bonnal, J.L.; Benahmed, M.; Cabon, F.; et al. Evidence for specific TRPM8 expression in human prostate secretory epithelial cells: Functional androgen receptor requirement. *Endocr. Relat. Cancer* **2005**, *12*, 367–382. [CrossRef] [PubMed]
18. Bidaux, G.; Flourakis, M.; Thebault, S.; Zholos, A.; Beck, B.; Gkika, D.; Roudbaraki, M.; Bonnal, J.L.; Mauroy, B.; Shuba, Y.; et al. Prostate cell differentiation status determines transient receptor potential melastatin member 8 channel subcellular localization and function. *J. Clin. Investig.* **2007**, *117*, 1647–1657. [CrossRef] [PubMed]
19. Asuthkar, S.; Elustondo, P.A.; Demirkhanyan, L.; Sun, X.; Baskaran, P.; Velpula, K.K.; Thyagarajan, B.; Pavlov, E.V.; Zakharian, E.; et al. The TRPM8 protein is a testosterone receptor: I. Biochemical evidence for direct TRPM8-testosterone interactions. *J. Biol. Chem.* **2015**, *290*, 2659–2669. [CrossRef] [PubMed]

20. Thebault, S.; Lemonnier, L.; Bidaux, G.; Flourakis, M.; Bavencoffe, A.; Gordienko, D.; Roudbaraki, M.; Delcourt, P.; Panchin, Y.; Shuba, Y.; et al. Novel Role of Cold/Menthol-sensitive Transient Receptor Potential Melastatine Family Member 8 (TRPM8) in the Activation of Store-operated Channels in LNCaP Human Prostate Cancer Epithelial Cells. *J. Biol. Chem.* **2005**, *280*, 39423–39435. [CrossRef] [PubMed]

21. Zhang, L.; Barritt, G.J. Evidence that TRPM8 Is an Androgen-Dependent Ca^{2+} Channel Required for the Survival of Prostate Cancer Cells. *Cancer Res.* **2004**, *64*, 8365–8373. [CrossRef] [PubMed]

22. Gkika, D.; Flourakis, M.; Lemonnier, L.; Prevarskaya, N. PSA reduces prostate cancer cell motility by stimulating TRPM8 activity and plasma membrane expression. *Oncogene* **2010**, *29*, 4611–4616. [CrossRef] [PubMed]

23. Déliot, N.; Constantin, B. Plasma membrane calcium channels in cancer: Alterations and consequences for cell proliferation and migration. *Biochim. Biophys. Acta Biomembr.* **2015**, *1848 (Pt B)*, 2512–2522. [CrossRef] [PubMed]

24. Mekahli, D.; Bultynck, G.; Parys, J.B.; Smedt, H.D.; Missiaen, L. Endoplasmic-Reticulum Calcium Depletion and Disease. *Cold Spring Harb. Perspect. Biol.* **2011**, *3*, a004317. [CrossRef] [PubMed]

25. Wang, Y.; Wang, X.; Yang, Z.; Zhu, G.; Chen, D.; Meng, Z. Menthol Inhibits the Proliferation and Motility of Prostate Cancer DU145 Cells. *Pathol. Oncol. Res.* **2012**, *18*, 903–910. [CrossRef] [PubMed]

26. Yang, Z.-H.; Wang, X.-H.; Wang, H.-P.; Hu, L.-Q. Effects of TRPM8 on the proliferation and motility of prostate cancer PC-3 cells. *Asian J. Androl.* **2009**, *11*, 157–165. [CrossRef] [PubMed]

27. Zhu, G.; Wang, X.; Yang, Z.; Cao, H.; Meng, Z.; Wang, Y.; Chen, D. Effects of TRPM8 on the proliferation and angiogenesis of prostate cancer PC-3 cells in vivo. *Oncol. Lett.* **2011**, *2*, 1213–1217. [PubMed]

28. Valero, M.L.; Mello de Queiroz, F.; Stühmer, W.; Viana, F.; Pardo, L.A. TRPM8 Ion Channels Differentially Modulate Proliferation and Cell Cycle Distribution of Normal and Cancer Prostate Cells. *PLoS ONE* **2012**, *7*, e51825. [CrossRef] [PubMed]

29. Valero, M.; Morenilla-Palao, C.; Belmonte, C.; Viana, F. Pharmacological and functional properties of TRPM8 channels in prostate tumor cells. *Pflügers Arch. Eur. J. Physiol.* **2011**, *461*, 99–114. [CrossRef] [PubMed]

30. Wertz, I.E.; Dixit, V.M. Characterization of Calcium Release-activated Apoptosis of LNCaP Prostate Cancer Cells. *J. Biol. Chem.* **2000**, *275*, 11470–11477. [CrossRef] [PubMed]

31. Peng, M.; Wang, Z.; Yang, Z.; Tao, L.; Liu, Q.; Yi, L.U.; Wang, X. Overexpression of short TRPM8 variant α promotes cell migration and invasion, and decreases starvation-induced apoptosis in prostate cancer LNCaP cells. *Oncol. Lett.* **2015**, *10*, 1378–1384. [CrossRef] [PubMed]

32. Bidaux, G.; Beck, B.; Zholos, A.; Gordienko, D.; Lemonnier, L.; Flourakis, M.; Roudbaraki, M.; Borowiec, A.S.; Fernández, J.; Delcourt, P.; et al. Regulation of activity of transient receptor potential melastatin 8 (TRPM8) channel by its short isoforms. *J. Biol. Chem.* **2012**, *287*, 2948–2962. [CrossRef] [PubMed]

33. Gkika, D.; Prevarskaya, N. TRP channels in prostate cancer: The good, the bad and the ugly? *Asian J. Androl.* **2011**, *13*, 673–676. [CrossRef] [PubMed]

34. Schlaepfer, D.D.; Mitra, S.K.; Ilic, D. Control of motile and invasive cell phenotypes by focal adhesion kinase. *Biochim. Biophys. Acta Mol. Cell Res.* **2004**, *1692*, 77–102. [CrossRef] [PubMed]

35. Liu, T.; Fang, Z.; Wang, G.; Shi, M.; Wang, X.; Jiang, K.; Yang, Z.; Cao, R.; Tao, H.; Wang, X.; et al. Anti-tumor activity of the TRPM8 inhibitor BCTC in prostate cancer DU145 cells. *Oncol. Lett.* **2016**, *11*, 182–188. [CrossRef] [PubMed]

36. Gkika, D.; Lemonnier, L.; Shapovalov, G.; Gordienko, D.; Poux, C.; Bernardini, M.; Bokhobza, A.; Bidaux, G.; Degerny, C.; Verreman, K.; et al. TRP channel-associated factors are a novel protein family that regulates TRPM8 trafficking and activity. *J. Cell Biol.* **2015**, *208*, 89–107. [CrossRef] [PubMed]

37. Schmidt, U.; Fuessel, S.; Koch, R.; Baretton, G.B.; Lohse, A.; Tomasetti, S.; Unversucht, S.; Froehner, M.; Wirth, M.P.; Meye, A. Quantitative multi-gene expression profiling of primary prostate cancer. *Prostate* **2006**, *66*, 1521–1534. [CrossRef] [PubMed]

38. Bai, V.U.; Murthy, S.; Chinnakannu, K.; Muhletaler, F.; Tejwani, S.; Barrack, E.R.; Kim, S.H.; Menon, M.; Veer Reddy, G.P. Androgen regulated TRPM8 expression: A potential mRNA marker for metastatic prostate cancer detection in body fluids. *Int. J. Oncol.* **2010**, *36*, 443–450. [PubMed]

39. Lashinger, E.S.R.; Steiginga, M.S.; Hieble, J.P.; Leon, L.A.; Gardner, S.D.; Nagilla, R.; Davenport, E.A.; Hoffman, B.E.; Laping, N.J.; Su, X. AMTB, a TRPM8 channel blocker: Evidence in rats for activity in overactive bladder and painful bladder syndrome. *Am. J. Physiol. Renal. Physiol.* **2008**, *295*, F803–F810. [CrossRef] [PubMed]

40. Colburn, R.W.; Matthews, J.M.; Qin, N.; Liu, Y.; Hutchinson, T.L.; Schneider, C.R.; Stone, D.J.; Lubin, M.; Pavlick, K.P.; Kenigs, S.; et al. Small-molecule TRPM8 antagonist JNJ-39267631 reverses neuropathy-induced cold allodynia in rats. In Proceedings of the 12th World Congress on Pain, Glasgow, UK, 17–22 August 2008.

41. Miller, S.; Rao, S.; Wang, W.; Liu, H.; Wang, J.; Gavva, N.R. Antibodies to the Extracellular Pore Loop of TRPM8 Act as Antagonists of Channel Activation. *PLoS ONE* **2014**, *9*, e107151. [CrossRef] [PubMed]

42. De Petrocellis, L.; Ligresti, A.; Schiano Moriello, A.; Iappelli, M.; Verde, R.; Stott, C.G.; Cristino, L.; Orlando, P.; Di Marzo, V. Non-THC cannabinoids inhibit prostate carcinoma growth in vitro and in vivo: Pro-apoptotic effects and underlying mechanisms. *Br. J. Pharmacol.* **2013**, *168*, 79–102. [CrossRef] [PubMed]

43. Knowlton, W.M.; Daniels, R.L.; Palkar, R.; McCoy, D.D.; McKemy, D.D. Pharmacological blockade of TRPM8 ion channels alters cold and cold pain responses in mice. *PLoS ONE* **2011**, *6*, e25894. [CrossRef] [PubMed]

44. Sherkheli, M.A.; Gisselmann, G.; Vogt-Eisele, A.K.; Doerner, J.F.; Hatt, H. Menthol derivative WS-12 selectively activates transient receptor potential melastatin-8 (TRPM8) ion channels. *Pak. J. Pharm. Sci.* **2008**, *21*, 370–378.

45. Duncan, D.; Stewart, F.; Frohlich, M.; Urdal, D. Preclinical evaluation of the TRPM8 ion channel agonist D-3263 for begnin prostatic hyperplasia. *J. Urol.* **2009**, *181*, 503. [CrossRef]

46. Zhang, X.; Mak, S.; Li, L.; Parra, A.; Denlinger, B.; Belmonte, C.; McNaughton, PA. Direct inhibition of the cold-activated TRPM8 ion channel by $G\alpha_q$. *Nat. Cell Biol.* **2012**, *14*, 851–858. [CrossRef] [PubMed]

47. Tang, Z.; Kim, A.; Masuch, T.; Park, K.; Weng, H.; Wetzel, C.; Dong, X. Pirt functions as an endogenous regulator of TRPM8. *Nat. Commun.* **2013**, *4*, 2179. [CrossRef] [PubMed]

48. Asuthkar, S.; Velpula, K.K.; Elustondo, P.A.; Demirkhanyan, L.; Zakharian, E. TRPM8 channel as a novel molecular target in androgen-regulated prostate cancer cells. *Oncotarget* **2015**, *6*, 17221–17236. [CrossRef] [PubMed]

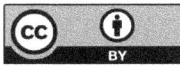

pharmaceuticals

MDPI

Review

Differential Activation of TRP Channels in the Adult Rat Spinal Substantia Gelatinosa by Stereoisomers of Plant-Derived Chemicals

Eiichi Kumamoto * and Tsugumi Fujita

Department of Physiology, Saga Medical School, 5-1-1 Nabeshima, Saga 849-8501, Japan; fujitat@cc.saga-u.ac.jp
* Correspondence: kumamote@cc.saga-u.ac.jp; Tel.: +81-952-34-2273; Fax: +81-952-34-2013

Academic Editors: Arpad Szallasi, Susan M. Huang and Jean Jacques Vanden Eynde
Received: 30 May 2016; Accepted: 25 July 2016; Published: 28 July 2016

Abstract: Activation of TRPV1, TRPA1 or TRPM8 channel expressed in the central terminal of dorsal root ganglion (DRG) neuron increases the spontaneous release of L-glutamate onto spinal dorsal horn lamina II (substantia gelatinosa; SG) neurons which play a pivotal role in regulating nociceptive transmission. The TRP channels are activated by various plant-derived chemicals. Although stereoisomers activate or modulate ion channels in a distinct manner, this phenomenon is not fully addressed for TRP channels. By applying the whole-cell patch-clamp technique to SG neurons of adult rat spinal cord slices, we found out that all of plant-derived chemicals, carvacrol, thymol, carvone and cineole, increase the frequency of spontaneous excitatory postsynaptic current, a measure of the spontaneous release of L-glutamate from nerve terminals, by activating TRP channels. The presynaptic activities were different between stereoisomers (carvacrol and thymol; (−)-carvone and (+)-carvone; 1,8-cineole and 1,4-cineole) in the extent or the types of TRP channels activated, indicating that TRP channels in the SG are activated by stereoisomers in a distinct manner. This result could serve to know the properties of the central terminal TRP channels that are targets of drugs for alleviating pain.

Keywords: TRPV1; TRPA1; TRPM8; plant-derived chemical; L-glutamate release; spinal dorsal horn; patch-clamp; rat

1. TRP Channels Involved in Nociceptive Transmission through Dorsal Root Ganglion Neurons

Cation-permeable transient receptor potential (TRP) channels expressed in dorsal root ganglion (DRG) neurons are involved in nociceptive transmission from the periphery (for a review see [1]). TRP channels, which are synthesized in the cell body of the DRG neuron, are transported to the peripheral and central terminals of the neuron by axonal transport. Among TRP channels involved in the nociceptive transmission, there are TRP vanilloid-1 (TRPV1), TRP ankyrin-1 (TRPA1) and TRP melastatin-8 (TRPM8) channels. The TRPA1 channel is found in a subset of rat DRG neurons in which it is co-expressed with the TRPV1, but not the TRPM8 channel [2,3]. They are activated by chemical substances and temperature (for reviews see [4,5]). For instance, in the peripheral terminal of the DRG neuron, the TRPV1 channel is activated by capsaicin (a natural pungent ingredient contained in red peppers), protons and noxious heat (>43 °C; [6]; for review see [7]); the TRPA1 channel by pungent compounds in mustard, cinnamon and garlic (allyl isothiocyanate (AITC), cinnamaldehyde and allicin, respectively), and noxious cold temperature (<17 °C; [2,8–10]); and the TRPM8 channel by menthol (a secondary alcohol contained in peppermint or other mint) and mild temperature (<25 °C; [11,12]). Such an activation depolarizes the membrane of the peripheral terminal, resulting in the production of action potentials. As a result, the nociceptive or temperature information is transferred to the spinal dorsal horn.

On the other hand, TRP channels in the central terminal of the DRG neuron are expressed in the superficial laminae of the dorsal horn, especially the substantia gelatinosa (SG; lamina II of Rexed; [13,14]). In support of this idea about TRP activation in the SG, many of plant-derived chemicals increase in SG neurons the frequency of spontaneous excitatory postsynaptic current (sEPSC), a measure of the spontaneous release of L-glutamate from nerve terminals, by activating TRPV1 channel [15–18], TRPA1 channel [19,20] and TRPM8 channel [21,22] (for a review see [23]). The SG neurons play a pivotal role in modulating nociceptive transmission from the periphery [24–26] and thus TRP channels in the SG are involved in its modulation. Their expressions in the SG have been shown by immunohistochemistry [27].

2. Spinal Substantia Gelatinosa Involved in Regulating Nociceptive Transmission

Nociceptive transmission in the SG is in origin not only monosynaptic from glutamatergic DRG neurons but also polysynaptic from glutamate-, GABA- and/or glycine-containing interneurons [28]. In support of the involvement of the SG in nociceptive transmission, a plastic change in glutamatergic inputs to SG neurons through DRG neurons occurred in hyperalgesic rats that were subject to either an intraplantar injection of complete Freund's adjuvant [29] or ovariectomy [30]. Endogenous and exogenous analgesics, which exhibit antinociception when administered intrathecally, hyperpolarize membranes of SG neurons and reduce the release of L-glutamate onto SG neurons from nerve terminals, both of which actions reduce the membrane excitability of the SG neurons [31]. For example, opioids ([32]; for a review see [33]), nociceptin [34,35], a $GABA_B$-receptor agonist baclofen [36,37], a μ-opioid receptor agonist tramadol [38], norepinephrine [39], serotonin [30,40], adenosine ([41,42]; for review see [43]), somatostatin [44,45], dopamine [46,47] and galanin [48] hyperpolarized membranes of rat SG neurons. Inhibition of the release of L-glutamate from nerve terminals onto rat SG neurons was produced by opioids ([49]; for review see [33]), nociceptin [50,51], baclofen [36,52,53], the endocannabinoid anandamide [16,54], norepinephrine [55], serotonin [30,40], adenosine ([41,56,57]; for a review see [43]) and galanin [48,58].

3. TRP Channels in Nociception

Much evidence demonstrates that TRP channels play a role in transferring nociceptive information. For example, neuropathic pain and hyperalgesia developed following excessive or ectopical expression of TRPV1 channel in the central nervous system (CNS) and peripheral nervous system, in both animals and humans [59–62]. Hyperalgesia in inflammatory pain models was reduced in TRPV1-knockout mice [63]. Nerve growth factor, which mediates inflammatory pain, upregulated the expression of TRPV1 channel in rat DRG neurons by an action of the small GTPase Ras [64]. Excessive expression of TRPV1 channel in primary-afferent fibers occurred in disease states including inflammatory disease and irritable bowel syndrome [65,66]. Peripheral inflammation upregulated TRPV1 channel involved in the enhancement of spontaneous excitatory transmission in rat SG neurons [67]. When intrathecally administrated, a powerful TRPV1 agonist resiniferatoxin (RTX, a component contained in the dried latex of the cactus-like plant; [68]) produced a prolonged antinociceptive response in dogs with bone cancer [69], possibly owing to a desensitization of TRPV1 channel. Selective inhibition of TRPV1 channel attenuated bone cancer pain in the mouse [70]. TRPV1 channel, which is a potential treatment target for cancer pain, was expressed in neurons that transfer information of this type of pain (for a review see [71]). Intrathecal application of a TRPV1 antagonist AS1928370 resulted in an inhibition of mechanical allodynia in a mouse model of neuropathic pain [72].

The TRPA1 agonist cinnamaldehyde evoked spontaneous pain, and induced mechanical hyperalgesia and cold hypoalgesia following its application to the forearm skin of human volunteers [73]. Moreover, TRPA1 channel was over-expressed in rat DRG neurons following peripheral inflammation and nerve injury, and cold hyperalgesia produced by inflammation and nerve injury was accompanied by the activation of the TRPA1 but not the TRPM8 channel [74]. Alternatively, TRPA1 channel was excessively expressed in the mouse spinal cord and DRG after peripheral inflammation occurred as a result of intraplantar injection of complete Freund's adjuvant; intrathecally-applied TRPA1 antagonist reversed hyperalgesia that occurred in mouse models of neuropathic pain [75].

TRPM8 channel is also involved in nociceptive transmission. Proudfoot et al. [76] have proposed the idea that TRPM8 activation in both peripheral and central terminals of adult rat DRG neurons produces the release of L-glutamate from its central terminal onto dorsal horn neurons expressing group II/III metabotropic glutamate receptors, the activation of which results in antinociception. In chronic constrictive nerve injury rat models, which exhibited cold allodynia in hindlimbs, compared with the sham group, TRPM8-immunoreactive DRG neurons increased in number, menthol-sensitive DRG neurons increased in number in neurons that responded to capsaicin, and membrane currents produced by menthol in DRG neurons enhanced in amplitude [77]. Kono et al. [78] have suggested an involvement of TRPM8 channel in acute peripheral hypersensitivity to cold in oxaliplatin (a third-generation platinum analog)-treated cancer patients. In adult mice, ($-$)-menthol and its derivative WS-12 (which activated TRPM8 channel in DRG neurons) inhibited acute thermal, capsaicin- and acrolein-induced nociceptive behavior in a manner sensitive to a nonselective opioid-receptor antagonist naloxone, suggesting an involvement of endogenous opioids in antinociception produced by TRPM8 activation [79].

In conclusion, the effects of the activation of TRPV1, TRPA1 or TRPM8 channel on nociceptive transmission appear to depend on the location of the TRP channels activated, i.e., the peripheral or central terminal of DRG neuron, or both of them. When antinociceptive drugs are administrated intrathecally, it would be necessary to consider the activation of TRP channels located in not only primary-afferent central terminal but also neuronal and glial cells in the CNS, because their expressions in the CNS have been reported [80,81].

4. Actions of Plant-Derived Stereoisomers on Spontaneous Excitatory Transmission in Substantia Gelatinosa Neurons

It is well-known that there is a difference among stereoisomers in their actions on voltage-gated ion channels and neurotransmitter receptors (see [82,83] for reviews). Activation of TRPA1 channel expressed in Chinese hamster ovary cells differs in efficacy between stereoisomers such as (+)-menthol and ($-$)-menthol [84]. In order to know whether such a difference between stereoisomers is seen in the SG, we examined the actions of plant-derived stereoisomers on spontaneous excitatory transmission in SG neurons with a focus on TRP activation by using transverse slice preparations dissected from the adult rat spinal cord [85].

4.1. Actions of Thymol and Carvacrol

Thymol (5-methyl-2-isopropylphenol, a compound where the cyclohexane ring of menthol is replaced by a benzene ring) differs only in the position of the -OH in the benzene ring from carvacrol (5-isopropyl-2-methylphenol; Figure 1A,B). Thymol and carvacrol are contained in thyme and oregano, respectively, and exhibit antinociception [86,87]. In all SG neurons tested, bath-applied thymol (1 mM) for 3 min increased the frequency of sEPSC with a small increase in its amplitude. The sEPSC frequency increase averaged to be 326% around 5 min (when a maximal effect was obtained) after the onset of thymol superfusion. Such a sEPSC frequency increase was concentration-dependent with the half-maximal effective concentration (EC_{50}) value of 0.18 mM (Figure 1C). In 77% of the neurons tested, thymol (1 mM) produced an outward current having the averaged peak amplitude of 16 pA at the V_H of -70 mV (see Figure 1E); remaining neurons had no outward currents [88].

Carvacrol exhibited similar actions to those of thymol. In 22% of the SG neurons tested, carvacrol (1 mM) superfused for 2 min produced an outward current, which was not accompanied by a change in sEPSC frequency, at -70 mV. On the other hand, 11% of the SG neurons produced no change in holding currents while exhibiting sEPSC frequency increase (see Figure 1Fa). In 63% of the neurons, both of the outward current and sEPSC frequency increase were produced [89].

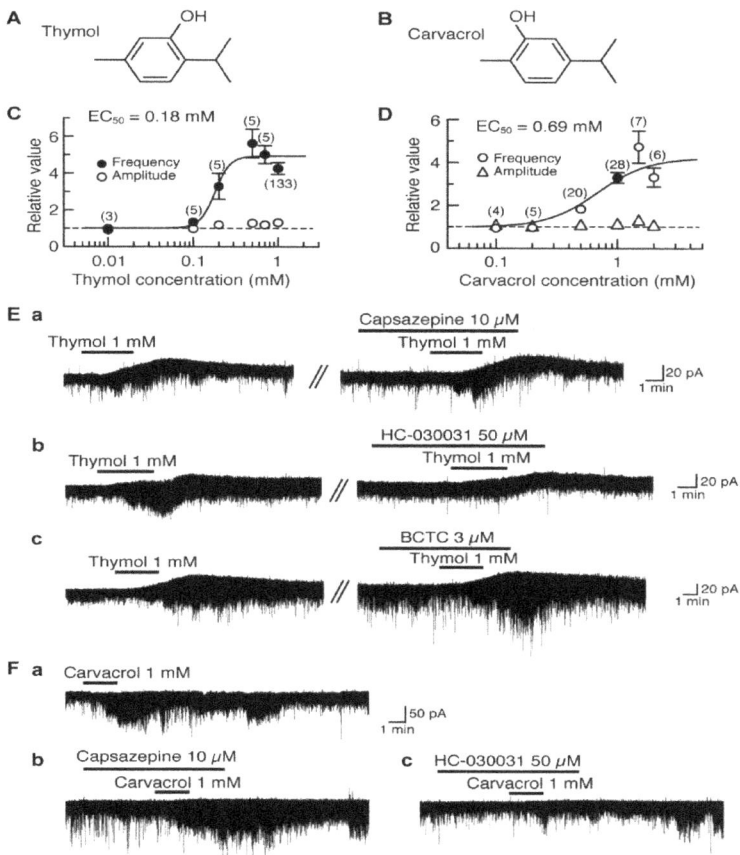

Figure 1. Effects of thymol and carvacrol on glutamatergic spontaneous excitatory transmission in rat substantia gelatinosa (SG) neurons. (**A,B**) The chemical structures of thymol (**A**) and carvacrol (**B**). (**C,D**) The frequency and amplitude of sEPSC under the action of thymol (**C**) or carvacrol (**D**), relative to those before drug superfusion, which were plotted against the logarithm of drug concentration. This thymol (carvacrol) effect was measured for 0.5 min around 5 min (3.5 min) after the beginning of its superfusion. The results in (**C**) were obtained from all neurons tested, while those in (**D**) were obtained from neurons where carvacrol (1 mM) increased sEPSC frequency > 5%. The continuous curves in (**C**) and (**D**) were drawn according to the Hill equation [half-maximal effective concentration (EC_{50}) and Hill coefficient (n_H) in (**C**) and (**D**): 0.18 mM, 4.9 and 0.69 mM, 2.1, respectively]. (**Ea–c**) Chart recordings showing sEPSCs and holding currents in the absence and presence of thymol in Krebs solution without (left) or with a TRPV1 antagonist capsazepine (**Ea**), a TRPA1 antagonist HC-030031 (**Eb**) or a TRPM8 antagonist BCTC (**Ec**; right). In each of (**Ea–c**), the right recording was obtained about 30 min after the left one from the same neuron. (**Fa–c**) Chart recordings showing sEPSCs in the absence and presence of carvacrol in Krebs solution without (**Fa**) and with capsazepine (**Fb**) or HC-030031 (**Fc**); these recordings were obtained from the same neuron at an interval of 30 min. In this and subsequent figures, value in parentheses indicates the number of neurons tested; each point with vertical bars represents the mean values and standard error of the mean (SEM); if the SEM of the values is less than the size of symbol, the vertical bar is not shown; control level (1) is indicated by horizontal dotted line; the duration of drug superfusion is shown by a horizontal bar above the chart recording. Holding potential (V_H) = −70 mV. This research was originally published in [88,89].

sEPSC frequency increase around 3.5 min (when a maximal effect was obtained) after the beginning of carvacrol superfusion averaged to be 262% with a small increase in its amplitude and the outward current had the averaged peak amplitude of 26 pA. Such a sEPSC frequency increase was concentration-dependent with the EC_{50} value of 0.69 mM (Figure 1D; [89]), a value larger than that of thymol. Thymol has an ability to activate TRP vanilloid-3 (TRPV3; [90]), TRPA1 [91] and TRPM8 channels [92] expressed in heterologous cells. On the other hand, carvacrol has been reported to activate TRPV3 and TRPA1 channels but not TRPV1 channel expressed in human embryonic kidney (HEK) or *Xenopus laevis* oocyte cells [90,91,93,94]. We next examined what types of TRP channel mediate the sEPSC frequency increases produced by thymol and carvacrol. The thymol activity was inhibited by a TRPA1 antagonist HC-030031 (50 μM; [95]) but not a TRPV1 antagonist capsazepine (10 μM; [96]) and a TRPM8 antagonist (4-(3-chloro- 2-pyridinyl)-*N*-[4-(1,1-dimethyl-ethyl)phenyl]-1-piperazinecarboxamide, BCTC, 3 μM; [97]; Figure 1E). BCTC at this concentration was effective in inhibiting sEPSC frequency increase produced by menthol in adult rat SG neurons [27]. As with thymol, the carvacrol activity was resistant to capsazepine (10 μM) while being depressed by HC-030031 (50 μM; Figure 1F). These results indicate an involvement of TRPA1 channel in the presynaptic activities of thymol and carvacrol. As distinct from these presynaptic actions, the outward currents produced by thymol and carvacrol were insensitive to capsazepine (10 μM), BCTC (3 μM) and HC-030031 (50 μM), indicating no involvement of TRP channels ([88,89]; for example see Figure 1E). The carvacrol current was inhibited in 10 mM-K^+ but not K^+-channel blockers (5 mM tetraethylammonium and 0.1 mM Ba^{2+})-containing and 11.0 mM-Cl^- Krebs solution, indicating an involvement of tetraethylammonium- and Ba^{2+}-insensitive K^+ channels [89]. It remains to be examined what types of ion channel are involved in the thymol current.

4.2. Actions of (−)-Carvone and (+)-Carvone

(−)-Carvone [(−)-2-methyl-5-(1-methylethenyl)-2-cyclohexenone; Figure 2A] contained in spearmint increased intracellular Ca^{2+} concentration in rat DRG neurons in a manner sensitive to capsazepine, indicating an involvement of TRPV1 channel [98]. A similar action of (−)-carvone was observed in HEK293 cells expressing human TRPV1 channel [98]. (+)-Carvone (a stereoisomer of (−)-carvone; Figure 2B) contained in caraway has been shown to have actions different from those of (−)-carvone in mouse locomotive [99] and anticonvulsive activities [100]. We examined the effects of (−)-carvone and (+)-carvone on glutamatergic spontaneous excitatory transmission with a focus on TRP activation. (−)-Carvone and (+)-carvone (each 1 mM) superfused for 2 min increased the frequency of sEPSC with a slight increase in its amplitude. Their sEPSC frequency increases averaged to be 299% and 284%, respectively, around 3 min (when a maximal effect was obtained) after the beginning of its superfusion. Such presynaptic activities of (−)-carvone and (+)-carvone were concentration-dependent with the EC_{50} values of 0.70 mM and 0.72 mM, respectively (Figure 2C,D).

(−)-Carvone and (+)-carvone (each 1 mM) did not produce any outward currents, as different from thymol and carvacrol. About 40% of the SG neurons tested produced a small inward current following the application of (−)-carvone or (+)-carvone [101], as seen by many kinds of TRPV1 agonists (capsaicin and RTX; [15,18]) and TRPA1 agonists (AITC, cinnamaldehyde and allicin; [19]).

The sEPSC frequency increase produced by (−)-carvone was resistant to HC-030031 (50 μM) while being inhibited by capsazepine (10 μM; Figure 2Ea,b). On the other hand, the sEPSC frequency increase produced by (+)-carvone was inhibited by HC-030031 (50 μM) while being resistant to capsazepine (10 μM; Figure 2Fa,b). These results indicate that (−)-carvone and (+)-carvone activate TRPV1 and TRPA1 channels, respectively, in the SG [101].

4.3. Actions of 1,8-Cineole and 1,4-Cineole

1,8-Cineole (1,3,3-trimethyl-2-oxabicylo[2.2.2]octane; Figure 3A), which is present in eucalyptus and rosemary, has various actions including antinociception [102]. As a minor component of plant extracts containing 1,8-cineole, there is its stereoisomer 1,4-cineole (1-methyl-4-(1-methylethyl)-

7-oxabicyclo[2.2.1]heptane; Figure 3B), which has on plant species an action which is different from that of 1,8-cineole [103].

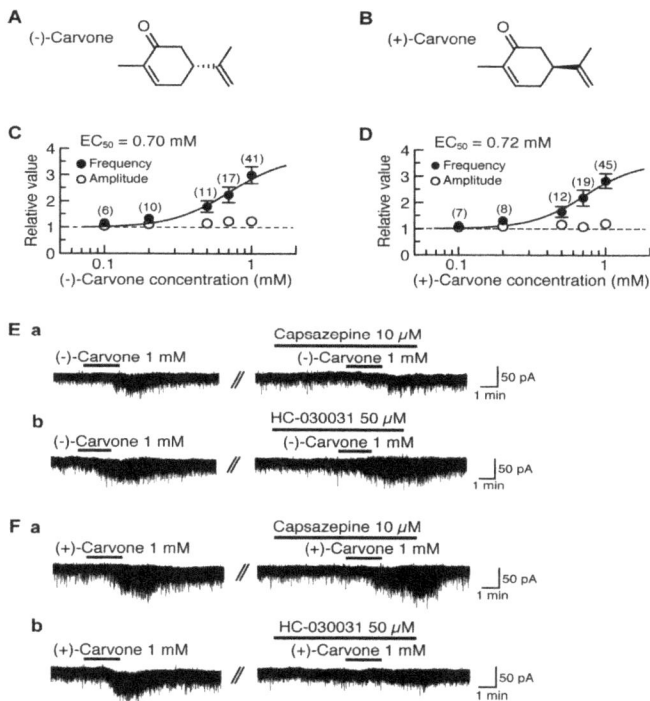

Figure 2. Effects of (−)-carvone and (+)-carvone on glutamatergic spontaneous excitatory transmission in rat SG neurons. (**A,B**) The chemical structures of (−)-carvone (**A**) and (+)-carvone (**B**). (**C,D**) The frequency and amplitude of sEPSC under the action of (−)-carvone (**C**) or (+)-carvone (**D**), relative to those before drug superfusion, which were plotted against the logarithm of drug concentration. This carvone effect was measured for 0.5 min around 3 min after the beginning of its superfusion. The continuous curves in (**C**) and (**D**) were drawn according to the Hill equation (EC_{50} and n_H in (**C**) and (**D**): 0.70 mM, 2.2 and 0.72 mM, 2.4, respectively). (**Ea,b,Fa,b**) Chart recordings showing sEPSCs in the absence and presence of (−)-carvone (**E**) or (+)-carvone (**F**) in Krebs solution without (left) and with capsazepine (**Ea,Fa**) or HC-030031 (**Eb,Fb**; right). In each of (**Ea,b,Fa,b**), the right recording was obtained about 20 min after the left one from the same neuron. $V_H = -70$ mV. This research was originally published in [101].

1,8-Cineole and 1,4-cineole have an ability to activate TRPM8 channel expressed heterologously in *Xenopus* oocytes [11] or HEK293 cells [104,105], although their efficacies are much less than that of the TRPM8 agonist menthol. We examined the effects of 1,8-cineole and 1,4-cineole on glutamatergic spontaneous excitatory transmission with a focus on TRP activation. As with (−)-carvone and (+)-carvone, bath-applied 1,8-cineole and 1,4-cineole for 3 min increased the frequency of sEPSC with a small increase in its amplitude. The sEPSC frequency increases produced by 1,8-cineole and 1,4-cineole (5 mM and 0.5 mM, respectively) averaged to be 159% and 226%, respectively, around 3.5 min (when a maximal effect was obtained) after the beginning of its superfusion. Such presynaptic actions of 1,8-cineole and 1,4-cineole were concentration-dependent with the EC_{50} values of 3.2 mM and 0.42 mM, respectively (Figure 3C,D).

The presynaptic activities of 1,8-cineole and 1,4-cineole were not accompanied by the production of outward current, as different from those of thymol and carvacrol. As with many kinds of TRPV1 and TRPA1 agonists [15,18,19] including (−)-carvone and (+)-carvone, 1,8-cineole and 1,4-cineole produced a small inward current (Figure 3E,F; [27]).

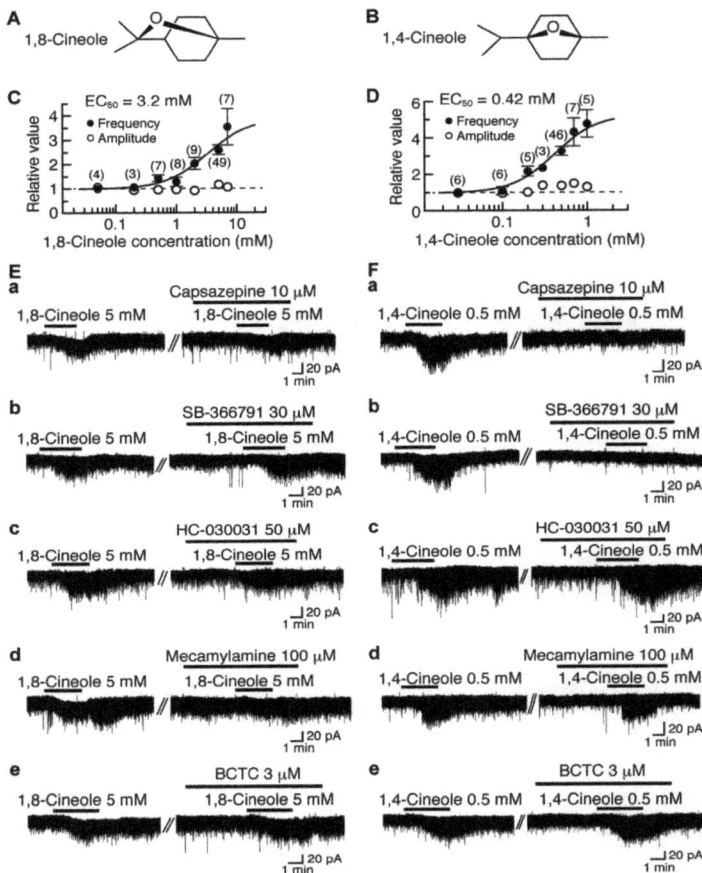

Figure 3. Effects of 1,8-cineole and 1,4-cineole on glutamatergic spontaneous excitatory transmission in rat SG neurons. (**A,B**) The chemical structures of 1,8-cineole (**A**) and 1,4-cineole (**B**). (**C,D**) The frequency and amplitude of sEPSC under the action of 1,8-cineole (**C**) or 1,4-cineole (**D**), relative to those before drug superfusion, which were plotted against the logarithm of drug concentration. This cineole effect was measured for 0.5 min around 3.5 min after the addition of its drug. The continuous curves in (**C**) and (**D**) were drawn according to the Hill equation (EC$_{50}$ and n$_H$ in (**C**) and (**D**): 3.2 mM, 1.3 and 0.42 mM, 1.7, respectively). (**Ea–e,Fa–e**) Chart recordings showing sEPSCs in the absence and presence of 1,8-cineole (**E**) or 1,4-cineole (**F**) in Krebs solution without (left) and with capsazepine (**a**), SB-366791 (**b**), HC-030031 (**c**), mecamylamine (**d**) or BCTC (**e**; right). In each of (**Ea–e,Fa–e**), the right recording was obtained about 20 min after the left one from the same neuron. V$_H$ = −70 mV. This research was originally published in [27].

The presynaptic action of 1,8-cineole was inhibited by HC-030031 (50 μM) and another TRPA1 antagonist mecamylamine (100 μM; which is known to be also a nicotinic acetylcholine-receptor antagonist [106]) while being resistant to capsazepine (10 μM) and another TRPV1 antagonist SB-366791 (30 μM; [67]; Figure 3Ea–d). On the contrary, 1,4-cineole's one was depressed by capsazepine (10 μM) and SB-366791 (30 μM) while being insensitive to HC-030031 (50 μM) and mecamylamine (100 μM; Figure 3Fa–d). BCTC (3 μM) did not affect the activities of 1,8-cineole and 1,4-cineole (Figure 3Ee,Fe). These results indicate that 1,8-cineole and 1,4-cineole activate TRPA1 and TRPV1 channels, respectively, in the SG.

5. Activation by Plant-Derived Stereoisomers of TRP Channels in the Substantia Gelatinosa in a Different Manner

Thymol and carvacrol, which are distinct only in the position of the -OH in the benzene ring (Figure 1A,B), activated the TRPA1 channel with EC_{50} values which differ four-fold from each other. Optic isomers, (−)-carvone and (+)-carvone (Figure 2A,B), activated TRPV1 and TRPA1 channels, respectively, with almost the same EC_{50} value. 1,8-Cineole and 1,4-cineole, which are different in the placement of the oxygen bridge (Figure 3A,B; where there is a free dimethyl side chain in 1,4-cineole but not 1,8-cineole [103]), activated TRPA1 and TRPV1 channels, respectively, with EC_{50} values eight-fold different from each other. The TRPV1 and TRPA1 activations resulted in an increase in spontaneous L-glutamate release from nerve terminals onto SG neurons. These results indicate that TRP channels in the SG have an ability to discriminate plant-derived stereoisomers from each other.

The stereoisomers mentioned in this review article are not endogenous ones that act on TRP channels located in the central terminals of DRG neurons under physiological conditions. There are several candidates for endogenous substances that activate TRP channels. For example, endogenous agonists for TRPV1 channel include endocannabinoids such as anandamide and lipoxygenase metabolites, which have structures similar to that of capsaicin which is not produced endogenously ([107,108]; for reviews see [7,109]). TRPV1 channel in the SG did not appear to be activated by anandamide [54] while anandamide-transport inhibitor AM404 activated the SG TRPV1 channel [110]. As candidates of endogenous TRPA1 activators, there is a potent and systemically active inhibitor of fatty acid amide hydrolase, 3'-carbamoylbiphenyl-3-yl cyclohexylcarbamate (URB597; [111]), a cyclopentane prostaglandin D_2 metabolite (15-deoxy-$\Delta^{12,14}$-prostaglandin J_2; [112]) or bradykinin [113]. To our knowledge, endogenous agonists for TRPM8 channel do not appear to be surely identified. Testosterone (a steroid hormone from the androgen group) has been recently reported to activate TRPM8 channel [114,115]. Although endogenous stereoisomers for TRP activation do not appear to be available, our findings about stereoisomers could serve to know the properties of the central terminal TRP channels.

Many of the properties of the TRP channels have been examined in the cell body of the primary-afferent neuron and in heterologous cell expressing the TRP channels. We have found out that a local anesthetic lidocaine, which acts on TRPV1 channel [116] and by a less extent on TRPA1 channel [117] in the cell body of primary-afferent neuron, activates TRPA1 but not TRPV1 channel in its central terminal [118]. The central terminal TRPV1 channel was activated by piperine (a pungent component of black pepper; [119]) but not olvanil (the synthetic oleic acid homologue of capsaicin; [120]), both of which compounds activated TRPV1 channel in the cell body of primary-afferent neuron [121,122]. Vanilloid compounds, eugenol (contained in clove) and zingerone (a pungent component of ginger), that reportedly activated TRPV1 channel in the cell body of primary-afferent neuron [121,123] were shown to activate the central terminal TRPA1 but not TRPV1 channel [124,125]. Based on their findings, we have proposed the idea that TRP channels located in the cell body and central terminal of the primary-afferent neuron have properties different from each other [23]. Such a difference may be due to a distinction between cell body and central terminal TRPA1 channels in terms of a functional interaction of TRPA1 channel and toll-like receptor-7 ([126]; see [125] for the other possibilities). It remains to be examined whether TRP channels in the cell body of DRG neuron are activated by plant-derived stereoisomers in a distinct manner.

TRPA1 channel in the central terminal of DRG neuron in the SG is activated by many plant-derived chemicals. Very recently, we have reported that citral, a mixture of geranial and neral, which is contained in lemongrass, activates TRPA1 channel in the SG [127]. Table 1 summarizes available values of EC_{50} for plant-derived chemicals in activating TRPV1 and TRPA1 channels in the adult rat SG. Their efficacy sequence for the TRPA1 activation was thymol (EC_{50} = 0.18 mM) > citral (0.58 mM) ⩾ carvacrol (0.69 mM) ⩾ (+)-carvone (0.72 mM) > zingerone (1.3 mM) > 1,8-cineole (3.2 mM) ⩾ eugenol (3.8 mM). This result could serve to know the property of central terminal TRPA1 channel that is a target of drugs for alleviating pain together with the above-mentioned results of stereoisomers.

Table 1. EC_{50} values for plant-derived chemicals in activating TRPV1 and TRPA1 channels in the adult rat SG.

Plant-Derived Chemicals	TRPV1 (mM)	TRPA1 (mM)	References
Resiniferatoxin	2.1×10^{-4}	–	[18]
Piperine	0.052	–	[120]
Eugenol	–	3.8	[124]
Zingerone	–	1.3	[125]
(−)-Carvone	0.70	–	[101]
(+)-Carvone	–	0.72	[101]
Carvacrol	–	0.69	[89]
Thymol	–	0.18	[88]
1,8-Cineole	–	3.2	[27]
1,4-Cineole	0.42	–	[27]
Cital	–	0.58	[127]

TRP activation in the SG is generally thought to be involved in nociception [1], because the enhancement of the spontaneous release of L-glutamate from nerve terminals onto SG neurons as a result of the TRP activation increases an excitability of the SG neurons, an action different from those of analgesic substances (see Section 2). However, antinociception produced by the intrathecal administration of acetaminophen has been attributed to TRPA1 activation in the superficial spinal dorsal horn [128]. AITC inhibited current responses recorded from SG neurons by using the in vivo patch-clamp technique [129] in response to pinch stimuli given to the skin [130]. It remains to be addressed whether TRPA1 activation in the SG results in nociception or antinociception.

Although the present review article mentions the actions of plant-derived stereoisomers on excitatory transmission, the regulation of nociceptive transmission in the SG is due to a modulation of not only excitatory but also GABAergic and/or glycinergic inhibitory transmissions [25,131,132]. It is possible that a modulation of inhibitory transmission by TRP activation is involved in nociceptive transmission. There is much evidence supporting the idea that inhibitory transmission enhancement in the spinal dorsal horn results in antinociception. First, the lack of GABA-synthesizing enzyme [133,134] and also reduction in the expression of K^+-Cl^- exporter KCC2, which causes inhibitory synaptic response to be excitatory [135], in the rat spinal dorsal horn leaded to nociception. Second, peripheral inflammation resulted in a reduced glycinergic transmission in rat spinal lamina I neurons [136]. Third, an increase in endogenous glycine due to glycine transporter-1 blockade produced an inhibitory effect on spinal nociceptive transmission ([137]; for reviews see [138,139]). Fourth, endogenous analgesics, acetylcholine, norepinephrine and serotonin, enhanced GABAergic and glycinergic inhibitory transmissions [140–145]. It appears to depend on the agonists used to activate TRP channels how TRP activation affects spontaneous inhibitory transmission in SG neurons. AITC and zingerone enhanced inhibitory transmission [19,125] while capsaicin and cinnamaldehyde did not [15,20]. It remains to be examined how plant-derived stereoisomers affect spontaneous inhibitory transmission.

Itch is partly similar to pain in the neuronal pathway and receptors involved, although they are distinct from each other in many points of neuronal transmissions. There is much evidence supporting the idea that TRPV1 and TRPA1 channels are involved in itch. For instance, a topical application of capsaicin to the skin produced itch [146,147]. It is thus likely that TRP channels located in the central terminal of a pruriceptive primary-afferent neuron are involved in the modulation of itch sensation. Although proteinase-activated receptor (PAR)-2 in the peripheral terminal of a primary-afferent neuron is involved in the production of itch [148,149], other types of PAR may play a role in modulating pruriceptive transmission in the spinal dorsal horn. Fujita et al. [150] have reported that PAR-1 activation presynaptically increases spontaneous excitatory transmission in adult rat SG neurons. The findings about plant-derived stereoisomers, mentioned in this review article, may serve to know how to modulate itch transmission in the spinal dorsal horn.

There are known to be species differences on the pharmacology of TRP channels. For example, Jordt and Julius [151] have found out that chicken TRPV1 channel has a much less sensitivity to capsaicin than rat one. Rat and human TRPV1 channels were about 100-fold more sensitive to capsaicin than rabbit one [152]. 4-Methyl-*N*-[2,2,2-trichloro-1-(4-nitro-phenylsulfanyl)-ethyl]-benzamide activated rat TRPA1 channel while blocking human TRPA1 activation by reactive and nonreactive agonists [153]. Caffeine inhibited human TRPA1 channel but activated mouse TRPA1 channel [154]. A967079 blocked mammalian TRPA1 channel [155], but failed to inhibit chicken TRPA1 channel [156]. It remains to be investigated whether a difference in TRP activation among plant-derived stereoisomers is seen in animal species other than rats.

6. Conclusions

Plant-derived chemical stereoisomers, i.e., thymol and carvacrol, (−)-carvone and (+)-carvone, or 1,8-cineole and 1,4-cineole, activated TRP channels in the SG in a manner different from each other in the extent and the types of TRP channels activated. TRP channels expressed in the central terminals of DRG neurons are thus suggested to have an ability to discriminate stereoisomers.

Acknowledgments: This study was partly supported by JSPS KAKENHI Grant Number 15K08673.

Conflicts of Interest: The authors declare no conflict of interest.

References

1. Patapoutian, A.; Tate, S.; Woolf, C.J. Transient receptor potential channels: Targeting pain at the source. *Nat. Rev. Drug Discov.* **2009**, *8*, 55–68. [CrossRef] [PubMed]
2. Story, G.M.; Peier, A.M.; Reeve, A.J.; Eid, S.R.; Mosbacher, J.; Hricik, T.R.; Earley, T.J.; Hergarden, A.C.; Andersson, D.A.; Hwang, S.W.; et al. ANKTM1, a TRP-like channel expressed in nociceptive neurons, is activated by cold temperatures. *Cell* **2003**, *112*, 819–829. [CrossRef]
3. Kobayashi, K.; Fukuoka, T.; Obata, K.; Yamanaka, H.; Dai, Y.; Tokunaga, A.; Noguchi, K. Distinct expression of TRPM8, TRPA1, and TRPV1 mRNAs in rat primary afferent neurons with Aδ/C-fibers and colocalization with Trk receptors. *J. Comp. Neurol.* **2005**, *493*, 596–606. [CrossRef] [PubMed]
4. Tominaga, M. TRP channels and nociception. In *Cellular and Molecular Mechanisms for the Modulation of Nociceptive Transmission in the Peripheral and Central Nervous Systems*; Kumamoto, E., Ed.; Research Signpost: Kelara, India, 2007; pp. 23–40.
5. Julius, D. TRP channels and pain. *Annu. Rev. Cell Dev. Biol.* **2013**, *29*, 355–384. [CrossRef] [PubMed]
6. Caterina, M.J.; Schumacher, M.A.; Tominaga, M.; Rosen, T.A.; Levine, J.D.; Julius, D. The capsaicin receptor: a heat-activated ion channel in the pain pathway. *Nature* **1997**, *389*, 816–824. [PubMed]
7. Caterina, M.J.; Julius, D. The vanilloid receptor: a molecular gateway to the pain pathway. *Annu. Rev. Neurosci.* **2001**, *24*, 487–517. [CrossRef] [PubMed]
8. Bandell, M.; Story, G.M.; Hwang, S.W.; Viswanath, V.; Eid, S.R.; Petrus, M.J.; Earley, T.J.; Patapoutian, A. Noxious cold ion channel TRPA1 is activated by pungent compounds and bradykinin. *Neuron* **2004**, *41*, 849–857. [CrossRef]
9. Jordt, S.E.; Bautista, D.M.; Chuang, H.H.; McKemy, D.D.; Zygmunt, P.M.; Högestätt, E.D.; Meng, I.D.; Julius, D. Mustard oils and cannabinoids excite sensory nerve fibres through the TRP channel ANKTM1. *Nature* **2004**, *427*, 260–265. [CrossRef] [PubMed]

10. Nilius, B.; Voets, T. TRP channels: a TR(I)P through a world of multifunctional cation channels. *Pflügers Arch.* **2005**, *451*, 1–10. [CrossRef] [PubMed]

11. McKemy, D.D.; Neuhausser, W.M.; Julius, D. Identification of a cold receptor reveals a general role for TRP channels in thermosensation. *Nature* **2002**, *416*, 52–58. [CrossRef] [PubMed]

12. Peier, A.M.; Moqrich, A.; Hergarden, A.C.; Reeve, A.J.; Andersson, D.A.; Story, G.M.; Earley, T.J.; Dragoni, I.; McIntyre, P.; Bevan, S.; et al. A TRP channel that senses cold stimuli and menthol. *Cell* **2002**, *108*, 705–715. [CrossRef]

13. Kumazawa, T.; Perl, E.R. Excitation of marginal and substantia gelatinosa neurons in the primate spinal cord: indications of their place in dorsal horn functional organization. *J. Comp. Neurol.* **1978**, *177*, 417–434. [CrossRef] [PubMed]

14. Sugiura, Y.; Lee, C.L.; Perl, E.R. Central projections of identified, unmyelinated (C) afferent fibers innervating mammalian skin. *Science* **1986**, *234*, 358–361. [CrossRef] [PubMed]

15. Yang, K; Kumamoto, E.; Furue, H.; Yoshimura, M. Capsaicin facilitates excitatory but not inhibitory synaptic transmission in substantia gelatinosa of the rat spinal cord. *Neurosci. Lett.* **1998**, *255*, 135–138. [CrossRef]

16. Morisset, V.; Urbán, L. Cannabinoid-induced presynaptic inhibition of glutamatergic EPSCs in substantia gelatinosa neurons of the rat spinal cord. *J. Neurophysiol.* **2001**, *86*, 40–48. [PubMed]

17. Baccei, M.L.; Bardoni, R.; Fitzgerald, M. Development of nociceptive synaptic inputs to the neonatal rat dorsal horn: glutamate release by capsaicin and menthol. *J. Physiol.* **2003**, *549*, 231–242. [CrossRef] [PubMed]

18. Jiang, C.-Y.; Fujita, T.; Yue, H.-Y.; Piao, L.-H.; Liu, T.; Nakatsuka, T.; Kumamoto, E. Effect of resiniferatoxin on glutamatergic spontaneous excitatory synaptic transmission in substantia gelatinosa neurons of the adult rat spinal cord. *Neuroscience* **2009**, *164*, 1833–1844. [CrossRef] [PubMed]

19. Kosugi, M.; Nakatsuka, T.; Fujita, T.; Kuroda, Y.; Kumamoto, E. Activation of TRPA1 channel facilitates excitatory synaptic transmission in substantia gelatinosa neurons of the adult rat spinal cord. *J. Neurosci.* **2007**, *27*, 4443–4451. [CrossRef] [PubMed]

20. Uta, D.; Furue, H.; Pickering, A.E.; Rashid, M.H.; Mizuguchi-Takase, H.; Katafuchi, T.; Imoto, K.; Yoshimura, M. TRPA1-expressing primary afferents synapse with a morphologically identified subclass of substantia gelatinosa neurons in the adult rat spinal cord. *Eur. J. Neurosci.* **2010**, *31*, 1960–1973. [CrossRef] [PubMed]

21. Suzuki, S.C.; Furue, H.; Koga, K.; Jiang, N.; Nohmi, M.; Shimazaki, Y.; Katoh-Fukui, Y.; Yokoyama, M.; Yoshimura, M.; Takeichi, M. Cadherin-8 is required for the first relay synapses to receive functional inputs from primary sensory afferents for cold sensation. *J. Neurosci.* **2007**, *27*, 3466–3476. [CrossRef] [PubMed]

22. Wrigley, P.J.; Jeong, H.-J.; Vaughan, C.W. Primary afferents with TRPM8 and TRPA1 profiles target distinct subpopulations of rat superficial dorsal horn neurones. *Br. J. Pharmacol.* **2009**, *157*, 371–380. [CrossRef] [PubMed]

23. Kumamoto, E.; Fujita, T.; Jiang, C.-Y. TRP channels involved in spontaneous L-glutamate release enhancement in the adult rat spinal substantia gelatinosa. *Cells* **2014**, *3*, 331–362. [CrossRef] [PubMed]

24. Melzack, R.; Wall, P.D. Pain mechanisms: a new theory. *Science* **1965**, *150*, 971–979. [CrossRef] [PubMed]

25. Willis, W.D., Jr.; Coggeshall, R.E. *Sensory Mechanisms of the Spinal Cord*, 2nd ed.; Plenum: New York, NY, USA, 1991.

26. Todd, A.J. Neuronal circuitry for pain processing in the dorsal horn. *Nat. Rev. Neurosci.* **2010**, *11*, 823–836. [CrossRef] [PubMed]

27. Jiang, C.-Y.; Wang, C.; Xu, N.-X.; Fujita, T.; Murata, Y.; Kumamoto, E. 1,8- and 1,4-cineole enhance spontaneous excitatory transmission by activating different types of transient receptor potential channels in the rat spinal substantia gelatinosa. *J. Neurochem.* **2016**, *136*, 764–777. [CrossRef] [PubMed]

28. Yoshimura, M.; Nishi, S. Blind patch-clamp recordings from substantia gelatinosa neurons in adult rat spinal cord slices: pharmacological properties of synaptic currents. *Neuroscience* **1993**, *53*, 519–526. [CrossRef]

29. Nakatsuka, T.; Park, J.-S.; Kumamoto, E.; Tamaki, T.; Yoshimura, M. Plastic changes in sensory inputs to rat substantia gelatinosa neurons following peripheral inflammation. *Pain* **1999**, *82*, 39–47. [CrossRef]

30. Ito, A.; Kumamoto, E.; Takeda, M.; Takeda, M.; Shibata, K.; Sagai, H.; Yoshimura, M. Mechanisms for ovariectomy-induced hyperalgesia and its relief by calcitonin: participation of 5-HT_{1A}-like receptor on C-afferent terminals in substantia gelatinosa of the rat spinal cord. *J. Neurosci.* **2000**, *20*, 6302–6308. [PubMed]

31. Fürst, S. Transmitters involved in antinociception in the spinal cord. *Brain Res. Bull.* **1999**, *48*, 129–141. [CrossRef]

32. Yoshimura, M.; North, R.A. Substantia gelatinosa neurones hyperpolarized *in vitro* by enkephalin. *Nature* **1983**, *305*, 529–530. [CrossRef] [PubMed]

33. Fujita, T.; Nakatsuka, T.; Kumamoto, E. Opioid receptor activation in spinal dorsal horn. In *Cellular and Molecular Mechanisms for the Modulation of Nociceptive Transmission in the Peripheral and Central Nervous Systems*; Kumamoto, E., Ed.; Research Signpost: Kelara, India, 2007; pp. 87–111.

34. Lai, C.C.; Wu, S.Y.; Dun, S.L.; Dun, N.J. Nociceptin-like immunoreactivity in the rat dorsal horn and inhibition of substantia gelatinosa neurons. *Neuroscience* **1997**, *81*, 887–891. [CrossRef]

35. Luo, C.; Kumamoto, E.; Furue, H.; Yoshimura, M. Nociceptin-induced outward current in substantia gelatinosa neurones of the adult rat spinal cord. *Neuroscience* **2001**, *108*, 323–330. [CrossRef]

36. Kangrga, I.; Jiang, M.; Randić, M. Actions of (−)-baclofen on rat dorsal horn neurons. *Brain Res.* **1991**, *562*, 265–275. [CrossRef]

37. Yang, K.; Kumamoto, E.; Furue, H.; Li, Y.-Q.; Yoshimura, M. Capsaicin induces a slow inward current which is not mediated by substance P in substantia gelatinosa neurons of the rat spinal cord. *Neuropharmacology* **2000**, *39*, 2185–2194. [CrossRef]

38. Koga, A.; Fujita, T.; Totoki, T.; Kumamoto, E. Tramadol produces outward currents by activating μ-opioid receptors in adult rat substantia gelatinosa neurones. *Br. J. Pharmacol.* **2005**, *145*, 602–607. [CrossRef] [PubMed]

39. Sonohata, M.; Furue, H.; Katafuchi, T.; Yasaka, T.; Doi, A.; Kumamoto, E.; Yoshimura, M. Actions of noradrenaline on substantia gelatinosa neurones in the rat spinal cord revealed by *in vivo* patch recording. *J. Physiol.* **2004**, *555*, 515–526. [CrossRef] [PubMed]

40. Abe, K.; Kato, G.; Katafuchi, T.; Tamae, A.; Furue, H.; Yoshimura, M. Responses to 5-HT in morphologically identified neurons in the rat substantia gelatinosa *in vitro*. *Neuroscience* **2009**, *159*, 316–324. [CrossRef] [PubMed]

41. Li, J.; Perl, E.R. Adenosine inhibition of synaptic transmission in the substantia gelatinosa. *J. Neurophysiol.* **1994**, *72*, 1611–1621. [PubMed]

42. Liu, T.; Fujita, T.; Kawasaki, Y.; Kumamoto, E. Regulation by equilibrative nucleoside transporter of adenosine outward currents in adult rat spinal dorsal horn neurons. *Brain Res. Bull.* **2004**, *64*, 75–83. [CrossRef] [PubMed]

43. Kumamoto, E.; Fujita, T. Role of adenosine in regulating nociceptive transmission in the spinal dorsal horn. In *Recent Research Developments in Physiology*; Pandalai, S.G., Ed.; Research Signpost: Kerala, India, 2005; Volume 3, pp. 39–57.

44. Jiang, N.; Furue, H.; Katafuchi, T.; Yoshimura, M. Somatostatin directly inhibits substantia gelatinosa neurons in adult rat spinal dorsal horn in vitro. *Neurosci. Res.* **2003**, *47*, 97–107. [CrossRef]

45. Nakatsuka, T.; Fujita, T.; Inoue, K.; Kumamoto, E. Activation of GIRK channels in substantia gelatinosa neurones of the adult rat spinal cord: a possible involvement of somatostatin. *J. Physiol.* **2008**, *586*, 2511–2522. [CrossRef] [PubMed]

46. Tamae, A.; Nakatsuka, T.; Koga, K.; Kato, G.; Furue, H.; Katafuchi, T.; Yoshimura, M. Direct inhibition of substantia gelatinosa neurones in the rat spinal cord by activation of dopamine D2-like receptors. *J. Physiol.* **2005**, *568*, 243–253. [CrossRef] [PubMed]

47. Taniguchi, W.; Nakatsuka, T.; Miyazaki, N.; Yamada, H.; Takeda, D.; Fujita, T.; Kumamoto, E.; Yoshida, M. *In vivo* patch-clamp analysis of dopaminergic antinociceptive actions on substantia gelatinosa neurons in the spinal cord. *Pain* **2011**, *152*, 95–105. [CrossRef] [PubMed]

48. Yue, H.-Y.; Fujita, T.; Kumamoto, E. Biphasic modulation by galanin of excitatory synaptic transmission in substantia gelatinosa neurons of adult rat spinal cord slices. *J. Neurophysiol.* **2011**, *105*, 2337–2349. [CrossRef] [PubMed]

49. Kohno, T.; Kumamoto, E.; Higashi, H.; Shimoji, K.; Yoshimura, M. Actions of opioids on excitatory and inhibitory transmission in substantia gelatinosa of adult rat spinal cord. *J. Physiol.* **1999**, *518*, 803–813. [CrossRef] [PubMed]

50. Liebel, J.T.; Swandulla, D.; Zeilhofer, H.U. Modulation of excitatory synaptic transmission by nociceptin in superficial dorsal horn neurones of the neonatal rat spinal cord. *Br. J. Pharmacol.* **1997**, *121*, 425–432. [CrossRef] [PubMed]

51. Luo, C.; Kumamoto, E.; Furue, H.; Chen, J.; Yoshimura, M. Nociceptin inhibits excitatory but not inhibitory transmission to substantia gelatinosa neurones of adult rat spinal cord. *Neuroscience* **2002**, *109*, 349–358. [CrossRef]

52. Ataka, T.; Kumamoto, E.; Shimoji, K.; Yoshimura, M. Baclofen inhibits more effectively C-afferent than Aδ-afferent glutamatergic transmission in substantia gelatinosa neurons of adult rat spinal cord slices. *Pain* **2000**, *86*, 273–282. [CrossRef]

53. Iyadomi, M.; Iyadomi, I.; Kumamoto, E.; Tomokuni, K.; Yoshimura, M. Presynaptic inhibition by baclofen of miniature EPSCs and IPSCs in substantia gelatinosa neurons of the adult rat spinal dorsal horn. *Pain* **2000**, *85*, 385–393. [CrossRef]

54. Luo, C.; Kumamoto, E.; Furue, H.; Chen, J.; Yoshimura, M. Anandamide inhibits excitatory transmission to rat substantia gelatinosa neurones in a manner different from that of capsaicin. *Neurosci. Lett.* **2002**, *321*, 17–20. [CrossRef]

55. Kawasaki, Y.; Kumamoto, E.; Furue, H.; Yoshimura, M. α_2 Adrenoceptor-mediated presynaptic inhibition of primary afferent glutamatergic transmission in rat substantia gelatinosa neurons. *Anesthesiology* **2003**, *98*, 682–689. [CrossRef] [PubMed]

56. Lao, L.-J.; Kumamoto, E.; Luo, C.; Furue, H.; Yoshimura, M. Adenosine inhibits excitatory transmission to substantia gelatinosa neurons of the adult rat spinal cord through the activation of presynaptic A_1 adenosine receptor. *Pain* **2001**, *94*, 315–324. [CrossRef]

57. Lao, L.-J.; Kawasaki, Y.; Yang, K.; Fujita, T.; Kumamoto, E. Modulation by adenosine of Aδ and C primary-afferent glutamatergic transmission in adult rat substantia gelatinosa neurons. *Neuroscience* **2004**, *125*, 221–231. [CrossRef] [PubMed]

58. Alier, K.A.; Chen, Y.; Sollenberg, U.E.; Langel, Ü.; Smith, P.A. Selective stimulation of GalR1 and GalR2 in rat *substantia gelatinosa* reveals a cellular basis for the anti- and pro-nociceptive actions of galanin. *Pain* **2008**, *137*, 138–146. [CrossRef] [PubMed]

59. Hudson, L.J.; Bevan, S.; Wotherspoon, G.; Gentry, C.; Fox, A.; Winter, J. VR1 protein expression increases in undamaged DRG neurons after partial nerve injury. *Eur. J. Neurosci.* **2001**, *13*, 2105–2114. [CrossRef] [PubMed]

60. Walker, K.M.; Urbán, L.; Medhurst, S.J.; Patel, S.; Panesar, M.; Fox, A.J.; McIntyre, P. The VR1 antagonist capsazepine reverses mechanical hyperalgesia in models of inflammatory and neuropathic pain. *J. Pharmacol. Exp. Ther.* **2003**, *304*, 56–62. [CrossRef] [PubMed]

61. Gavva, N.R.; Tamir, R.; Qu, Y.; Klionsky, L.; Zhang, T.J.; Immke, D.; Wang, J.; Zhu, D.; Vanderah, T.W.; Porreca, F.; et al. AMG 9810 [(E)-3-(4-t-butylphenyl)-N-(2,3-dihydrobenzo[b][1,4] dioxin-6-yl)acrylamide], a novel vanilloid receptor 1 (TRPV1) antagonist with antihyperalgesic properties. *J. Pharmacol. Exp. Ther.* **2005**, *313*, 474–484. [CrossRef] [PubMed]

62. Culshaw, A.J.; Bevan, S.; Christiansen, M.; Copp, P.; Davis, A.; Davis, C.; Dyson, A.; Dziadulewicz, E.K.; Edwards, L.; Eggelte, H.; et al. Identification and biological characterization of 6-aryl-7-isopropylquinazolinones as novel TRPV1 antagonists that are effective in models of chronic pain. *J. Med. Chem.* **2006**, *49*, 471–474. [CrossRef] [PubMed]

63. Davis, J.B.; Gray, J.; Gunthorpe, M.J.; Hatcher, J.P.; Davey, P.T.; Overend, P.; Harries, M.H.; Latcham, J.; Clapham, C.; Atkinson, K.; et al. Vanilloid receptor-1 is essential for inflammatory thermal hyperalgesia. *Nature* **2000**, *405*, 183–187. [CrossRef] [PubMed]

64. Bron, R.; Klesse, L.J.; Shah, K.; Parada, L.F.; Winter, J. Activation of Ras is necessary and sufficient for upregulation of vanilloid receptor type 1 in sensory neurons by neurotrophic factors. *Mol. Cell. Neurosci.* **2003**, *22*, 118–132. [CrossRef]

65. Yiangou, Y.; Facer, P.; Dyer, N.H.C.; Chan, C.L.H.; Knowles, C.; Williams, N.S.; Anand, P. Vanilloid receptor 1 immunoreactivity in inflamed human bowel. *Lancet* **2001**, *357*, 1338–1339. [CrossRef]

66. Chan, C.L.H.; Facer, P.; Davis, J.B.; Smith, G.D.; Egerton, J.; Bountra, C.; Williams, N.S.; Anand, P. Sensory fibres expressing capsaicin receptor TRPV1 in patients with rectal hypersensitivity and faecal urgency. *Lancet* **2003**, *361*, 385–391. [CrossRef]

67. Lappin, S.C.; Randall, A.D.; Gunthorpe, M.J.; Morisset, V. TRPV1 antagonist, SB-366791, inhibits glutamatergic synaptic transmission in rat spinal dorsal horn following peripheral inflammation. *Eur. J. Pharmacol.* **2006**, *540*, 73–81. [CrossRef] [PubMed]

68. Szallasi, A.; Blumberg, P.M. Resiniferatoxin, a phorbol-related diterpene, acts as an ultrapotent analog of capsaicin, the irritant constituent in red pepper. *Neuroscience* **1989**, *30*, 515–520. [CrossRef]
69. Brown, D.C.; Iadarola, M.J.; Perkowski, S.Z.; Erin, H.; Shofer, F.; Laszlo, K.J.; Olah, Z.; Mannes, A.J. Physiologic and antinociceptive effects of intrathecal resiniferatoxin in a canine bone cancer model. *Anesthesiology* **2005**, *103*, 1052–1059. [CrossRef] [PubMed]
70. Ghilardi, J.R.; Röhrich, H.; Lindsay, T.H.; Sevcik, M.A.; Schwei, M.J.; Kubota, K.; Halvorson, K.G.; Poblete, J.; Chaplan, S.R.; Dubin, A.E.; et al. Selective blockade of the capsaicin receptor TRPV1 attenuates bone cancer pain. *J. Neurosci.* **2005**, *25*, 3126–3131. [CrossRef] [PubMed]
71. Prevarskaya, N.; Zhang, L.; Barritt, G. TRP channels in cancer. *Biochim. Biophys. Acta* **2007**, *1772*, 937–946. [CrossRef] [PubMed]
72. Watabiki, T.; Kiso, T.; Tsukamoto, M.; Aoki, T.; Matsuoka, N. Intrathecal administration of AS1928370, a transient receptor potential vanilloid 1 antagonist, attenuates mechanical allodynia in a mouse model of neuropathic pain. *Biol. Pharm. Bull.* **2011**, *34*, 1105–1108. [CrossRef] [PubMed]
73. Namer, B.; Seifert, F.; Handwerker, H.O.; Maihöfner, C. TRPA1 and TRPM8 activation in humans: effects of cinnamaldehyde and menthol. *NeuroReport* **2005**, *16*, 955–959. [CrossRef] [PubMed]
74. Obata, K.; Katsura, H.; Mizushima, T.; Yamanaka, H.; Kobayashi, K.; Dai, Y.; Fukuoka, T.; Tokunaga, A.; Tominaga, M.; Noguchi, K. TRPA1 induced in sensory neurons contributes to cold hyperalgesia after inflammation and nerve injury. *J. Clin. Investig.* **2005**, *115*, 2393–2401. [CrossRef] [PubMed]
75. da Costa, D.S.M.; Meotti, F.C.; Andrade, E.L.; Leal, P.C.; Motta, E.M.; Calixto, J.B. The involvement of the transient receptor potential A1 (TRPA1) in the maintenance of mechanical and cold hyperalgesia in persistent inflammation. *Pain* **2010**, *148*, 431–437. [CrossRef] [PubMed]
76. Proudfoot, C.J.; Garry, E.M.; Cottrell, D.F.; Rosie, R.; Anderson, H.; Robertson, D.C.; Fleetwood-Walker, S.M.; Mitchell, R. Analgesia mediated by the TRPM8 cold receptor in chronic neuropathic pain. *Curr. Biol.* **2006**, *16*, 1591–1605. [CrossRef] [PubMed]
77. Xing, H.; Chen, M.; Ling, J.; Tan, W.; Gu, J.G. TRPM8 mechanism of cold allodynia after chronic nerve injury. *J. Neurosci.* **2007**, *27*, 13680–13690. [CrossRef] [PubMed]
78. Kono, T.; Satomi, M.; Suno, M.; Kimura, N.; Yamazaki, H.; Furukawa, H.; Matsubara, K. Oxaliplatin-induced neurotoxicity involves TRPM8 in the mechanism of acute hypersensitivity to cold sensation. *Brain Behav.* **2012**, *2*, 68–73. [CrossRef] [PubMed]
79. Liu, B.; Fan, L.; Balakrishna, S.; Sui, A.; Morris, J.B.; Jordt, S.-E. TRPM8 is the principal mediator of menthol-induced analgesia of acute and inflammatory pain. *Pain* **2013**, *154*, 2169–2177. [CrossRef] [PubMed]
80. Edwards, J.G. TRPV1 in the central nervous system: synaptic plasticity, function, and pharmacological implications. *Prog. Drug Res.* **2014**, *68*, 77–104. [PubMed]
81. Zygmunt, P.M.; Högestätt, E.D. TRPA1. *Handb. Exp. Pharmacol.* **2014**, *222*, 583–630. [PubMed]
82. Soudijn, W.; van Wijngaarden, I.; IJzerman, A.P. Stereoselectivity of drug-receptor interactions. *IDrugs* **2003**, *6*, 43–56.
83. Valenzuela, C.; Moreno, C.; de la Cruz, A.; Macías, Á.; Prieto, Á.; González, T. Stereoselective interactions between local anesthetics and ion channels. *Chirality* **2012**, *24*, 944–950. [CrossRef] [PubMed]
84. Karashima, Y.; Damann, N.; Prenen, J.; Talavera, K.; Segal, A.; Voets, T.; Nilius, B. Bimodal action of menthol on the transient receptor potential channel TRPA1. *J. Neurosci.* **2007**, *27*, 9874–9884. [CrossRef] [PubMed]
85. Yang, K.; Li, Y.-Q.; Kumamoto, E.; Furue, H.; Yoshimura, M. Voltage-clamp recordings of postsynaptic currents in substantia gelatinosa neurons in vitro and its applications to assess synaptic transmission. *Brain Res. Protoc.* **2001**, *7*, 235–240. [CrossRef]
86. Baser, K.H.C. Biological and pharmacological activities of carvacrol and carvacrol bearing essential oils. *Curr. Pharm. Des.* **2008**, *14*, 3106–3119. [CrossRef] [PubMed]
87. Angeles-López, G.; Pérez-Vásquez, A.; Hernández-Luis, F.; Déciga-Campos, M.; Bye, R.; Linares, E.; Mata, R. Antinociceptive effect of extracts and compounds from *Hofmeisteria schaffneri*. *J. Ethnopharmacol.* **2010**, *131*, 425–432. [CrossRef] [PubMed]
88. Xu, Z.-H.; Wang, C.; Fujita, T.; Jiang, C.-Y.; Kumamoto, E. Action of thymol on spontaneous excitatory transmission in adult rat spinal substantia gelatinosa neurons. *Neurosci. Lett.* **2015**, *606*, 94–99. [CrossRef] [PubMed]

89. Luo, Q.-T.; Fujita, T.; Jiang, C.-Y.; Kumamoto, E. Carvacrol presynaptically enhances spontaneous excitatory transmission and produces outward current in adult rat spinal substantia gelatinosa neurons. *Brain Res.* **2014**, *1592*, 44–54. [CrossRef] [PubMed]

90. Xu, H.; Delling, M.; Jun, J.C.; Clapham, D.E. Oregano, thyme and clove-derived flavors and skin sensitizers activate specific TRP channels. *Nat. Neurosci.* **2006**, *9*, 628–635. [CrossRef] [PubMed]

91. Lee, S.P.; Buber, M.T.; Yang, Q.; Cerne, R.; Cortés, R.Y.; Sprous, D.G.; Bryant, R.W. Thymol and related alkyl phenols activate the hTRPA1 channel. *Br. J. Pharmacol.* **2008**, *153*, 1739–1749. [CrossRef] [PubMed]

92. Ortar, G.; Morera, L.; Moriello, A.S.; Morera, E.; Nalli, M.; Di Marzo, V.; De Petrocellis, L. Modulation of thermo-transient receptor potential (thermo-TRP) channels by thymol-based compounds. *Bioorg. Med. Chem. Lett.* **2012**, *22*, 3535–3539. [CrossRef] [PubMed]

93. Vogt-Eisele, A.K.; Weber, K.; Sherkheli, M.A.; Vielhaber, G.; Panten, J.; Gisselmann, G.; Hatt, H. Monoterpenoid agonists of TRPV3. *Br. J. Pharmacol.* **2007**, *151*, 530–540. [CrossRef] [PubMed]

94. de la Roche, J.; Eberhardt, M.J.; Klinger, A.B.; Stanslowsky, N.; Wegner, F.; Koppert, W.; Reeh, P.W.; Lampert, A.; Fischer, M.J.M.; Leffler, A. The molecular basis for species-specific activation of human TRPA1 protein by protons involves poorly conserved residues within transmembrane domains 5 and 6. *J. Biol. Chem.* **2013**, *288*, 20280–20292. [CrossRef] [PubMed]

95. McNamara, C.R.; Mandel-Brehm, J.; Bautista, D.M.; Siemens, J.; Deranian, K.L.; Zhao, M.; Hayward, N.J.; Chong, J.A.; Julius, D.; Moran, M.M.; et al. TRPA1 mediates formalin-induced pain. *Proc. Natl. Acad. Sci. USA* **2007**, *104*, 13525–13530. [CrossRef] [PubMed]

96. Urban, L.; Dray, A. Capsazepine, a novel capsaicin antagonist, selectively antagonises the effects of capsaicin in the mouse spinal cord in vitro. *Neurosci. Lett.* **1991**, *134*, 9–11. [CrossRef]

97. Madrid, R.; Donovan-Rodríguez, T.; Meseguer, V.; Acosta, M.C.; Belmonte, C.; Viana, F. Contribution of TRPM8 channels to cold transduction in primary sensory neurons and peripheral nerve terminals. *J. Neurosci.* **2006**, *26*, 12512–12525. [CrossRef] [PubMed]

98. Gonçalves, J.C.R.; Silveira, A.L.; de Souza, H.D.N.; Nery, A.A.; Prado, V.F.; Prado, M.A.M.; Ulrich, H.; Araújo, D.A.M. The monoterpene (−)-carvone: a novel agonist of TRPV1 channels. *Cytometry Part A* **2013**, *83*, 212–219. [CrossRef] [PubMed]

99. Buchbauer, G.; Jäger, W.; Gruber, A.; Dietrich, H. R-(+)- and S-(−)-carvone: influence of chirality on locomotion activity in mice. *Flavour Fragr. J.* **2005**, *20*, 686–689. [CrossRef]

100. de Sousa, D.P.; de Farias Nóbrega, F.F.; de Almeida, R.N. Influence of the chirality of (R)-(−)- and (S)-(+)-carvone in the central nervous system: a comparative study. *Chirality* **2007**, *19*, 264–268. [CrossRef] [PubMed]

101. Kang, Q.; Jiang, C.-Y.; Fujita, T.; Kumamoto, E. Spontaneous L-glutamate release enhancement in rat substantia gelatinosa neurons by (−)-carvone and (+)-carvone which activate different types of TRP channel. *Biochem. Biophys. Res. Commun.* **2015**, *459*, 498–503. [CrossRef] [PubMed]

102. Liapi, C.; Anifantis, G.; Chinou, I.; Kourounakis, A.P.; Theodosopoulos, S.; Galanopoulou, P. Antinociceptive properties of 1,8-cineole and β-pinene, from the essential oil of *Eucalyptus camaldulensis* leaves, in rodents. *Planta Med.* **2007**, *73*, 1247–1254. [CrossRef] [PubMed]

103. Romagni, J.G.; Allen, S.N.; Dayan, F.E. Allelopathic effects of volatile cineoles on two weedy plant species. *J. Chem. Ecol.* **2000**, *26*, 303–313. [CrossRef]

104. Behrendt, H.-J.; Germann, T.; Gillen, C.; Hatt, H.; Jostock, R. Characterization of the mouse cold-menthol receptor TRPM8 and vanilloid receptor type-1 VR1 using a fluorometric imaging plate reader (FLIPR) assay. *Br. J. Pharmacol.* **2004**, *141*, 737–745. [CrossRef] [PubMed]

105. Takaishi, M.; Fujita, F.; Uchida, K.; Yamamoto, S.; Sawada Shimizu, M.; Hatai Uotsu, C.; Shimizu, M.; Tominaga, M. 1,8-Cineole, a TRPM8 agonist, is a novel natural antagonist of human TRPA1. *Mol. Pain* **2012**, *8*, 86. [CrossRef] [PubMed]

106. Talavera, K.; Gees, M.; Karashima, Y.; Meseguer, V.M.; Vanoirbeek, J.A.J.; Damann, N.; Everaerts, W.; Benoit, M.; Janssens, A.; Vennekens, R.; et al. Nicotine activates the chemosensory cation channel TRPA1. *Nat. Neurosci.* **2009**, *12*, 1293–1299. [CrossRef] [PubMed]

107. Zygmunt, P.M.; Petersson, J.; Andersson, D.A.; Chuang, H.-h.; Sørgård, M.; Di Marzo, V.; Julius, D.; Högestätt, E.D. Vanilloid receptors on sensory nerves mediate the vasodilator action of anandamide. *Nature* **1999**, *400*, 452–457. [PubMed]

108. Hwang, S.W.; Cho, H.; Kwak, J.; Lee, S.-Y.; Kang, C.-J.; Jung, J.; Cho, S.; Min, K.H.; Suh, Y.-G.; Kim, D.; et al. Direct activation of capsaicin receptors by products of lipoxygenases: endogenous capsaicin-like substances. *Proc. Natl. Acad. Sci. USA* **2000**, *97*, 6155–6160. [CrossRef] [PubMed]

109. Starowicz, K.; Niga, S.; Di Marzo, V. Biochemistry and pharmacology of endovanilloids. *Pharmacol. Ther.* **2007**, *114*, 13–33. [CrossRef] [PubMed]

110. Yue, H.-Y.; Fujita, T.; Kawasaki, Y.; Kumamoto, E. AM404 enhances the spontaneous release of L-glutamate in a manner sensitive to capsazepine in adult rat substantia gelatinosa neurones. *Brain Res.* **2004**, *1018*, 283–287. [CrossRef] [PubMed]

111. Niforatos, W.; Zhang, X.-F.; Lake, M.R.; Walter, K.A.; Neelands, T.; Holzman, T.F.; Scott, V.E.; Faltynek, C.R.; Moreland, R.B.; Chen, J. Activation of TRPA1 channels by the fatty acid amide hydrolase inhibitor 3'-carbamoylbiphenyl-3-yl cyclohexylcarbamate (URB597). *Mol. Pharmacol.* **2007**, *71*, 1209–1216. [CrossRef] [PubMed]

112. Cruz-Orengo, L.; Dhaka, A.; Heuermann, R.J.; Young, T.J.; Montana, M.C.; Cavanaugh, E.J.; Kim, D.; Story, G.M. Cutaneous nociception evoked by 15-delta PGJ2 via activation of ion channel TRPA1. *Mol. Pain* **2008**, *4*, 30. [CrossRef] [PubMed]

113. Wang, H.; Kohno, T.; Amaya, F.; Brenner, G.J.; Ito, N.; Allchorne, A.; Ji, R.-R.; Woolf, C.J. Bradykinin produces pain hypersensitivity by potentiating spinal cord glutamatergic synaptic transmission. *J. Neurosci.* **2005**, *25*, 7986–7992. [CrossRef] [PubMed]

114. Asuthkar, S.; Elustondo, P.A.; Demirkhanyan, L.; Sun, X.; Baskaran, P.; Velpula, K.K.; Thyagarajan, B.; Pavlov, E.V.; Zakharian, E. The TRPM8 protein is a testosterone receptor: I. Biochemical evidence for direct TRPM8-testosterone interactions. *J. Biol. Chem.* **2015**, *290*, 2659–2669. [CrossRef] [PubMed]

115. Asuthkar, S.; Demirkhanyan, L.; Sun, X.; Elustondo, P.A.; Krishnan, V.; Baskaran, P.; Velpula, K.K.; Thyagarajan, B.; Pavlov, E.V.; Zakharian, E. The TRPM8 protein is a testosterone receptor: II. Functional evidence for an ionotropic effect of testosterone on TRPM8. *J. Biol. Chem.* **2015**, *290*, 2670–2688. [CrossRef] [PubMed]

116. Leffler, A.; Fischer, M.J.; Rehner, D.; Kienel, S.; Kistner, K.; Sauer, S.K.; Gavva, N.R.; Reeh, P.W.; Nau, C. The vanilloid receptor TRPV1 is activated and sensitized by local anesthetics in rodent sensory neurons. *J. Clin. Investig.* **2008**, *118*, 763–776. [CrossRef] [PubMed]

117. Leffler, A.; Lattrell, A.; Kronewald, S.; Niedermirtl, F.; Nau, C. Activation of TRPA1 by membrane permeable local anesthetics. *Mol. Pain* **2011**, *7*, 62. [CrossRef] [PubMed]

118. Piao, L.-H.; Fujita, T.; Jiang, C.-Y.; Liu, T.; Yue, H.-Y.; Nakatsuka, T.; Kumamoto, E. TRPA1 activation by lidocaine in nerve terminals results in glutamate release increase. *Biochem. Biophys. Res. Commun.* **2009**, *379*, 980–984. [CrossRef] [PubMed]

119. Szallasi, A. Piperine: researchers discover new flavor in an ancient spice. *Trends Pharmacol. Sci.* **2005**, *26*, 437–439. [CrossRef] [PubMed]

120. Yang, L.; Fujita, T.; Jiang, C.-Y.; Piao, L.-H.; Yue, H.-Y.; Mizuta, K.; Kumamoto, E. TRPV1 agonist piperine but not olvanil enhances glutamatergic spontaneous excitatory transmission in rat spinal substantia gelatinosa neurons. *Biochem. Biophys. Res. Commun.* **2011**, *410*, 841–845. [CrossRef] [PubMed]

121. Liu, L.; Simon, S.A. Similarities and differences in the currents activated by capsaicin, piperine, and zingerone in rat trigeminal ganglion cells. *J. Neurophysiol.* **1996**, *76*, 1858–1869. [PubMed]

122. Liu, L.; Lo, Y.-C.; Chen, I.-J.; Simon, S.A. The responses of rat trigeminal ganglion neurons to capsaicin and two nonpungent vanilloid receptor agonists, olvanil and glyceryl nonamide. *J. Neurosci.* **1997**, *17*, 4101–4111. [PubMed]

123. Yang, B.H.; Piao, Z.G.; Kim, Y.-B.; Lee, C.-H.; Lee, J.K.; Park, K.; Kim, J.S.; Oh, S.B. Activation of vanilloid receptor 1 (VR1) by eugenol. *J. Dent. Res.* **2003**, *82*, 781–785. [CrossRef] [PubMed]

124. Inoue, M.; Fujita, T.; Goto, M.; Kumamoto, E. Presynaptic enhancement by eugenol of spontaneous excitatory transmission in rat spinal substantia gelatinosa neurons is mediated by transient receptor potential A1 channels. *Neuroscience* **2012**, *210*, 403–415. [CrossRef] [PubMed]

125. Yue, H.-Y.; Jiang, C.-Y.; Fujita, T.; Kumamoto, E. Zingerone enhances glutamatergic spontaneous excitatory transmission by activating TRPA1 but not TRPV1 channels in the adult rat substantia gelatinosa. *J. Neurophysiol.* **2013**, *110*, 658–671. [CrossRef] [PubMed]

126. Park, C.-K.; Xu, Z.-Z.; Berta, T.; Han, Q.; Chen, G.; Liu, X.-J.; Ji, R.-R. Extracellular microRNAs activate nociceptor neurons to elicit pain via TLR7 and TRPA1. *Neuron* **2014**, *82*, 47–54. [CrossRef] [PubMed]

127. Zhu, L.; Fujita, T.; Jiang, C.-Y.; Kumamoto, E. Enhancement by citral of glutamatergic spontaneous excitatory transmission in adult rat substantia gelatinosa neurons. *NeuroReport* **2016**, *27*, 166–171. [CrossRef] [PubMed]

128. Andersson, D.A.; Gentry, C.; Alenmyr, L.; Killander, D.; Lewis, S.E.; Andersson, A.; Bucher, B.; Galzi, J.-L.; Sterner, O.; Bevan, S.; et al. TRPA1 mediates spinal antinociception induced by acetaminophen and the cannabinoid Δ^9-tetrahydrocannabiorcol. *Nat. Commun.* **2011**, *2*, 551. [CrossRef] [PubMed]

129. Furue, H.; Narikawa, K.; Kumamoto, E.; Yoshimura, M. Responsiveness of rat substantia gelatinosa neurones to mechanical but not thermal stimuli revealed by *in vivo* patch-clamp recording. *J. Physiol.* **1999**, *521*, 529–535.

130. Yamanaka, M.; Taniguchi, W.; Nishio, N.; Hashizume, H.; Yamada, H.; Yoshida, M.; Nakatsuka, T. *In vivo* patch-clamp analysis of the antinociceptive actions of TRPA1 activation in the spinal dorsal horn. *Mol. Pain* **2015**, *11*, 20. [CrossRef] [PubMed]

131. Todd, A.J.; Watt, C.; Spike, R.C.; Sieghart, W. Colocalization of GABA, glycine and their receptors at synapses in the rat spinal cord. *J. Neurosci.* **1996**, *16*, 974–982. [PubMed]

132. Coggeshall, R.E.; Carlton, S.M. Receptor localization in the mammalian dorsal horn and primary afferent neurons. *Brain Res. Rev.* **1997**, *24*, 28–66. [CrossRef]

133. Moore, K.A.; Kohno, T.; Karchewski, L.A.; Scholz, J.; Baba, H.; Woolf, C.J. Partial peripheral nerve injury promotes a selective loss of GABAergic inhibition in the superficial dorsal horn of the spinal cord. *J. Neurosci.* **2002**, *22*, 6724–6731. [PubMed]

134. Kohno, T. A role of spinal inhibition in neuropathic pain. In *Cellular and Molecular Mechanisms for the Modulation of Nociceptive Transmission in the Peripheral and Central Nervous Systems*; Kumamoto, E., Ed.; Research Signpost: Kelara, India, 2007; pp. 131–145.

135. Coull, J.A.M.; Boudreau, D.; Bachand, K.; Prescott, S.A.; Nault, F.; Sik, A.; de Koninck, P.; de Koninck, Y. Trans-synaptic shift in anion gradient in spinal lamina I neurons as a mechanism of neuropathic pain. *Nature* **2003**, *424*, 938–942. [CrossRef] [PubMed]

136. Müller, F.; Heinke, B.; Sandkühler, J. Reduction of glycine receptor-mediated miniature inhibitory postsynaptic currents in rat spinal lamina I neurons after peripheral inflammation. *Neuroscience* **2003**, *122*, 799–805. [CrossRef] [PubMed]

137. Tanabe, M.; Takasu, K.; Yamaguchi, S.; Kodama, D.; Ono, H. Glycine transporter inhibitors as a potential therapeutic strategy for chronic pain with memory impairment. *Anesthesiology* **2008**, *108*, 929–937. [CrossRef] [PubMed]

138. Sandkühler, J. Models and mechanisms of hyperalgesia and allodynia. *Physiol. Rev.* **2009**, *89*, 707–758. [CrossRef] [PubMed]

139. Zeilhofer, H.U.; Wildner, H.; Yévenes, G.E. Fast synaptic inhibition in spinal sensory processing and pain control. *Physiol. Rev.* **2012**, *92*, 193–235. [CrossRef] [PubMed]

140. Baba, H.; Kohno, T.; Okamoto, M.; Goldstein, P.A.; Shimoji, K.; Yoshimura, M. Muscarinic facilitation of GABA release in substantia gelatinosa of the rat spinal dorsal horn. *J. Physiol.* **1998**, *508*, 83–93. [CrossRef] [PubMed]

141. Baba, H.; Goldstein, P.A.; Okamoto, M.; Kohno, T.; Ataka, T.; Yoshimura, M.; Shimoji, K. Norepinephrine facilitates inhibitory transmission in substantia gelatinosa of adult rat spinal cord (part 2): effects on somatodendritic sites of GABAergic neurons. *Anesthesiology* **2000**, *92*, 485–492. [CrossRef] [PubMed]

142. Baba, H.; Shimoji, K.; Yoshimura, M. Norepinephrine facilitates inhibitory transmission in substantia gelatinosa of adult rat spinal cord (part 1): effects on axon terminals of GABAergic and glycinergic neurons. *Anesthesiology* **2000**, *92*, 473–484. [CrossRef] [PubMed]

143. Takeda, D.; Nakatsuka, T.; Papke, R.; Gu, J.G. Modulation of inhibitory synaptic activity by a non-$\alpha 4\beta 2$, non-$\alpha 7$ subtype of nicotinic receptors in the substantia gelatinosa of adult rat spinal cord. *Pain* **2003**, *101*, 13–23. [CrossRef]

144. Fukushima, T.; Ohtsubo, T.; Tsuda, M.; Yanagawa, Y.; Hori, Y. Facilitatory actions of serotonin type 3 receptors on GABAergic inhibitory synaptic transmission in the spinal superficial dorsal horn. *J. Neurophysiol.* **2009**, *102*, 1459–1471. [CrossRef] [PubMed]

145. Liu, T.; Fujita, T.; Kumamoto, E. Acetylcholine and norepinephrine mediate GABAergic but not glycinergic transmission enhancement by melittin in adult rat substantia gelatinosa neurons. *J. Neurophysiol.* **2011**, *106*, 233–246. [CrossRef] [PubMed]

146. Bíró, T.; Tóth, B.I.; Marincsák, R.; Dobrosi, N.; Géczy, T.; Paus, R. TRP channels as novel players in the pathogenesis and therapy of itch. *Biochim. Biophys. Acta* **2007**, *1772*, 1004–1021. [CrossRef] [PubMed]

147. Sikand, P.; Shimada, S.G.; Green, B.G.; LaMotte, R.H. Similar itch and nociceptive sensations evoked by punctate cutaneous application of capsaicin, histamine and cowhage. *Pain* **2009**, *144*, 66–75. [CrossRef] [PubMed]

148. Akiyama, T.; Carstens, E. Neural processing of itch. *Neuroscience* **2013**, *250*, 697–714. [CrossRef] [PubMed]

149. Liu, T.; Ji, R.-R. New insights into the mechanisms of itch: are pain and itch controlled by distinct mechanisms? *Pflügers Arch.* **2013**, *465*, 1671–1685. [CrossRef] [PubMed]

150. Fujita, T.; Liu, T.; Nakatsuka, T.; Kumamoto, E. Proteinase-activated receptor-1 activation presynaptically enhances spontaneous glutamatergic excitatory transmission in adult rat substantia gelatinosa neurons. *J. Neurophysiol.* **2009**, *102*, 312–319. [CrossRef] [PubMed]

151. Jordt, S.-E.; Julius, D. Molecular basis for species-specific sensitivity to "hot" chili peppers. *Cell* **2002**, *108*, 421–430. [CrossRef]

152. Gavva, N.R.; Klionsky, L.; Qu, Y.; Shi, L.; Tamir, R.; Edenson, S.; Zhang, T.J.; Viswanadhan, V.N.; Toth, A.; Pearce, L.V.; et al. Molecular determinants of vanilloid sensitivity in TRPV1. *J. Biol. Chem.* **2004**, *279*, 20283–20295. [CrossRef] [PubMed]

153. Chen, J.; Zhang, X.-F.; Kort, M.E.; Huth, J.R.; Sun, C.; Miesbauer, L.J.; Cassar, S.C.; Neelands, T.; Scott, V.E.; Moreland, R.B.; et al. Molecular determinants of species-specific activation or blockade of TRPA1 channels. *J. Neurosci.* **2008**, *28*, 5063–5071. [CrossRef] [PubMed]

154. Nagatomo, K.; Kubo, Y. Caffeine activates mouse TRPA1 channels but suppresses human TRPA1 channels. *Proc. Natl. Acad. Sci. USA* **2008**, *105*, 17373–17378. [CrossRef] [PubMed]

155. Chen, J.; Joshi, S.K.; DiDomenico, S.; Perner, R.J.; Mikusa, J.P.; Gauvin, D.M.; Segreti, J.A.; Han, P.; Zhang, X.-F.; Niforatos, W.; et al. Selective blockade of TRPA1 channel attenuates pathological pain without altering noxious cold sensation or body temperature regulation. *Pain* **2011**, *152*, 1165–1172. [CrossRef] [PubMed]

156. Banzawa, N.; Saito, S.; Imagawa, T.; Kashio, M.; Takahashi, K.; Tominaga, M.; Ohta, T. Molecular basis determining inhibition/activation of nociceptive receptor TRPA1 protein: a single amino acid dictates species-specific actions of the most potent mammalian TRPA1 antagonist. *J. Biol. Chem.* **2014**, *289*, 31927–31939. [CrossRef] [PubMed]

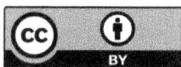

pharmaceuticals

MDPI

Review

Role of TRPM7 in Cancer: Potential as Molecular Biomarker and Therapeutic Target

Nelson S. Yee

Division of Hematology-Oncology, Department of Medicine, PennState Health Milton S. Hershey Medical Center, Program of Experimental Therapeutics, PennState Cancer Institute, The Pennsylvania State University College of Medicine, 500 University Drive, Hershey, PA 17033, USA; nyee@pennstatehealth.psu.edu; Tel.: +1-717-531-0003

Academic Editor: Arpad Szallasi
Received: 2 January 2017; Accepted: 29 March 2017; Published: 5 April 2017

Abstract: The transient receptor potential melastatin-subfamily member 7 (TRPM7) is a ubiquitously expressed ion channel with intrinsic kinase activity. Molecular and electrophysiological analyses of the structure and activity of TRPM7 have revealed functional coupling of its channel and kinase activity. Studies have indicated the important roles of TRPM7 channel-kinase in fundamental cellular processes, physiological responses, and embryonic development. Accumulating evidence has shown that TRPM7 is aberrantly expressed and/or activated in human diseases including cancer. TRPM7 plays a variety of functional roles in cancer cells including survival, cell cycle progression, proliferation, growth, migration, invasion, and epithelial-mesenchymal transition (EMT). Data from a study using mouse xenograft of human cancer show that TRPM7 is required for tumor growth and metastasis. The aberrant expression of TRPM7 and its genetic mutations/polymorphisms have been identified in various types of carcinoma. Chemical modulators of TRPM7 channel produced inhibition of proliferation, growth, migration, invasion, invadosome formation, and markers of EMT in cancer cells. Taken together, these studies suggest the potential value of exploiting TRPM7 channel-kinase as a molecular biomarker and therapeutic target in human malignancies.

Keywords: transient receptor potential; TRP; TRPM7; ion channel; cancer; biomarker; therapeutic target

---

1. Introduction

Ion channels play oncogenic and tumor suppressive roles in the pathogenesis of malignant neoplasms, and they have been implicated in the various hallmarks of cancer [1]. The transient receptor potential (TRP) superfamily of protein function as channels that control passage of various ions across biological membranes [2]. Activation of TRP channels typically results in transmembrane flow of cations such as Ca^{2+} and Mg^{2+} and, consequently, modulation of the associated signaling pathways. By detecting changes in various physical and chemical stimuli, TRP channels act as cellular sensors and transducers and mediate a variety of physiological responses [3]. Of the eight sub-families in the vertebral TRP family, the melastatin-subfamily (TRPM) possesses unique structural motifs and share common architectural features [4]. Growing evidence has shown that the TRPM7 member plays crucial roles in cellular processes, embryonic development, and human diseases, particularly cancer [5–8]. Accumulating data suggest the potential value of TRPM7 as a molecular biomarker and therapeutic target in human malignancies [5,8,9].

The biochemical and electrophysiological properties of TRPM7 have been determined by in vitro assays, and the functional roles of TRPM7 have been studied in cultured cells and model organisms. Under physiological conditions, TRPM7 is a divalent cation-selective channel, and it possesses protein serine/threonine kinase activity [10–12]. The TRPM7 channel-kinase is ubiquitously expressed [13]. Spanning over 134.34 kb on the long arm of chromosome 15, the human *TRPM7* gene consists of 39 exons, and four transcripts of its nine splice variants encode protein. The full-length human TRPM7 transcript contains 7263 nucleotides, and the encoded protein is composed of 1865 amino acids (MW 210 kDa) [14]. The basic structural features of the TRPM7 protein are shown in Figure 1. As a regulator of ionic homeostasis, the TRPM7 channel preferentially permits the flow of Mg^{2+} and Ca^{2+}, and the Mg^{2+} influx through the TRPM7 channel in certain cell types can lead to altered intracellular levels of Ca^{2+} [12,15,16]. The physiologically essential divalent metal cations (Zn^{2+}, Mn^{2+}, Co^{2+}) as well as environmentally toxic metals (Ni^{2+}, Cd^{2+}, Ba^{2+}, Sr^{2+}) are also permeable through the TRPM7 channel [10,12,17]. In addition, as a member of the atypical protein kinase family called alpha-kinases [18], TRPM7 can autophosphorylate its serine and threonine residues [19]. The roles of the channel and kinase activities in the physiological functions of TRPM7 depend on the cell types and the molecular context.

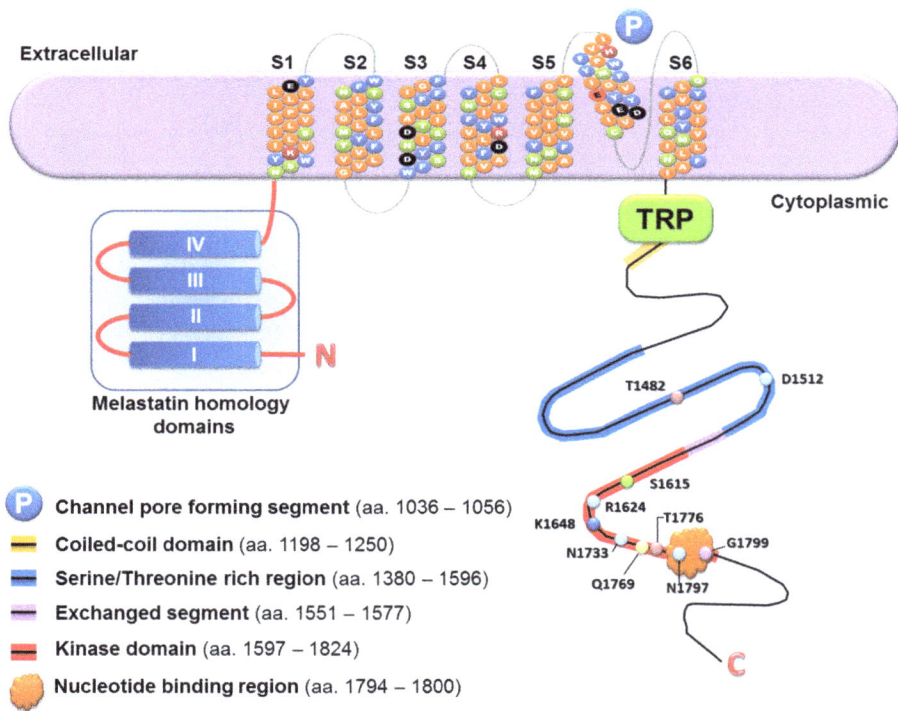

Figure 1. A schematic diagram to illustrate the protein structure of TRPM7 channel-kinase.

The TRPM7 protein contains six transmembrane segments (S1 to S6), each about 21 amino acid (aa.) residues in length. The amino (N) and carboxyl (C) terminal components embrace the transmembrane segments. The channel pore (P) is shown slightly off plane and formed between S5 and S6. The two negatively charged amino acids (E1047 and E1052) in the pore forming loop are important for Ca^{2+} and Mg^{2+} permeability as well as pH sensitivity of the channel. Selected amino acid residues are shown and they play important roles in the functions of TRPM7 channel and kinase. The numbers of the amino acid residues correspond to human TRPM7 protein. This figure is adapted from *Cells* 2014, *3*, 751–777 with permission from the publisher [5].

Experimental analyses of TRPM7 channel-kinase have revealed the molecular features that are important for its physiological responses and biological functions of TRPM7 in normal and cancerous cells. In vitro studies using site-directed mutagenesis in combination with electrophysiological and biochemical studies have generated insights into the molecular basis underlying the TRPM7 channel-kinase activities. Moreover, the amino acid residues of the TRPM7 protein that modulates its kinase activity, the sites of autophosphorylation and substrate binding, and their functional significance have been determined [5,20]. A growing body of data have supported diverse roles of TRPM7 in cellular proliferation, survival, differentiation, growth, and migration [5,21,22]. Studies using model organisms have revealed the crucial roles of TRPM7 in embryogenesis as well as the requirement of TRPM7 for development and functions of melanocytes, skeleton, thymus, nervous system, kidney, exocrine pancreas, urinary bladder, and megakaryocytes/platelets [5,23–26]. Accumulating evidence indicates that the TRPM7 channel-kinase plays oncogenic and tumor suppressing roles in various types of malignant tumors.

This purpose of this article is to discuss the emerging roles of the TRPM7 channel-kinase in various human malignancies, and the potential of exploiting TRPM7 as a cancer biomarker and therapeutic target. In this article, I will provide a review of the expression of TRPM7 in cancer, the roles of TRPM7 in cancer cells including proliferation, survival, migration, invasion, and epithelial-mesenchymal transition, as well as the role of TRPM7 in tumor growth and metastasis. The findings of TRPM7 genetic polymorphisms and mutations in various carcinoma will be presented. A list of chemicals that modulate TRPM7 expression and/or channel activity will be summarized. Finally, I will discuss the potential of developing TRPM7 channel-kinase as a molecular biomarker and therapeutic target for achieving the goal of precision oncology.

2. Roles of TRPM7 in Human Cancer

The TRPM7 channel-kinase has been implicated in a variety of human malignant tumors. In certain carcinoma examined, TRPM7 is aberrantly over-expressed in cell lines and/or tissues. Consistent with the functional roles of TRPM7 in the normal cell types and during organogenesis, numerous studies have shown that TRPM7 regulates cellular proliferation, survival, cell cycle progression, migration, and invasion in cancer cell lines. The signaling mechanisms underlying the biological functions of TRPM7 have been elucidated, and how aberrant expression and activity of TRPM7 contributes to neoplasia has begun to be understood. The expression and functional roles of TRPM7 in human malignant diseases are summarized in Table 1.

The functional roles of TRPM7 were examined by using RNA interference-mediated inhibition of TRPM7 expression or by using chemical inhibitors of TRPM7 channel activities as indicated. RNA interference is generally target-specific, though the extent of inhibition and the stability of the interfering agents are issues of potential concern. While the chemical inhibitors are relatively specific for TRPM7 activity, they may produce "off-target" effects depending on their concentrations being used. This table is adapted and modified from *Cells* 2014, *3*, 751–777 with permission from the publisher [5].

Table 1. Expression and roles of TRPM7 channels in various human malignancies.

Cancer	Expression	Functional roles of TRPM7	References
Pancreatic adenocarcinoma	- Increased in human pancreatic adenocarcinoma tissues and cell lines. - Increased in chronic pancreatitis, pancreatic intra-epithelial neoplasms	- Required for cellular proliferation and cell cycle progression involving Mg^{2+}. - Required for preventing replicative senescence. - Required for cell migration involving Mg^{2+}. - Required for cell invasion.	[9,27–31]
Breast carcinoma	- Over-expression in human breast carcinoma tissues and cell lines - Increased expression in infiltrating ductal carcinoma with microcalcifications - Somatic mutation T720S (Thr→Ser) in a breast infiltrating ductal carcinoma	- Required for cancer cell proliferation in vitro. - Required for cancer cell migration in vitro and tumor metastasis in a mouse xenograft model. - Waixenicin A, TRPM7 blocker, inhibits growth and survival of breast cancer cells MCF-7. - TRPM7 involved in estrogen receptor-negative metastatic breast cancer cells migration through kinase domain. - Involved in ginsenoside Rd-induced apoptosis in cells. - Involved in epithelial mesenchymal transition. - TRPM7 mediates migration and invasion of breast cancer cells (MDA-MB-435) involving phosphorylation of Src and MAPK.	[32–40]
Gastric carcinoma	- Expressed in human gastric adenocarcinoma cell lines (AGS, MKN-1, MKN-45, SNU-1, SNU-484) - Somatic mutation M830V (Met→Val) in gastric adenocarcinoma	- Required for cell survival involving Mg^{2+}. - Waixenicin A, TRPM7 blocker, inhibits growth and survival of gastric cancer cells AGS. - Involved in ginsenoside Rd-induced apoptosis AGS cells.	[37,38,40–43]
Head and neck Carcinoma	- Expressed in FaDu cells and SCC-25 cells. - High expression in 5-8F cells, low expression in 6-10B cells	- Required for cell growth and proliferation. - Required for migration of nasopharyngeal carcinoma cells (5-8F and 6-10B). - Proliferation of FaDu hypopharyngeal squamous cells (FaDu) inhibited by midazolam that targets TRPM7.	[44–46]
Retinoblastoma	- Existence in 5-8F cells	- Required for cell proliferation. - Required for 5-8F cell migration.	[47]
Melanoma	- Expressed in cell lines	- Not reported.	[48,49]
Lung carcinoma	- Expressed in A549 cells	- Required for migration of A549 cells.	[50]
Erythroleukemia	- TRPM7-like currents in cell lines	- Not reported.	[51]

Table 1. *Cont.*

Cancer	Expression	Functional roles of TRPM7	References
Colon cancer	- TRPM7 (Thr1482Ile) polymorphism	- TRPM7 (Thr1482Ile) polymorphism associated with elevated risk of both adenomatous and hyperplastic polyps. - Individuals with TRPM7 (Thr1482Ile) polymorphism with a high Ca:Mg ratio intake in diet at a relatively high risk of developing adenoma and hyperplastic polyps.	[52]
Leukemia	- Not reported	- Waixenicin inhibits T cell leukemia (Jurkat T lymphocytes) and rat basophilic leukemia cells (RBL1) through blocking TRPM7 channel activity.	[53]
Neuroblastoma	- Not reported	- In mouse neuroblastoma cells (N1E-115), TRPM7 promotes formation of Ca^{2+} sparking and invadosome by affecting actomyosin contractility independent from Ca^{2+} influx. - In vivo and in vitro studies using N1E-115 cells, TRPM7 promotes tumor metastasis in a mouse xenograft model and cell migration in Boyden chamber.	[54,55]
Ovarian carcinoma	- Somatic mutation S406C (Ser→Cys) in ovarian serous carcinoma	- Not reported.	[40]
Prostate cancer	- Expressed in human prostate cancer cell line DU145	- Increased Ca^{2+} to Mg^{2+} ratio in prostate cancer cells enhances TRPM7-mediated currents and promotes cellular entry of Ca^{2+}, leading to increase in cell proliferation.	[56]
Glioblastoma	- Over-expressed in human glioblastoma cell line U87	- Carvacrol inhibits TRPM7 and suppresses glioblastoma cell proliferation, migration, and invasion - Xylokeletal B inhibits TRPM7 and suppresses glioblastoma cell proliferation and migration through PI3K/Akt and MEK/ERK signaling - Midazolam inhibits TRPM7-mediated current and suppresses TRPM7 expression, and induces cell cycle arrest and impairs proliferation	[57–59]

2.1. Expression of TRPM7 in Cancer

While it is ubiquitously expressed in normal tissues and cells, TRPM7 is aberrantly over-expressed in various types of malignant neoplasms (Table 1). Studies have demonstrated increased expression of TRPM7 in a panel of human pancreatic adenocarcinoma cells and tissues [9,27–31]. For each histological type of pancreatic tumors, the proportions of samples with corresponding TRPM7 expression levels have been reported [31]. The expression levels of TRPM7 in pancreatic adenocarcinoma tissues were found to positively correlate with the primary tumor size and tumor stages. These results suggest that aberrant over-expression of TRPM7 is associated with pancreatic tumor growth and metastasis. Besides pancreatic cancer, TRPM7 is aberrantly over-expressed in the cell lines and tissues of breast cancer [33] and glioblastoma [57]. Somatic mutations or polymorphisms of TRPM7 have been identified in breast carcinoma [40], gastric carcinoma [40], colon carcinoma [52], and ovarian carcinoma [40]. While the significance of those mutations and polymorphisms of TRPM7 remains to be determined, the Thr1482Ile polymorphism was shown to be associated with elevated dietary $Ca^{2+}:Mg^{2+}$ ratio and risk of colonic polyps [52].

2.2. Roles of TRPM7 in Proliferation of Cancer

The proliferative role of TRPM7 has been demonstrated in a variety of malignant tumors including pancreatic adenocarcinoma, breast carcinoma, head/neck carcinoma, retinoblastoma, and glioblastoma. In studies using human pancreatic adenocarcinoma cell lines, TRPM7 channels have been shown to be necessary for maintaining proliferation and preventing replicative senescence [9,27,30]. Additionally, downregulation of TRPM7 in human pancreatic cancer cells led to inhibition of proliferation by arresting the cells in the G_0/G_1 and G_2/M phases of the cell cycle; these effects could be reversed by Mg^{2+} supplementation [9,27,30,31]. Moreover, small interfering RNA mediated silencing of TRPM7 induced senescence-associated β-galactosidase in pancreatic adenocarcinoma cells, suggesting a novel role of ion channels in replicative senescence of cancer [30]. Besides pancreatic cancer, TRPM7 is required for proliferation of cancer cells derived from a variety of malignant tumors. These include breast carcinoma [33], head/neck carcinoma [45], retinoblastoma [47], prostate carcinoma [56], T cell leukemia and rat basophilic leukemia [53], hypopharyngeal squamous cell carcinoma [46], and glioblastoma [57–59]. These results indicate that TRPM7 is required for proliferation of cancer cells and support a potential role of TRPM7 channels in tumor growth.

2.3. Roles of TRPM7 in Survival of Cancer Cells

A pro-survival role of TRPM7 channels has been demonstrated in various cancer cells, including pancreatic adenocarcinoma, gastric carcinoma, and breast carcinoma. In pancreatic cancer cells, small interfering RNA (siRNA)-induced knockdown of TRPM7 induced cell death without causing apoptosis [30]. In gastric cancer cells, TRPM7 is required for Mg^{2+}-dependent cell survival, and involved in ginsenoside Rd-induced apoptosis [41–43]. In breast cancer cells, TRPM7 in involved in ginsenoside Rd-induced apoptosis [37]. Results of these studies suggest the mechanisms that mediate TRPM7-induced cell death may depend on the cell types; however, they support a role of TRPM7 in promoting survival of cancer cells and tumor growth.

2.4. Roles of TRPM7 in Migration and Invasion of Cancer Cells

Downregulation of TRPM7 in human cancer cells impaired cell migration and invasion; these effects could be reversed by Mg^{2+} supplementation. TRPM7 is required for cell migration in breast carcinoma that involves the kinase domain of TRPM7 as well as phosphorylation of Src and MAPK [32,34,36]. Similarly, TRPM7 is required for cell migration in nasopharyngeal carcinoma [44] and lung carcinoma [50]. In pancreatic adenocarcinoma, TRPM7 is required for Mg^{2+}-dependent cell migration [9,28] and cell invasion [31]. These results indicate that TRPM7-regulated Mg^{2+} homeostasis and the associated signaling are required for migration and invasion of cancer cells, and support a potential role of TRPM7 channels in tumor metastasis.

2.5. Role of TRPM7 in Epithelial-Mesenchymal Transition

Functional expression of TRPM7 plays a regulatory role in epithelial-mesenchymal transition (EMT), which represents a tumor microenvironment-induced invasive phenotype adopted by cancer cells in metastasis. Epidermal growth factor (EGF)- or hypoxia-induced EMT is associated with a transient elevation of intracellular Ca^{2+} and activation of signal transducer and activator of transcription 3 (STAT3). Silencing of TRPM7 in a breast cancer cell line (MDA-MB468) produced suppression of EGF-induced expression of vimentin and phosphorylation of STAT3, which are markers of EMT [39]. These data suggest that TRPM7 channel is involved in EMT and tumor metastasis.

2.6. Roles of TRPM7 in Cancer Growth and Metastasis

In vivo studies have provided insights into the roles of TRPM7 in tumorigenesis. Using a mouse xenograft model of human breast carcinoma, TRPM7 has been shown to be required for tumor metastasis [32]. This process involves TRPM7-mediated modification of focal adhesion number, cell–cell adhesion and polarized cell movement through regulation of myosin II–based cellular tension. These data are consistent with the in vitro evidence for the requirement of TRPM7 in cancer cell migration and invasion and supportive of a mechanosensory role of TRPM7 in tumor metastasis.

2.7. Signaling Mechanisms for Functional Roles TRPM7 in Cancer

The signaling pathways and the mechanisms that mediate the various cellular effects of TRPM7 in cancer cells have been elucidated. Depending on the cell types, the TRPM7 channel–kinase may interact and modulate the signaling pathways that mediate the effects of mitogens and inflammatory cytokines [22,27,50,58,60–67]. In a working model (Figure 2), the TRPM7 channel-kinase acts as a cellular sensor of the physical and chemical stimuli such as mechanical stretch, oxidative stress, changes in cell volume or osmolar gradient, and alterations in extracellular or cytosolic pH. It also acts as a signal transducer by controlling ionic fluxes and modulating the mitogen- and cytokine-induced signaling pathways. Hypothetically, aberrantly expressed TRPM7 and dysregulated homeostasis of Mg^{2+} and Ca^{2+} in cancer cells modulate the epidermal growth factor (EGF)- or other mitogen-induced signaling pathways. These lead to perturbation of the signaling mediators and nuclear events, resulting in uncontrolled proliferation, survival, growth, and invasion of cancer cells.

The TRPM7 channel and kinase are constitutively active in resting cells. In response to physicochemical stimuli in the extracellular medium and in the cytosol, conduction of Mg^{2+} and Ca^{2+} through the TRPM7 channel can be positively or negatively regulated. The TRPM7 kinase can auto-phosphorylate itself and also phosphorylate various substrates in the cytocol. The resultant perturbation of ionic homeostasis and series of phosphorylation events produce activation or inhibition of the signaling molecules downstream of epidermal growth factor or other cytokines. Those signaling events induce transcription and translation of the cell cycle regulators, senescence-associated genes, and motility factors. These lead to a number of biological processes including cellular survival, proliferation, differentiation, growth, adhesion, rounding, migration, and invasion. Such cellular effects underlie TRPM7 channel-kinase mediated functions in physiological responses, embryonic development, and diseases such as cancer. This figure is adapted and modified from *Cells* 2014, 3, 751–777 with permission from the publisher [5].

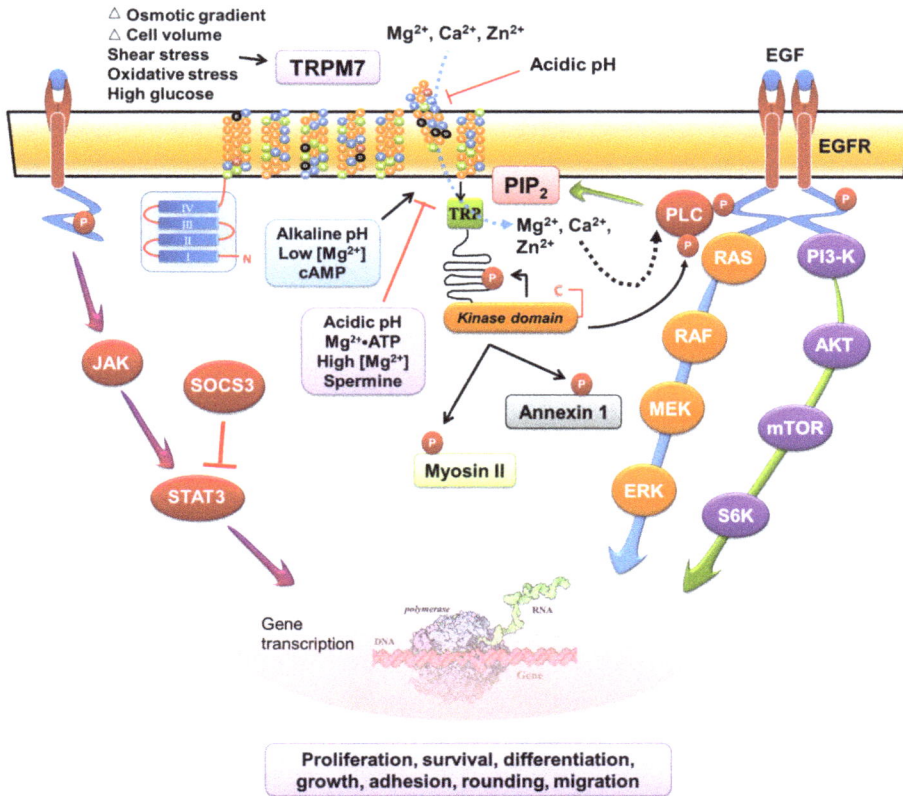

Figure 2. A working model of the signaling mechanisms that mediate the functional roles of TRPM7.

3. TRPM7 Channel as Molecular Biomarker and Therapeutic Target in Cancer

The findings of over-expression of TRPM7 protein and genetic mutations/polymorphisms in the TRPM7 gene in (pre)malignant diseases suggest the potential of exploiting it as a cancer biomarker. In pancreatic adenocarcinoma, a positive correlation was identified between the aberrant over-expression of TRPM7 and the tumor size/stages [31]. Results from the epidemiological study demonstrate that the TRPM7 variant T1482I, which was previously identified in patients with neurodegenerative diseases, is associated with dietary intake of Ca^{2+}/Mg^{2+} and formation of the pre-malignant colonic adenoma/polyps [52]. Moreover, somatic mutations in TRPM7 have been identified in breast carcinoma (T720S, Thr->Ser), gastric carcinoma (M830V, Met->Val), and ovarian carcinoma (S406C, Ser->Cys) [40]. While the functional significance of these mutations remain to be determined, these data suggest the potential of exploiting TRPM7 as a molecular biomarker for prevention, early detection, and prognostication of cancer.

Furthermore, the aberrant expression and/or activity of TRPM7 in malignant tumors offer the opportunity of targeting TRPM7 for treatment of patients with cancer. A number of chemicals that modulate the expression and channel activity of TRPM7 have been identified and characterized [68]. These are not only valuable research tools to probe the mechanisms underlying the electrophysiological and cellular functions of TRPM7, but also potential therapeutic agents for various diseases, particularly cancer (Table 2).

Table 2. Chemical modulators of TRPM7 channel activities as potential anti-cancer therapeutics.

Chemicals	Effects on TRPM7	Types of Cancer (Cell Lines)	Cellular Effects	References
Midazolam	Reduces expression of TRPM7, blocks TRPM7 channel activity (TRPM7 currents)	Human hypopharyngeal squamous cell carcinoma (FaDu), human glioma (MGR2)	Inhibits growth and proliferation with cell cycle arrest	[46,59]
Ginsenoside Rg3	Blocks TRPM7 channel activity (TRPM7 currents)	Human gastric adenocarcinoma (AGS)	Inhibits growth and survival (MTT-based viability assay: IC_{50} of 350 μM)	[42]
Ginsenoside Rd	Inhibits TRPM7 channel activity (TRPM7 currents)	Human breast adenocarcinoma (MCF-7), Human gastric adenocarcinoma (AGS)	Inhibits proliferation and survival (MTT-based viability assay: IC_{50} of 154 μM in MCF-7; IC_{50} of 131 μM in AGS)	[37]
Waixenicin A	Inhibits TRPM7 channel activity (TRPM7 currents: IC_{50} of 7 μM in 0 $[Mg^{2+}]_i$; 16 nM in 700 uM $[Mg^{2+}]_i$)	T cell leukemia (Jurkat), Rat basophilic leukemia (RBL1), Human gastric adenocarcinoma (AGS), Human breast adenocarcinoma (MCF-7), Mouse neuroblastoma (N1E-115)	Inhibits proliferation, inhibits invadosome formation	[38,53,54]
Carvacrol	Inhibits TRPM7 channel activity	Human glioblastoma (U87)	Inhibits survival, migration, and invasion (MTT-based viability assay: IC_{50} of 561 μM)	[57]
Xyloketal B	Inhibits TRPM7 channel activity (TRPM7 currents)	Human glioblastoma (U251)	Inhibits survival, proliferation and migration (MTT-based viability assay: IC_{50} of 287 μM)	[58]
NS8593	Inhibits TRPM7 channel activity (TRPM7 currents: IC_{50} 1.6 μM in $[Mg^{2+}]_i$, IC_{50} of 5.9 uM in 300 μM $[Mg^{2+}]_i$)	Human breast carcinoma (MDA-MB468)	Inhibits epidermal growth factor-induced vimentin expression (epithelial-mesenchymal transition)	[39,69]

Those chemical modulators can inhibit the TRPM7 channel activity and/or expression have been studied [37–39,42,46,53,54,57–59,69–76]. These inhibitors of TRPM7 channels include non-specific channel blockers, compounds derived from natural sources, and synthetic compounds. Most of their inhibitory actions are reversible at the concentrations tested and their IC_{50} values in the μM range. The chemical inhibitors of TRPM7 have been extensively used to study the mechanisms of the TRPM7 channel and kinase, and some of them show potential for therapeutic application.

On the other hand, a set of small molecule chemicals that activate the TRPM7 channel has been identified and characterized [77]. Among these TRPM7 agonists, the δ–opioid receptor antagonist, naltriben, has been studied in detail. It was proposed that naltriben is a positive gating modulator of a TRPM7 channel, with a reversible stimulatory effect on the TRPM7 channel that is independent of $[Mg^{2+}]_{ic}$, and an EC_{50} 20.7 μM [77]. In a recent report, two positive modulators of TRPM7, mibefradil and NNC 50-0396, have been recovered from a high throughout screen [78]. Mifebradil was shown to reversibly activate TRPM7-mediated Ca^{2+} entry and whole cell currents. In contrast to naltriben, mifebradil activates the TRPM7 channel only at physiological $[Mg^{2+}]_{ic}$. These TRPM7 channel agonists will be useful tools to study the mechanistic actions of TRPM7, and their biological effects and potential medical applications remain to be determined.

Some of the TRPM7 modulators have been tested in cancer cells, such as a clinically used anesthetic (midazolam), naturally occurring compounds (ginsenoside Rg3, ginsenoside Rd, waixenicin A, carvacrol, and xyloketal B), and the synthetic compound NS8593. The chemically induced blockade of TRPM7 expression or its channel activity produces a variety of cellular effects including inhibition of cancer cell survival, proliferation, migration, invasion, and invadosome formation (Table 2). This suggests the potential value of developing these chemical modulators of TRPM7 into anti-cancer therapeutics.

4. Conclusions

TRPM7 is a ubiquitously expressed ion channel with intrinsic kinase activity that plays regulatory roles in a variety of cellular processes, physiological responses, early development, organogenesis, and human diseases, particularly cancer. Experimental evidence implicates important roles of the TRPM7 channel-kinase in the hallmarks of cancer, including uncontrolled cell cycle progression, survival, proliferation, growth, migration, invasion, epithelial-mesenchymal transition, and metastasis. While the functions mediated by TRPM7 in cancer appear to depend on the organ involved, the signaling mechanisms that mediate the functional roles of TRPM7 are related to the cellular and molecular context.

Future studies are indicated to understand how the TRPM7 channel-kinase sensing the physical and chemical changes inside the cells and in the microenvironment contributes to neoplasia. Animal models are urgently needed to determine the mechanistic roles of TRPM7 channel-kinase in the multistep process of carcinogenesis, such as tumor initiation, growth, invasion, and metastasis. The aberrant expression of TRPM7 and its genetic mutations/polymorphisms in malignant tumors suggest the opportunity for developing it as a clinical biomarker for prevention and early detection of cancer. Pharmacological inhibition of the TRPM7 channel in conjunction with genetic silencing of TRPM7 expression have not only provided mechanistic understanding of the biological functions of TRPM7, but also offer new hope for developing targeted therapeutics for achieving the goal of precision oncology.

Acknowledgments: The research work conducted in the author's Laboratory of Pancreatic Development and Cancer was supported by The Pennsylvania State University Physician Scientist Stimulus Package, the National Institute of Health (K08 DK 60529-05, R03 DK 071960-03, P30 NCI), the Pilot Grant in Translational Research from The University of Iowa Carver College of Medicine, the American Cancer Society Institutional Research Grant, and the Fraternal Order of Eagles Art Ehrmann Cancer Fund.

Conflicts of Interest: The author declares no conflict of interest.

References

1. Yee, N.S. Ion channels. In *Encyclopedia of Cancer*, 3rd ed.; Springer: Berlin/Heidelberg, Germany, 2014; pp. 1–4.
2. Pedersen, S.F.; Owsianik, G.; Nilius, B. TRP channels: An overview. *Cell Calcium* **2005**, *38*, 233–252.
3. Owsianik, G.; D'Hoedt, D.; Voets, T.; Nilius, B. Structure-function relationship of the TRP channel superfamily. *Rev. Physiol. Biochem. Pharmacol.* **2006**, *156*, 61–90. [PubMed]
4. Fleig, A.; Penner, R. The TRPM ion channel subfamily: Molecular, biophysical and functional features. *Trends Pharmacol. Sci.* **2004**, *25*, 633–639. [CrossRef] [PubMed]
5. Yee, N.S.; Kazi, A.A.; Yee, R.K. Cellular and developmental biology of TRPM7 channel-kinase: Implicated roles in cancer. *Cells* **2014**, *3*, 751–777. [CrossRef] [PubMed]
6. Fleig, A.; Chubanov, V. TRPM7. Mammalian Transient Receptor Potential (TRP) Cation Channels. In *Handbook of Experimental Pharmacology*; Nilius, B., Flockerzi, V., Eds.; Springer: Berlin/Heidelberg, Germany, 2014; p. 521.
7. Cabezas-Bratesco, D.; Brauchi, S.; Gonzales-Teuber, V.; Steinberg, X.; Valencia, I.; Colenso, C. The different roles of the channel-kinases TRPM6 and TRPM7. *Curr. Med. Chem.* **2015**, *22*, 2943–2953. [CrossRef] [PubMed]
8. Gautier, M.; Perriere, M.; Monet, M.; Vanlaeys, A.; Korichneva, I.; Dhennin-Duthille, I.; Ouadid-Ahidouch, H. Recent advances in oncogenic roles of the TRPM7 chanzyme. *Curr. Med. Chem.* **2016**, *23*, 4092–4107.
9. Yee, N.S.; Chan, A.S.; Yee, J.D.; Yee, R.K. TRPM7 and TRPM8 ion channels in pancreatic adenocarcinoma: Potential roles as cancer biomarkers and targets. *Scientifica* **2012**. [CrossRef] [PubMed]
10. Nadler, M.J.; Hermosura, M.C.; Inabe, K.; Perraud, A.L.; Zhu, Q.; Stokes, A.; Kurosaki, T.; Kinet, J.P.; Penner, R.; Scharenberg, A.M.; et al. LTRPC7 is a Mg.ATP-regulated divalent cation channel required for cell viability. *Nature* **2001**, *411*, 590–595. [CrossRef] [PubMed]
11. Runnels, L.W.; Yue, L.; Clapham, D.E. TRP-PLIK, a bifunctional protein with kinase and ion channel activities. *Science* **2001**, *291*, 1043–1047. [CrossRef] [PubMed]
12. Schmitz, C.; Perraud, A.L.; Johnson, C.O.; Inabe, K.; Smith, M.K.; Penner, R.; Kurosaki, T.; Fleig, A. Scharenberg, A.M. Regulation vertebrate cellular Mg^{2+} homeostasis by TRPM7. *Cell* **2003**, *114*, 191–200.
13. Fonfria, E.; Murdock, P.R.; Cusdin, F.S.; Benham, C.D.; Kelsell, R.E.; McNulty, S. Tissue distribution profiles of the human TRPM cation channel family. *J. Recept. Signal Transduct. Res.* **2006**, *26*, 159–178.
14. Kraft, R.; Harteneck, C. The mammalian melastatin-related transient receptor potential cation channels: An overview. *Pflügers Arch.* **2005**, *451*, 204–211. [CrossRef] [PubMed]
15. Aarts, M.; Iihara, K.; Wei, W.L.; Xiong, Z.G.; Arundine, M.; Cerwinski, W.; MacDonald, J.F.; Tymianski, M. A key role for TRPM7 channels in anoxic neuronal death. *Cell* **2003**, *115*, 863–877. [CrossRef]
16. Wei, C.; Wang, X.; Chen, M.; Ouyang, K.; Song, L.S.; Cheng, H. Calcium flickers steer cell migration. *Nature* **2009**, *457*, 901–905. [CrossRef] [PubMed]
17. Monteilh-Zoller, M.K.; Hermosura, M.C.; Nadler, M.J.; Scharenberg, A.M.; Penner, R.; Fleig, A. TRPM7 provides an ion channel mechanism for cellular entry of tract metal ions. *J. Gen. Physiol.* **2003**, *121*, 49–60.
18. Fujiwara, Y.; Minor, D.L., Jr. X-ray crystal structure of a TRPM assembly domain reveals an antiparallel four-stranded coiled-coil. *J. Mol. Biol.* **2008**, *383*, 854–870. [CrossRef] [PubMed]
19. Matsushita, M.; Kozak, J.A.; Shimizu, Y.; McLachlin, D.T.; Yamaguchi, H.; Wei, F.Y.; Tomizawa, K.; Matsui, H.; Chait, B.T.; Cahalan, M.D.; et al. Channel function is dissociated from the intrinsic kinase activity and autophosphorylation of TRPM7/chak1. *J. Biol. Chem.* **2005**, *280*, 20793–20803. [CrossRef] [PubMed]
20. Kaitsuka, T.; Katagiri, C.; Beesetty, P.; Nakamura, K.; Hourani, S.; Tomizawa, K.; Kozak, J.A.; Matsushita, M. Inactivation of TRPM7 kinase activity does not impair its channel function in mice. *Sci. Rep.* **2014**, *4*, 5718.
21. Schilling, T.; Miralles, F.; Eder, C. TRPM7 regulates proliferation and polarization of macrophages. *J. Cell Sci.* **2014**, *127*, 4561–4566. [CrossRef] [PubMed]
22. Zeng, Z.; Leng, T.; Feng, X.; Sun, H.; Inoue, K.; Zhu, L.; Xiong, Z-G. Silencing TRPM7 in mouse cortical astrocytes impairs cell proliferation and migration via ERK and JNK signaling pathways. *PLoS ONE* **2015**, *10*, e0119912. [CrossRef] [PubMed]
23. Sah, R.; Mesirca, P.; Van den Boogert, M.; Rosen, J.; Mably, J.; Mangoni, M.E.; Clapham, D.E. Ion channel-kinase TRPM7 is required for maintaining cardiac automaticity. *Proc. Natl. Acad. Sci. USA* **2013**, E3037–E3046. [CrossRef] [PubMed]

24. Ryazanova, L.V.; Hu, Z.; Suzuki, S.; Chubanov, V.; Fleig, A.; Ryazanov, A. Elucidating the role of the TRPM7 alpha-kinase: TRPM7 kinase inactivation leads to magnesium deprivation resistance phenotype in mice. *Sci. Rep.* **2014**, *4*, 7599. [CrossRef] [PubMed]
25. Watanabe, M.; Suzuki, Y.; Uchida, K.; Miyazaki, N.; Murata, K.; Matsumoto, S.; Kakizaki, H.; Tominaga, M. TRPM7 protein contributes to intercellular junction formation in mouse urothelium. *J. Biol. Chem.* **2015**, *290*, 29882–29892. [CrossRef] [PubMed]
26. Stritt, S.; Nurden, P.; Favier, R.; Favier, M.; Ferioli, S.; Gotru, S.K.; van Eeuwik, J.M.M.; Schulze, H.; Nurden, A.T.; Lambert, M.P.; et al. Defects in TRPM7 channel function deregulate thrombopoiesis and cytoskeletal architecture. *Nat. Commun.* **2016**, *7*, 11097. [CrossRef] [PubMed]
27. Yee, N.S.; Zhou, W.; Liang, I.-C. Transient receptor potential ion channel TRPM7 regulates exocrine pancreatic epithelial proliferation by Mg^{2+}-sensitive Socs3a signaling in development and cancer. *Dis. Mod. Mech.* **2011**, *4*, 240–254. [CrossRef] [PubMed]
28. Rybarczyk, P.; Gautier, M.; Hague, F.; Dhennin-Duthille, I.; Chatelain, D.; Kerr-Conte, J.; Pattou, F; Regimbeau, J.M.; Sevestre, H.; Ouadid-Ahidouch, H. Transient receptor potential melastatin-related 7 channel is overexpressed in human pancreatic ductal adenocarcinomas and regulates human pancreatic cancer cell migration. *Int. J. Cancer* **2012**, *131*, E851–E861. [CrossRef] [PubMed]
29. Yee, N.S.; Yee, R.K. Ion channels as novel pancreatic cancer biomarkers and targets. In *New Advances on Disease Biomarkers and Molecular Targets in Biomedicine*; Lee, N.P.-Y., Ed.; Springer: New York, NY, USA, 2013.
30. Yee, N.S.; Zhou, W.; Lee, M.; Yee, R.K. Targeted silencing of TRPM7 ion channel induces replicative senescence and produces enhanced cytotoxicity with gemcitabine in pancreatic adenocarcinoma. *Cancer Lett.* **2012**, *318*, 99–105. [CrossRef] [PubMed]
31. Yee, N.S.; Kazi, A.A.; Li, Q.; Yang, Z.; Berg, A.; Yee, R.K. Aberrant over-expression of TRPM7 ion channels in pancreatic cancer: Required for cancer cell invasion and implicated in tumor growth and metastasis. *Biol. Open* **2015**, *4*, 507–514. [CrossRef] [PubMed]
32. Middelbeek, J.; Kuipers, A.J.; Henneman, L.; Visser, D.; Eidhof, I.; van Horssen, R.; Wieringa, B.; Canisius, S.V.; Zwart, W.; Wessels, L.F.; et al. TRPM7 is required for breast tumor cell metastasis. *Cancer Res.* **2012**, *72*, 4250–4261. [CrossRef] [PubMed]
33. Guilbert, A.; Gautier, M.; Dhennin-Duthille, I.; Haren, N.; Sevestre, H.; Ouadid-Ahidouch, H. Evidence that TRPM7 is required for breast cancer cell proliferation. *Am. J. Physiol. Cell Physiol.* **2009**, *297*, C493–C502. [CrossRef] [PubMed]
34. Guilbert, A.; Gautier, M.; Dhennin-Duthille, I.; Rybarczyk, P.; Sahni, J.; Sevestre, H.; Scharenberg, A.M.; Ouadid-Ahidouch, H. Transient receptor potential melastatin 7 is involved in oestrogen receptor-negative metastatic breast cancer cells migration through its kinase domain. *Eur. J. Cancer* **2013**, *49*, 3694–3707. [CrossRef] [PubMed]
35. Mandavilli, S.; Singh, B.B.; Sahmoun, A.E. Serum calcium levels, TRPM7, TRPC1, microcalcifications, and breast cancer using breast imaging reporting and data system scores. *Breast Cancer* **2012**, *2013*, 1–7.
36. Meng, X.; Cai, C.; Wu, J.; Cai, S.; Ye, C.; Chen, H.; Yang, Z.; Zeng, H.; Shen, Q.; Zou, F. TRPM7 mediates breast cancer cell migration and invasion through the MAPK pathway. *Cancer Lett.* **2013**, *333*, 96–102. [CrossRef] [PubMed]
37. Kim, B.J. Involvement of melastatin type transient receptor potential 7 channels in ginsenoside Rd- induced apoptosis in gastric and breast cancer cells. *J. Ginseng Res.* **2013**, *37*, 201–209. [CrossRef] [PubMed]
38. Kim, B.J.; Nam, J.H.; Kwon, Y.K.; So, I.; Kim, S.J. The role of waixenicin A as transient receptor potential melastatin 7 blocker. *Basic Clin. Pharmacol. Toxicol.* **2013**, *112*, 83–89. [CrossRef] [PubMed]
39. Davis, F.M.; Azimi, I.; Faville, R.A.; Peters, A.A.; Jalink, K.; Putney, J.W., Jr.; Goodhill, G.J.; Thompson, E.W.; Roberts-Thomson, S.J.; monteith, G.R. Induction of epitheial-mesenchymal transition (EMT) in breast cancer cells is calcium signal dependent. *Oncogene* **2014**, *33*, 2307–2316. [CrossRef] [PubMed]
40. Greenman, C.; Stephens, P.; Smith, R.; Dalgliesh, G.L.; Hunter, C.; Bignell, G.; Davies, H.; Teague, J.; Butler, A.; Stevens, C.; et al. Patterns of somatic mutation in human cancer genomes. *Nature* **2007**, *446*, 153–158. [CrossRef] [PubMed]
41. Kim, B.J.; Kim, S.Y.; Lee, S.; Jeon, J.H.; Matsui, H.; Kwon, Y.K.; Kim, S.J.; So, I. The role of transient receptor potential channel blockers in human gastric cancer cell viability. *Can. J. Physiol. Pharmacol.* **2012**, *990*, 175–186. [CrossRef] [PubMed]

42. Kim, B.J.; Nah, S.Y.; Jeon, J.H.; So, I.; Kim, S.J. Transient receptor potential melastatin 7 channels are involved in ginsenoside Rg3-induced apoptosis in gastric cancer cells. *Basic Clin. Pharmacol. Toxicol.* **2011**, *109*, 233–239. [CrossRef] [PubMed]
43. Kim, B.J.; Park, E.J.; Lee, J.H.; Jeon, J.H.; Kim, S.J.; So, I. Suppression of transient receptor potential melastatin 7 channel induces cell death in gastric cancer. *Cancer Sci.* **2008**, *99*, 2502–2509. [CrossRef] [PubMed]
44. Chen, J.P.; Luan, Y.; You, C.X.; Chen, X.H.; Luo, R.C.; Li, R. TRPM7 regulates the migration of human nasopharyngeal carcinoma cell by mediating Ca^{2+} influx. *Cell Calcium* **2010**, *47*, 425–432. [CrossRef] [PubMed]
45. Jiang, J.; Li, M.H.; Inoue, K.; Chu, X.P.; Seeds, J.; Xiong, Z.G. Transient receptor potential melastatin 7-like current in human head and neck carcinoma cells: Role in cell proliferation. *Cancer Res.* **2007**, *67*, 10929–10938. [CrossRef] [PubMed]
46. Dou, Y.; Li, Y.; Chen, J.; Wu, S.; Xiao, X.; Xie, S.; Tang, L.; Yan, M.; Wang, Y.; Lin, J.; et al. Inhibition of cancer cell proliferation by midazolam by targeting transient receptor potential melastatin 7. *Oncol. Lett.* **2013**, *5*, 1010–1016. [PubMed]
47. Hanano, T.; Hara, Y.; Shi, J.; Morita, H.; Umebayashi, C.; Mori, E.; Sumimoto, H.; Ito, Y.; Mori, Y.; Inoue, R. Involvement of TRPM7 in cell growth as a spontaneously activated Ca^{2+} entry pathway in human retinoblastoma cells. *J. Pharmacol. Sci.* **2004**, *95*, 403–419. [CrossRef] [PubMed]
48. McNeill, M.S.; Paulsen, J.; Bonde, G.; Burnright, E.; Hsu, M.Y.; Cornell, R.A. Cell death of melanophores in zebrafish trpm7 mutant embryos depends on melanin synthesis. *J. Investig. Dermatol.* **2007**, *127*, 2020–2030. [CrossRef] [PubMed]
49. Guo, H.; Carlson, J.A.; Slominski, A. Role of TRPM in melanocytes and melanoma. *Exp. Dermatol.* **2012**, *21*, 650–654. [CrossRef] [PubMed]
50. Gao, H.; Chen, X.; Du, X.; Guan, B.; Liu, Y.; Zhang, H. EGF enhances the migration of cancer cells by up-regulation of TRPM7. *Cell Calcium* **2011**, *50*, 559–568. [CrossRef] [PubMed]
51. Mason, M.J.; Schaffner, C.; Floto, R.A.; Teo, Q.A. Constitutive expression of a Mg^{2+}-inhibited K$^+$ current and a TRPM7-like current in human erythroleukemia cells. *Am. J. Physiol. Cell Physiol.* **2012**, *302*, C853–C867. [CrossRef] [PubMed]
52. Dai, Q.; Shrubsole, M.J.; Ness, R.M.; Schlundt, D.; Cai, Q.; Smalley, W.E.; Li, M.; Shyr, Y.; Zheng, W. The relation of magnesium and calcium intakes and a genetic polymorphism in the magnesium transporter to colorectal neoplasia risk. *Am. J. Clin. Nutr.* **2007**, *86*, 743–751. [PubMed]
53. Zierler, S.; Yao, G.; Zhang, Z.; Kuo, W.C.; Porzgen, P.; Penner, R.; Horgen, F.D.; Fleig, A. Waixenicin A inhibits cell proliferation through magnesium-dependent block of transient receptor potential melastatin 7 (TRPM7) channels. *J. Biol. Chem.* **2011**, *286*, 39328–39335. [CrossRef] [PubMed]
54. Visser, D.; Langeslag, M.; Kedziora, K.M.; Klarenbeek, J.; Kamermans, A.; Horgen, F.D.; Fleig, A.; van Leeuwen, F.N.; Jalink, K. TRPM7 triggers Ca^{2+} sparks and invadosome formation in neuroblastoma cells. *Cell Calcium* **2013**, *54*, 404–415. [CrossRef] [PubMed]
55. Middlebeek, J.; Visser, D.; Henneman, L.; Kamermans, A.; Kuipers, A.J.; Hoogerbrugge, P.M.; Jalink, K.; van Leeuwen, F.N. TRPM7 maintains progenitor-like features of neuroblastoma cells: Implications for metastasis formation. *Oncotarget* **2015**, *6*, 8760–8776. [CrossRef] [PubMed]
56. Sun, Y.; Selvaraj, S.; Varma, A.; Derry, S.; Sahmoun, A.E.; Singh, B.B. Increase in serum Ca^{2+}/Mg^{2+} ratio promotes proliferation of prostate cancer cells by activating TRPM7 channels. *J. Biol. Chem.* **2013**, *288*, 255–263. [CrossRef] [PubMed]
57. Chen, W.L.; Barszczyk, A.; Turlova, E.; Deurloo, M.; Liu, B.; Yang, B.B.; Rutka, J.T.; Feng, Z.P.; Sun, H.S. Inhibition of TRPM7 by carvacrol suppresses glioblastoma cell proliferation, migration and invasion. *Oncotarget* **2015**, *6*, 16321–16340. [CrossRef] [PubMed]
58. Chen, W.L.; Turlova, E.; Sun, C.L.; Kim, J.S.; Huang, S.; Zhong, X.; Guan, Y.Y.; Wang, G.L.; Rutka, J.T.; Feng, Z.P.; et al. Xyloketal B suppresses glioblastoma cell proliferation and migration in vitro through inhibiting TRPM7-regulated PI3K/Akt and MEK/ERK signaling pathways. *Mar. Drugs* **2015**, *13*, 2505–2525. [CrossRef] [PubMed]
59. Chen, J.; Dou, Y.; Zheng, X.; Leng, T.; Lu, X.; Ouyang, Y.; Sun, H.; Xing, F.; Mai, J.; Gu, J.; et al. TRPM7 channel inhibition mediates midazolam-induced proliferation loss in human malignant glioma. *Tumour Biol.* **2016**, *37*, 14721–14731. [CrossRef] [PubMed]

60. Runnels, L.W.; Yue, L.; Clapham, D.E. The TRPM7 channel is inactivated by PIP_2 hydrolysis. *Nat. Cell Biol.* **2002**, *4*, 329–336. [CrossRef] [PubMed]

61. Dorovkov, M.V.; Ryazanov, A.G. Phosphorylation of annexin I by TRPM7 channel-kinase. *J. Biol. Chem.* **2004**, *279*, 50643–50646. [CrossRef] [PubMed]

62. Jin, J.; Desai, B.N.; Navarro, B.; Donovan, A.; Andrews, N.C.; Clapham, D.E. Deletion of Trpm7 disrupts embryonic development and thymopoiesis without altering Mg^{2+} homeostasis. *Science* **2008**, *322*, 756–760. [CrossRef] [PubMed]

63. Sahni, J.; Scharenberg, A.M. TRPM7 ion channels are required for sustained phosphoinositide 3-kinase signaling in lymphocytes. *Cell Metab.* **2008**, *8*, 84–93. [CrossRef] [PubMed]

64. Sahni, J.; Tamura, R.; Sweet, I.R.; Scharenberg, A.M. TRPM7 regulates quiescent/proliferative metabolic transitions in lymphocytes. *Cell Cycle* **2010**, *9*, 3565–3574. [CrossRef] [PubMed]

65. Clark, K.; Middlebeek, J.; Lasonder, E.; Dulyaninova, N.G.; Morrice, N.A.; Ryazanov, A.G.; Bresnick, A.R.; Figdor, C.G.; van Leeuwen, F.N. TRPM7 regulates myosin IIA filament stability and protein localization by heavy chain phosphorylation. *J. Mol. Biol.* **2008**, *378*, 790–803. [CrossRef] [PubMed]

66. Inoue, K.; Xiong, Z.-G. Silencing of TRPM7 promotes growth/proliferation and nitric oxide production of vascular endothelial cells via the ERK pathway. *Cardiovasc. Res.* **2009**, *83*, 547–557. [CrossRef] [PubMed]

67. Liu, M.; Inoue, K.; Leng, T.; Guo, S.; Xiong, Z.G. Trpm7 channels regulate glioma stem cell through stat3 and notch signaling pathways. *Cell. Signal.* **2014**, *26*, 2773–2781. [CrossRef] [PubMed]

68. Chubanov, V.; Schafer, S.; Ferioli, S.; Gudermann, T. Natural and Synthetic Modulators of the TRPM7 Channel. *Cells* **2014**, *3*, 1089–1101. [CrossRef] [PubMed]

69. Chubanov, V.; Schnitzler, M.M.; Meißner, M.; Schäfer, S.; Abstiens, K.; Hofmann, T.; Gudermann, T. Natural and synthetic modulators of SK (Kca2) potassium channels inhibit magnesium-dependent activity of the kinase-coupled cation channel TRPM7. *Br. J. Pharmacol.* **2012**, *166*, 1357–1376. [CrossRef] [PubMed]

70. Prakriya, M.; Lewis, R.S. Separation and characterization of currents through store-operated crac channels and Mg^{2+}-Inhibited Cation (MIC) channels. *J. Gen. Physiol.* **2002**, *119*, 487–507. [CrossRef] [PubMed]

71. Li, M.; Jiang, J.; Yue, L. Functional characterization homo- and heteromeric channel kinases TRPM6 and TRPM7. *J. Gen. Physiol.* **2006**, *127*, 525–537. [CrossRef] [PubMed]

72. Kozak, J.A.; Kerschbaum, H.H; Cahalan, M.D. Distinct properties of crac and mic channels in RBL cells. *J. Gen. Physiol.* **2002**, *120*, 221–235. [CrossRef] [PubMed]

73. Chen, X.; Numata, T.; Li, M.; Mori, Y.; Orser, B.A.; Jackson, M.F.; Xiong, Z.G.; MacDonald, J.F. The modulation of TRPM7 currents by nafamostat mesilate depends directly upon extracellular concentrations of divalent cations. *Mol. Brain* **2010**, *3*, 38. [CrossRef] [PubMed]

74. Parnas, M.; Peters, M.; Dadon, D.; Lev, S.; Vertkin, I.; Slutsky, I.; Minke, B. Carvacrol is a novel inhibitor of Drosophila TRPL and mammalian TRPM7 channels. *Cell Calcium* **2009**, *45*, 300–309. [CrossRef] [PubMed]

75. Chen, H.C.; Xie, J.; Zhang, Z.; Su, L.T.; Yue, L.; Runnels, L.W. Blockade of TRPM7 channel activity and cell death by inhibitors of 5-lipoxygenase. *PLoS ONE* **2010**, *5*, e11161. [CrossRef] [PubMed]

76. Qin, X.; Yue, Z.; Sun, B.; Yang, W.; Xie, J.; Ni, E.; Feng, Y.; Mahmood, R.; Zhang, Y.; Yue, L. Sphingosine and FTY720 are potent inhibitors of the transient receptor potential melastatin 7 (TRPM7) channels. *Br. J. Pharmacol.* **2013**, *168*, 1294–1312. [CrossRef] [PubMed]

77. Hofmann, T.; Schäfer, S.; Linseisen, M.; Sytik, L.; Gudermann, T.; Chubanov, V. Activation of TRPM7 channels by small molecules under physiological conditions. *Pflugers Arch.* **2014**, *466*, 2177–2189. [CrossRef] [PubMed]

78. Schäfer, S.; Ferioli, S.; Hofmann, T.; Sierler, S.; Gudermann, T.; Chubanov, V. Mibefradil represents a new class of benzimidazole TRPM7 channel agonists. *Pflugers Arch.* **2016**, *468*, 623–634. [CrossRef] [PubMed]

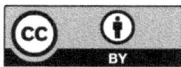

pharmaceuticals

MDPI

Review

TRP Channels as Therapeutic Targets in Diabetes and Obesity

Andrea Zsombok [1,2,*] and Andrei V. Derbenev [1]

[1] Department of Physiology, School of Medicine, Tulane University, New Orleans, LA 70112, USA; aderben@tulane.edu

[2] Department of Medicine, Endocrinology Section, School of Medicine, Tulane University, New Orleans, LA 70112, USA

* Correspondence: azsombo@tulane.edu; Tel.: +1-504-988-2597

Academic Editors: Arpad Szallasi and Susan M. Huang
Received: 3 June 2016; Accepted: 11 August 2016; Published: 17 August 2016

Abstract: During the last three to four decades the prevalence of obesity and diabetes mellitus has greatly increased worldwide, including in the United States. Both the short- and long-term forecasts predict serious consequences for the near future, and encourage the development of solutions for the prevention and management of obesity and diabetes mellitus. Transient receptor potential (TRP) channels were identified in tissues and organs important for the control of whole body metabolism. A variety of TRP channels has been shown to play a role in the regulation of hormone release, energy expenditure, pancreatic function, and neurotransmitter release in control, obese and/or diabetic conditions. Moreover, dietary supplementation of natural ligands of TRP channels has been shown to have potential beneficial effects in obese and diabetic conditions. These findings raised the interest and likelihood for potential drug development. In this mini-review, we discuss possibilities for better management of obesity and diabetes mellitus based on TRP-dependent mechanisms.

Keywords: TRPV1; TRPM; TRPA1; obesity; diabetes mellitus; metabolism; glucose homeostasis

1. Introduction

The World Health Organization estimates that obesity doubled between 1980 and 2014, with 39% of adults being overweight and 13% being obese in 2014. In the United States the statistics are similarly alarming, more than one-third of the adults are obese and 17% of youth are also obese [1,2]. The consequences of obesity are severe including higher mortality rate, hypertension, dyslipidemia, heart disease, stroke, type 2 diabetes mellitus (T2DM), and many more.

Among the various pathophysiological conditions, T2DM is very prevalent and affects approximately 10% of the population worldwide. Lifestyle changes including weight loss can result in better glucose management; however, lifestyle changes require disciplined behavior and frequent monitoring. Unfortunately, patients often give up before reaching their goals or detectable results. In recent years, bariatric surgery has emerged as an effective treatment for improvement or remission of T2DM; however, due to the invasiveness of the procedure and potential surgical complications, bariatric surgery is not the most feasible solution. The most common treatments are still pharmacological interventions. Current pharmacological treatments mainly target the end organs by increasing insulin secretion from pancreatic beta cells (e.g., sulfonylureas), increasing tissue sensitivity to insulin (e.g., metformin), modulating the glucagon-like peptide 1 (GLP-1) system, preventing glucose reabsorption in the kidneys (SGLT2 inhibitors) or administering insulin. Despite the existing treatments, new therapeutic interventions are in great demand, therefore, every new idea, pathway, receptor, or compound (natural or synthetic) which has the potential of developing a new class of drugs for weight and/or glucose management receives attention.

Members of the transient receptor potential (TRP) family have been identified as key contributors in many physiological and pathophysiological conditions [3]. TRP channels were identified in numerous metabolically important tissues. Members of the canonical (TRPC), melastatin (TRPM), ankyrin (TRPA1), and vanilloid (TRPV) subfamilies were found to be expressed in the pancreas [3,4], liver, gastrointestinal tract [5], skeletal muscle, kidney [6–8], adipose tissue [9–12], heart [13–15], vasculature [16–18], and nervous system [19,20], including autonomic centers of the brain [21,22]. Despite that TRP channels and their natural ligands received considerable attention in the field of obesity and diabetes [4,23–28], their role in many of the metabolic processes are still debated and under investigation. This mini-review summarizes findings demonstrating functional roles of TRP channels in obese and diabetic conditions.

2. TRPV1 for the Prevention and Treatment of Obesity and Diabetes Mellitus

TRPV1 is one of the most studied TRP channels even in the context of obesity and diabetes mellitus. TRPV1, the first described member of the vanilloid subfamily, was cloned in 1997 [29]. It is a nonselective cation channel with permeability to Ca^{2+}. In the past decades TRPV1 was extensively researched and investigated as potential drug target for a variety of applications [23,30,31]. Numerous findings related to TRPV1 including its structure, species-related differences, topology, agonists, antagonists, cellular mechanisms, and pharmacological applicability can be found elsewhere including in a review by Nilius and Szallasi [23]. TRPV1 is activated by a variety of exogenous and endogenous ligands [23,32]. Among the well-known exogenous ligands, capsaicin—the pungent ingredient of hot peppers—is investigated the most for its beneficial effects on body weight and metabolism. Capsaicin-binding site of TRPV1 is intracellular [33]. Activation of TRPV1 results in influx of cations and leads to depolarization of the cell [34,35]. Capsaicin specifically binds to TRPV1; however, we have to keep in mind that capsaicin is able to cause disruption in the organization of membranes due to its localization in the lipid bilayer [36–38]. This might have important implications for delivery of drug molecules and may result in a TRPV1-independent effect.

Among the numerous physiological functions, TRPV1 has been proposed to have functional roles in a variety of metabolically important tissues including the pancreas [39,40], gastrointestinal tract [41], adipose tissue [9,12], and nervous system [21,42]. In this section, based on human and animal model studies, we provide a brief overview of TRPV1's potential for improvement of obese and diabetic conditions.

2.1. Dietary Interventions and Possible Mechanisms in Human and Animal Model Studies

Ingredients of spices, such as capsaicin in red peppers, are well-known for a variety of effects. Recently, Nilius and Appendino published a detailed overview about the beneficial science of spices, focusing on TRPs [28], while in this section we summarize dietary interventions and potential underlying mechanisms related to TRPV1.

Previous studies in male human subjects examined the effects of red pepper diet and demonstrated a trend for increased energy expenditure (EE), significantly higher carbohydrate oxidation, and lower lipid oxidation [43]. This increased EE immediately after a red pepper containing meal was proposed to be due to beta-adrenergic stimulation [43]. Increased carbohydrate oxidation and elevated epinephrine and norepinephrine levels following dietary red pepper ingestion were confirmed in men by another study [44].

In Japanese female subjects, diet-induced thermogenesis and lipid oxidation was higher following red pepper diet compared to the control diet [45]. On the other hand, Matsumoto and co-workers found that diet-induced thermogenesis was increased in the age- and height-matched lean control group; however, there was no thermogenic response detected in the obese group [46]. The study demonstrated that despite the identical resting sympathovagal activities, reduced sympathetic responsiveness to the capsaicin diet exists in obese females. This reduced sympathetic responsiveness likely leads to impairment of the diet-induced thermogenic response and could be an important factor in the development of obesity in female subjects [46].

A crossover study with male and female participants also aimed to determine the effect of a capsaicin-containing lunch on EE and hormone levels [47]. This study revealed increased GLP-1 levels and a decreasing trend in ghrelin levels; however, no effect on satiety, EE, and peptide YY levels were observed [47]. The negative finding on satiety was in disagreement with a previous study from the same group, in which significantly higher feelings of satiety were seen after capsaicin supplementation over two days compared to placebo [48]. The authors suggested that the satiety feeling observed after capsaicin need to be built up, and the postprandial state may mask the effects of capsaicin in general [47,48].

Many of the studies demonstrating beneficial findings of capsaicin investigated a single meal in a small group of lean subjects [45,49], while other studies focused on determining the effects of weeks long chili diet. The effect of daily ingestion of chili pepper for four weeks was investigated on the resistance of serum lipoproteins to oxidation in healthy men and women [50]. The rate of oxidation was lower following the chili pepper diet compared to the bland diet, suggesting that regular consumption of the chili diet for an extended period inhibits oxidation of serum lipoproteins; however, in addition to capsaicin, other ingredients of chili pepper can contribute to these findings [50].

On the other hand, the same group revealed no obvious beneficial or harmful effects on metabolic and vascular parameters, but suggested that four week long chili consumption may reduce resting heart rate and increase effective myocardial perfusion pressure time in men [51].

A crossover intervention study by the same group used two dietary periods of four weeks each and measured EE, serum insulin, C-peptide, and glucose levels following a bland meal after bland diet, a chili meal after bland diet, and a chili meal after chili-containing diet and suggested that regular consumption of chili may attenuate postprandial hyperinsulinemia [52].

Lejeune and co-workers revealed no difference in body weight maintenance after body weight loss following capsaicin consumption for multiple weeks compared to the placebo group [53]. However, substrate oxidation was affected by capsaicin, which was consistent with the observation of a short-term study by Yoshioka [54].

In general, as demonstrated by the abovementioned examples, in human subjects there are controversial findings regarding capsaicin containing diets, and clearly more detailed studies are necessary to make a conclusion about the dietary effects of capsaicin and TRPV1-activating supplements. We also have to note that many variables including age, metabolic status, postprandial state, sex, the diet itself (e.g., chili pepper vs. capsaicin), and many more can profoundly influence or even mask the metabolic effects in the above-discussed human studies.

Despite that the animal model studies are more mechanistic, they also revealed controversial findings about the metabolic effects of TRPV1 activation. Major dietary and topical interventions in obese and diabetic conditions were recently reviewed in more detail [4,26]. Briefly, it has been reported that TRPV1 activation with capsaicin prevented adipogenesis and obesity [9]. The study verified TRPV1 expression in 3T3-L1-preadipocytes and visceral adipose tissue from mice and humans. The findings revealed that capsaicin dose-dependently increased intracellular calcium in 3T3-L1-preadipocytes, which indicates inhibition of preadipocytes' differentiation. The capsaicin-dependent calcium increase was significantly lower in mature adipocytes compared to preadipocytes, which was consistent with the observed TRPV1 downregulation during adipogenesis [9]. This study also revealed that both db/db and ob/ob mice have lower TRPV1 expression in their visceral adipose tissue compared with the lean controls. Indeed, lower TRPV1 expression was determined in visceral and subcutaneous adipose tissue of obese men compared to lean men [9]. These observations suggest that downregulation of TRPV1 in visceral adipose tissue is a common finding both in animal models of obesity and diabetes, and in human subjects.

Dietary capsaicin (0.01%) did not affect the body weight of mice on normal chow diet; however, dietary supplementation of capsaicin to high fat diet (HFD) treated mice prevented obesity, which was not observed in TRPV1 knockout mice [9]. The prevention of obesity was associated with small adipocyte size and increased TRPV1 expression. These findings suggest that activation of TRPV1 triggers calcium influx, and leads to prevention of adipogenesis and TRPV1 downregulation that may result in attenuation of obesity in mice kept on HFD.

A more recent study evaluated the effect of dietary capsaicin (0.01%) on browning of white adipose tissue (WAT) [55]. Capsaicin diet prevented the weight gain of wild type mice on HFD, while this effect was not observed in TRPV1 knockout mice. HFD downregulated the expression of TRPV1 in epididymal and subcutaneous fat pads, and the capsaicin diet prevented this downregulation and caused browning of WAT. The prevention of obesity was associated with increased uncoupling protein 1 (UCP1) expression levels, and increased sirtuin-1 expression and activity. These findings were due to TRPV1-dependent increase of Ca^{2+} and phosphorylation of CaMKII and AMPK. TRPV1 activation elevated metabolic and ambulatory activities and induced browning of WAT likely via peroxisome proliferator-activated receptor gamma (PPAR-γ)/PRDM-16 interaction [55]. These results suggest that TRPV1 activation could be used to promote browning of WAT and thus decrease obesity (Table 1).

Table 1. Transient receptor potential (TRP) channels and their potential role in metabolism.

Title	TRPV1	TRPA1	TRPM2	TRPM3	TRPM5
Natural ligands for dietary interventions	capsaicin; red pepper; chili; capsaicinoids; capsiate	cinnamon; cinnamaldehyde; AITC			
Synthetic small molecule modulators	BCTC [56]; AZV1 [57]; AMG 517	methyl syringate [58]; glibenclamide [59]		CIM0216 [60]	
Pancreas	insulin + [40]	insulin + [59,61]	insulin + [62,63]	insulin + [60,64,65]	insulin + [66]
GI hormones and GI tract	GLP-1 + [47] ghrelin − [47]	GLP-1 + [67] ghrelin − [68]; peptide YY [58]; gastric and gut motility − [58,68]			GLP-1 + [69]
WAT	adipogenesis − [9]; browning + [12,55]; fat oxidation + [45,70]; leptin − [70,71]; adiponectin + [72]	fat oxidation + [68]; leptin − [73]			
BAT	thermogenesis + [12,45,46,71]	thermogenesis + [73,74]			
Nervous system	satiety + [48]; neuronal excitability + [21,22,42]; gene expression [71]	gene expression [73]	neuronal excitability [75]		neuronal excitability + [76]

AITC: allyl isothiocyanate; GLP-1: glucagon-like peptide 1; +: increase, −: decrease.

We have to mention that in addition to TRPV1, TRPV3 and TRPV4 have been shown to have functional roles in adipocytes. Recently, higher expression of TRPV3 was found in adipocytes when compared to other TRPVs. Activation of TRPV3 was shown to prevent lipid accumulation and adipogenesis by inhibiting the phosphorylation of insulin receptor substrate 1 and the expression of PPAR-γ [77]. Moreover, HFD-treated, db/db, and ob/ob mice had reduced TRPV3 expression in their visceral adipose tissue, whereas chronic treatment with TRPV3 agonists prevented adipogenesis and weight gain in HFD-treated mice [77].

In contrast, Ye and co-workers found that TRPV1, TRPV2, and TRPV4 mRNA are expressed in 3TT-F442A adipocytes, but their study showed a lack of TRPV3 mRNA. TRPV4 was expressed at the highest level [78], which confirmed previous observations revealing TRPV4 expression in adipose tissue [79]. Furthermore, Ye's paper determined that TRPV4 is a negative regulator of oxidative metabolism and it controls proinflammatory gene programming. In TRPV4 knockout mice the subcutaneous adipose tissue showed higher UCP1 mRNA and protein expression levels compared to controls. Elevated EE was found in the TRPV4 knockout mice, which was associated with the elevated thermogenic gene programming. In addition, TRPV4 knockout mice were protected from diet-induced obesity and insulin resistance [78]. Taken together, strong evidence suggests that TRPVs including TRPV1, TRPV3, and TRPV4 likely have important functional roles in adipocytes.

The effect of dietary hot pepper (1%) was determined to be beneficial to attenuate diet-induced obesity in rabbits [80]. TRPV1 mRNA was detected in various tissues of the rabbit with high similarity to human TRPV1. Rabbits fed with dietary hot pepper consumed similar amount of food; however, the hot pepper fed group gained less weight compared to the control group. This was associated with decreased adipose tissue and ratio of adipose tissue to body weight [80]. On the other hand, previous studies found that rabbits are insensitive to capsaicin and do not have resiniferatoxin binding sites [81]. It was later found that two amino acid substitutions in rabbit TRPV1 render the protein >100-fold less sensitive to vanilloids and RTX [82]. Therefore, it is debatable that the beneficial effects of dietary hot pepper observed by Yu [80] are mediated by capsaicin-dependent TRPV1 activation.

Male C57Bl/6 mice were kept on HFD for ten weeks and then received capsaicin (0.015%) supplement [70]. Dietary capsaicin resulted in lower fasting glucose, insulin, and leptin levels. In addition, it also attenuated the impairment of glucose tolerance, likely by reducing inflammatory responses and increasing fatty acid oxidation [70]. In another study by the same group, genetically obese diabetic mice (KKAy) were subjected to an HFD for two weeks then received capsaicin [72]. Dietary capsaicin reduced fasting glucose, insulin, and triglyceride levels, while adiponectin levels and its receptor expression were increased and inflammatory gene expression was decreased, resulting in reduced metabolic dysregulation.

In Swiss albino mice the effect of three month long treatment with capsaicin (2 mg/kg) plus HFD were compared with control diet and HFD [71]. The results demonstrated that capsaicin supplementation to HFD modulated hypothalamic satiety genes, altered gut microbial composition, induced browning of subcutaneous WAT, and increased thermogenesis in brown adipose tissue (BAT). Capsaicin-treated mice on HFD gained less weight than mice on HFD only. Fasting glucose levels were not different among the groups, whereas leptin and TNFα levels were decreased in the capsaicin-treated mice compared with the HFD group [71]. Hypothalamic expression of TRPV1 was downregulated in HDF mice and capsaicin treatment increased TRPV1 expression. Anorectic genes including peptide YY, brain-derived neurotrophic factor (BDNF) and CART prepropeptide were enhanced in capsaicin-treated HDF mice compared with HFD mice, while expression of orexigenic genes were reduced following capsaicin in the diet, with the exception of melanin-concentrating hormone receptor 1, hypocretin (orexin), and neuropeptide Y (NPY) [71]. The authors hypothesized that capsaicin activates vagal TRPV1 or afferent nerves in the gastrointestinal tract and thus influences hypothalamic TRPV1 and other genes' expression.

Furthermore, TRPV1 is also known to modulate insulin secretion and pancreatic function, including development of islet inflammation and type 1 diabetes mellitus. These findings were described and reviewed earlier in detail [23–26,39,83].

2.2. Behind the Scene: Activating or Antagonizing TRPV1 for Treating Obesity and Diabetes Mellitus

Despite that various studies investigated TRPV1 activation, it is not clear whether activation or inhibition would be a better approach for the modulation of metabolism. Capsaicin-desensitized rats were protected from obesity despite atrophied BAT [11,84,85]. The body weight of capsaicin-desensitized rats was significantly lower 14 and 32 weeks after treatment. The lower body weight was associated with reduced food intake, smaller epididymal and retroperitoneal WAT depots, smaller interscapular BAT, decreased total protein, UCP, and cytochrome oxidase in BAT; however, the resting metabolic rate and colonic temperature of the groups were not different [11].

On the other hand, adult male rats, which were neonatally treated with capsaicin, did not differ in body weight, basal plasma leptin, or fasting leptin, insulin, adiponectin, and corticosterone levels [86]. Glucose levels following intravenous glucose tolerance tests were similar in the capsaicin-treated and vehicle-treated rats [86]. However, the capsaicin-treated rats displayed reduced plasma insulin and corticosterone responses, indicating increased insulin sensitivity and lower plasma corticosterone levels [86]. The increased insulin sensitivity was also supported by euglycemic hyperinsulinemic clamp studies [87]. Koopmans and co-workers suggested that adult rats with neonatal capsaicin treatment exhibit decreased corticosterone levels, which could contribute to amplified insulin action during hyperglycemia [86].

Studies using TRPV1 knockout mice also revealed conflicting results. On one hand, TRPV1 knockout mice gained less weight following HFD compared with wild-type mice [88]. In this study wild-type and TRPV1 knockout mice had similar energy intake, but TRPV1 knockout mice had greater thermogenic capacity. In contrast, in a more recent study TRPV1 knockout mice kept on HFD became more obese than the wild-type mice kept on the same HFD [89]. TRPV1 knockout mice on HFD were significantly heavier than the wild-type mice after one month of HFD, which was mainly due to increased whole-body fat mass. Indirect calorimetry demonstrated increased food intake of TRPV1 knockout mice on day 3. Decreased physical activity was observed during the night-cycle, which was consistent with reduced night-cycle energy expenditure rates in TRPV1 knockout mice [89]. TRPV1 knockout mice also developed more severe insulin and leptin resistance and they exhibited dysfunctional hypothalamic leptin signaling.

Marshall and co-workers investigated metabolic and cardiovascular parameters and found that wild-type and TRPV1 knockout mice gain a similar amount of weight on HFD [27]. In wild-type mice, HFD was associated with increased mean arterial pressure, which was not observed in TRPV1 knockout mice. Furthermore, parameters of vascular hypertrophy showed an increase in wild-type mice on HFD compared with TRPV1 knockout mice on HFD and mice on normal chow [27]. In the HFD-treated groups, baseline glucose levels showed an increasing trend, and impaired glucose tolerance was observed. Interestingly, glucose levels normalized faster in TRPV1 knockout mice, which was indicated by the area under the curve. Interleukin 10 and 1β levels were significantly elevated in wild-type, but not in TRPV1 knockout mice [27]. Based on their findings the authors suggested that TRPV1 deletion may be protective against obesity-induced hypertension, and that TRPV1 may contribute to the development of cardiometabolic disturbances. The role of TRP channels in the cardiovascular system can be found elsewhere [90].

Promising findings have been identified with TRPV1 antagonists. Since agonists can prevent TRPV1 signaling by desensitizing the receptor [17], TRPV1 antagonists may influence TRPV1 signaling by antagonizing the receptor, and thus improve obese and/or diabetic conditions. BCTC *N*-(4-tertiarybutylphenyl)-4-(3-chloropyridin-2-yl)tetrahydropyrazine-1(2*H*)-carbox-amide, a TRPV1 antagonist has been shown to inhibit TRPV1 signaling in cultured cells and was found to decrease inflammation and neuropathic pain in vivo [91,92]. Tanaka and co-workers investigated the effect of BCTC on whole-body glucose and lipid metabolism in ob/ob mice and compared the effect of BCTC with pioglitazone, an insulin sensitizer [56]. The insulin-resistant, hyperinsulinemic ob/ob mice were treated with BCTC or pioglitazone twice a day for four weeks. Plasma glucose levels were decreased with a high dose BCTC (100 mg/kg) and the decrease was similar to pioglitazone. Plasma insulin levels showed a dose-dependent decreasing trend following BCTC treatment, but significance was observed only in the pioglitazone group [56]. Plasma triglyceride levels were significantly lower both in the BCTC and pioglitazone-treated mice, which was accompanied with a decreasing trend in calcitonin gene-related peptide. The oral glucose tolerance test indicated that BCTC increased insulin secretion, but likely in a different way than pioglitazone, even though glucose tolerance was improved by both drugs [56]. The authors also reported that BCTC did not alter insulin or glucose levels in normoglycemic control mice, indicating that inhibiting TRPV1 could be more important during the diabetic condition [56]. In summary, BCTC was shown to improve insulin resistance, which may be due to inhibiting TRPV1 in adipocytes and skeletal muscle. On the other hand, increased insulin secretion was associated with BCTC in diabetic ob/ob mice. These findings suggest that BCTC may have a dual effect by improving insulin resistance and enhancing insulin secretion in ob/ob mice. We also have to note that BCTC is an antagonist of TRPM8 and we cannot exclude a possible effect and/or interaction with TRPM8 channels [93].

More recently, at the European Association for the Study of Diabetes 2015, a novel TRPV1 antagonist, AZV1 by Astra Zeneca, was shown to improve insulin sensitivity in ob/ob mice [57]. Mice were treated daily with the TRPV1 antagonist AZV1 or vehicle for eight days. Body weight of TRPV1 antagonist-treated mice was not different compared with vehicle-treated mice; however, the glucose control of ob/ob mice was improved. Glucose levels, homeostatic model assessment and fructosamine levels of the TRPV1 antagonist-treated mice were significantly decreased compared with vehicle-treated mice. Moreover, increased liver weight was observed in the TRPV1 antagonist treated mice [57]. The data demonstrated that AZV1 was well-tolerated without effects on food intake or body weight, but it exerted an antidiabetic effect, which may be due to improved insulin sensitivity. Findings from these two studies suggest that TRPV1 antagonism could be useful for the treatment of type 2 diabetes mellitus; however, we have to note that these antagonist studies did not investigate potential temperature changes.

Taken together, the beneficial effects of TRPV1 could be valuable; however, there are numerous unanswered questions about the mechanisms underlying the findings. These include sensitization vs. desensitization, important cell types/tissues/pathways underlying the effects (e.g., pancreatic beta cells vs. sensory nerves), or the contribution of the sympathetic nervous system.

3. Role of TRPM Channels in Metabolism

Members of the TRPM family have highly variable permeability to Ca^{2+} and they lack the N-terminal ankyrin repeats [23,94]. TRPM channels including TRPM2, TRPM3, TRPM4, and TRPM5 were identified as candidates to play a role in the regulation of metabolism [4].

Comprehensive metabolic studies were conducted to determine insulin sensitivity of TRPM2 knockout mice [95]. TRPM2 knockout mice were more insulin-sensitive due to increased glucose metabolism in the heart. TRPM2 knockout mice exerted increased EE and elevated expression levels of metabolic genes including peroxisome proliferator-activated receptor alpha (PPARα) and PPARγ co-activator-1 alpha and 1 beta in WAT resulting in resistance to HFD. The hyperinsulinemic euglycemic clamp studies showed that TRPM2 knockout mice are more insulin-sensitive and have elevated Akt and glycogen synthase kinase 3β phosphorylation in the heart, and reduced inflammation in the liver and adipose tissue [95]. These findings demonstrated that TRPM2 likely plays an important role in whole-body metabolism.

TRPM2, in addition to TRPM3, TRPM4, and TRPM5, was described in rodent insulinoma cell lines and in mouse islets. Moreover, transcripts of TRPM2, TRPM4 and TRPM5 have been identified in human islets [96,97], suggesting that they may have an important functional role in the regulation of pancreatic function and insulin secretion. TRPM2 is activated by a variety of stimuli including reactive oxygen species (e.g., H_2O_2), glucose, and incretins [62,98,99]. In TRPM2 knockout mice plasma insulin levels were reduced and glucose clearance was impaired. This was associated with decreased insulin secretion initiated by incretins and glucose, and was supported by the observation that in the β cells of TRPM2 knockout mice the increase of intracellular Ca^{2+} was impaired following stimulation with incretins or insulin [99]. Since TRPM2 activity can be modulated by adenine dinucleotides, intracellular Ca^{2+} levels, and incretin-induced PKA phosphorylation, the regulation of TRPM2 can be more complex; however, it is undoubtedly an important mechanism for insulin secretion [62]. Involvement of TRPM2 in type 1 and type 2 diabetes mellitus has been suggested and the current hypotheses, including impairment in insulin secretion due to dysfunction of TRPM2, have been discussed in detail previously [63].

TRPM3 is important for Zn^{2+} entry in β cells and might contribute to insulin synthesis [100]. This is supported by recent studies, which demonstrated expression of TRPM3 in rat pancreatic INS-1 insulinoma cells and in mouse pancreatic islets [101]. Previously it had been revealed that pregnenolone sulfate, a canonical TRPM3 agonist, induces Ca^{2+} influx. The increase of Ca^{2+} is due to activation of TRPM3 and L-type Ca^{2+} channels, and upregulation of genes, which lead to insulin secretion [64,65]. Recently, the roles of TRPM3 and L-type Ca^{2+} channels were clarified [101]. The authors concluded that both TRPM3 and L-type Ca^{2+} channels are necessary for the pregnenolone sulfate mediated gene stimulation in INS-1 cells cultured in low-glucose medium. These data suggest that activation of TRPM3 following pregnenolone sulfate stimulation leads to an initial Ca^{2+} influx followed by activation of L-type Ca^{2+} channels [65,101].

More recently, a synthetic small-molecule TRPM3 agonist, CIM0216, has been shown to stimulate insulin release [60]. Pregnenolone sulfate, the well-known agonist of TRPM3 and CIM0216, caused Ca^{2+} increase in pancreatic islets and a dose-dependent increase of insulin release. The increase of insulin release was not observed in TRPM3-deficient islets, further confirming the findings [60].

TRPM4 has been identified in several β cell lines suggesting non-species specific TRPM4 expression [102]. TRPM4 currents were characterized with a biphasic pattern following Ca^{2+} perfusion; however, the activation and inactivation time varied among cell lines. Inhibition of TRPM4 decreased the magnitude of Ca^{2+} signals, and it has been shown that blockade of TRPM4 decreased glucose stimulated insulin secretion in INS-1 cells [103]. Marigo and co-workers suggested that in β cells, TRPM4 may have a critical role in the regulation of membrane potential oscillations during glucose stimulation [102,103]. In contrast, TRPM4 knockout mice did not show differences in glucose tolerance test and glucose-induced insulin secretion from isolated islets compared to wild-type mice [104,105]. In addition, TRPM4 was proposed to be involved in glucagon secretion [105].

TRPM5 is important for the Ca^{2+} activated cation current in pancreatic β cells since this current was reduced in TRPM5 knockout mice [66]. TRPM5 is suggested to play crucial role during glucose stimulation, and it is likely responsible for the fast glucose-induced oscillations of membrane potential and Ca^{2+} [66]. These fast oscillations are more efficient to trigger insulin release [106]. Furthermore, impaired glucose tolerance was observed in TRPM5 knockout mice, supporting an important role for TRPM5 in the regulation of metabolism [66]. Its role in the control of metabolism is further demonstrated by the existence of TRPM5 in the enteroendocrine cells in the gastrointestinal tract. Specifically, TRPM5 is expressed in the GLP-1 secreting L-cells, which are important for controlling proper glucose homeostasis [69].

In addition, TRPM5 plays a role in taste signaling, and TRPM5 knockout mice develop severe impairment in sweet, bitter, and umami taste signaling [107–109]. Interestingly, members of taste signaling pathways including TRPM5 were identified in gastrointestinal L-cells, suggesting that sweet taste signaling is directly involved in the release of GLP-1, and thus can have an important role in glucose-mediated control of metabolism [69]. Manipulation of taste is also an approach of pharmacological interventions for obesity prevention, and TRPM5 has been investigated for potential taste modifications; details can be found elsewhere [110,111]. In addition, TRPM2, TRPM4, and TRPM5 channels are identified in the brain and may play a role in neuronal excitability, cell death, or neurodegeneration; however, their functional role in autonomic centers has not been described [19,75,76] (Table 1).

4. Implications for TRPA1

TRPA1, currently the only member of the ankyrin family, was named after the high number of ankyrin repeats. TRPA1 is a voltage-dependent, Ca^{2+}-permeable cation channel. Like many of the TRP channels, TRPA1 is also modulated by herbal compounds, suggesting the potential for alternative dietary therapies. One of the natural compounds activating TRPA1 is cinnamon, a widely used spice, which originates from the bark of trees of the *Cinnamomum* genus. In one study, cinnamon treatment has been shown to improve the glucose and lipid profiles of type 2 diabetic patients [112], while other studies showed moderate improvement of glucose levels [113] or no effect [114]. We have to note that age, sex, length of the disease, and many other variables may play a role in the outcome of the human studies; therefore, it is too early to make a conclusion regarding the dietary benefits of cinnamon.

One of the main ingredients of cinnamon is cinnamaldehyde, which is a potent agonist of TRPA1. Cinnamaldehyde effect was associated with inhibition of ghrelin secretion and gastric emptying, whereas improved insulin sensitivity was observed [68]. In mice fed with high-fat high-sucrose diet, cinnamaldehyde ingestion was associated with reduced visceral adipose tissue [115] and increased fatty acid oxidation [68]. Recently it was shown that cinnamaldehyde (10 mg/kg) administration prevented the increase of weight gain caused by HFD [73]. Serum leptin levels and leptin/ghrelin ratio, a marker of weight gain, were decreased in the cinnamaldehyde-treated HFD groups. In addition, cinnamaldehyde treatment increased the expression levels of anorexigenic genes including pro-opiomelanocortin, urocortin, BDNF, and cholecystokinin [73]. The study also determined that cinnamaldehyde prevented visceral WAT accumulation, increased BAT activity and reduced inflammation, but did not affect gut microbial composition. Improved fasting blood glucose levels and glucose tolerance were observed in ob/ob mice following cinnamon extract treatment [116]. This was associated with improved insulin sensitivity, locomotor activity and improved brain activity.

Allyl isothiocyanate (AITC), an ingredient of mustard, horseradish, and wasabi, is also a potent TRPA1 agonist. It has been shown that intravenous injection of AITC induces adrenalin secretion. This response was attenuated in the presence of cholinergic blockers, suggesting activation of the adrenal sympathetic nerve through the central nervous system [117]. AITC increased thermogenesis and expression of UPC1 [74]. Recently, dietary AITC was reported to protect against free fatty acid induced insulin resistance, and it increased mitochondrial activity in skeletal muscle cells [118]. Dietary AITC reduced diet-induced obesity in C57Bl/6 mice and improved blood lipid profile compared to HFD-treated mice. AITC also reduced high fat induced hepatic steatosis and decreased hyperglycemia, hyperinsulinemia, HbA1C levels and ameliorated insulin resistance [118]. These findings suggest that activation of TRPA1 likely have beneficial effects; however, further studies are necessary to reveal the exact underlying mechanisms.

Multiple methodological approaches were used to reveal TRPA1 expression in rat pancreatic cells [61]. Expression of TRPA1 was confirmed in beta, but not in glucagon-secreting alpha cells, and activation of TRPA1 stimulated insulin release synergistically with ATP-dependent potassium channel (K_{ATP}) blockade [61]. The latter is further supported with the findings that glibenclamide, a widely used K_{ATP} channel inhibitor is an agonist of TRPA1 [59], and it has been suggested that the synergistic effect of TRPA1 and K_{ATP} channels underlies the hyperinsulinism in patients with glibenclamide treatment.

Similar to TRPM5, TRPA1 is expressed in L-cells and TRPA1 agonist administration into the duodenum or by gavage increased GLP-1 secretion [67]. On the other hand, the effect was not eliminated in TRPA1 knockout mice. GLP-1 levels did not change following activation of TRPA1 despite elevation of peptide YY, and reduced gastric emptying and food intake [58]. In dogs, following AITC, gastric and jejunum motility was increased, and this effect was prevented with ruthenium red [119]. The potential role of TRPA1 on pancreatic, adipose tissue, and the autonomic nervous system and its importance as a dietary supplement has been recently reviewed [26].

5. Conclusions

TRP channels are expressed in many tissues and organs important for the maintenance of whole body metabolism. Results from dietary supplementation of TRP ligands (e.g., capsaicin) are controversial, either showing beneficial effects on body weight, metabolism, and hormone levels, or no effects. The target tissue of the dietary supplementation is not entirely clear since many tissues including the adipose tissue, the pancreas, and even the central nervous system could be modulated by the components of the diet. TRP channels have benefits; however, currently it is not clear whether activation or inhibition, central or peripheral mechanisms, diet or topical administration, or even which tissue/organ is the most critical. In summary, further research is needed before final conclusions are available, but undoubtedly TRP channels are good potential targets for weight and diabetes management.

Acknowledgments: The authors acknowledge funding support from the National Institutes of Health (R01 DK099598 for AZs and HL122829 for AVD).

Conflicts of Interest: The authors declare no conflict of interest.

References

1. Ogden, C.L.; Carroll, M.D.; Kit, B.K.; Flegal, K.M. Prevalence of childhood and adult obesity in the United States, 2011–2012. *JAMA* **2014**, *311*, 806–814. [CrossRef] [PubMed]
2. Ogden, C.L.; Carroll, M.D.; Fryar, C.D.; Flegal, K.M. Prevalence of obesity among adults and youth: United States, 2011–2014. *NCHS Data Brief* **2015**, *219*, 1–8. [PubMed]
3. Jacobson, D.A.; Philipson, L.H. TRP channels of the pancreatic β cell. *Handb. Exp. Pharmacol.* **2007**, 409–424. [CrossRef]
4. Zhu, Z.; Luo, Z.; Ma, S.; Liu, D. TRP channels and their implications in metabolic diseases. *Pflug. Arch.* **2011**, *461*, 211–223. [CrossRef] [PubMed]
5. Yu, X.; Yu, M.; Liu, Y.; Yu, S. TRP channel functions in the gastrointestinal tract. *Semin. Immunopathol.* **2016**, *38*, 385–396. [CrossRef] [PubMed]
6. Kunert-Keil, C.; Bisping, F.; Kruger, J.; Brinkmeier, H. Tissue-specific expression of TRP channel genes in the mouse and its variation in three different mouse strains. *BMC Genom.* **2006**, *7*, 159. [CrossRef] [PubMed]
7. Feng, N.H.; Lee, H.H.; Shiang, J.C.; Ma, M.C. Transient receptor potential vanilloid type 1 channels act as mechanoreceptors and cause substance p release and sensory activation in rat kidneys. *Am. J. Physiol. Ren. Physiol.* **2008**, *294*, F316–F325. [CrossRef] [PubMed]
8. Tomilin, V.; Mamenko, M.; Zaika, O.; Pochynyuk, O. Role of renal TRP channels in physiology and pathology. *Semin. Immunopathol.* **2016**, *38*, 371–383. [CrossRef] [PubMed]
9. Zhang, L.L.; Liu, D.Y.; Ma, L.Q.; Luo, Z.D.; Cao, T.B.; Zhong, J.; Yan, Z.C.; Wang, L.J.; Zhao, Z.G.; Zhu, S.J.; et al. Activation of transient receptor potential vanilloid type-1 channel prevents adipogenesis and obesity. *Circ. Res.* **2007**, *100*, 1063–1070. [CrossRef] [PubMed]
10. Lee, G.R.; Shin, M.K.; Yoon, D.J.; Kim, A.R.; Yu, R.; Park, N.H.; Han, I.S. Topical application of capsaicin reduces visceral adipose fat by affecting adipokine levels in high-fat diet-induced obese mice. *Obesity* **2013**, *21*, 115–122. [CrossRef] [PubMed]
11. Cui, J.; Himms-Hagen, J. Long-term decrease in body fat and in brown adipose tissue in capsaicin-desensitized rats. *Am. J. Physiol.* **1992**, *262*, R568–R573. [PubMed]
12. Baboota, R.K.; Singh, D.P.; Sarma, S.M.; Kaur, J.; Sandhir, R.; Boparai, R.K.; Kondepudi, K.K.; Bishnoi, M. Capsaicin induces "brite" phenotype in differentiating 3T3-L1 preadipocytes. *PLoS ONE* **2014**, *9*, e103093.
13. Zvara, A.; Bencsik, P.; Fodor, G.; Csont, T.; Hackler, L., Jr.; Dux, M.; Furst, S.; Jancso, G.; Puskas, L.G.; Ferdinandy, P. Capsaicin-sensitive sensory neurons regulate myocardial function and gene expression pattern of rat hearts: A DNA microarray study. *FASEB J.* **2006**, *20*, 160–162. [CrossRef] [PubMed]
14. Watanabe, H.; Murakami, M.; Ohba, T.; Ono, K.; Ito, H. The pathological role of transient receptor potential channels in heart disease. *Circ. J.* **2009**, *73*, 419–427. [CrossRef] [PubMed]
15. Thilo, F.; Liu, Y.; Schulz, N.; Gergs, U.; Neumann, J.; Loddenkemper, C.; Gollasch, M.; Tepel, M. Increased transient receptor potential vanilloid type 1 (TRPV1) channel expression in hypertrophic heart. *Biochem. Biophys. Res. Commun.* **2010**, *401*, 98–103. [CrossRef] [PubMed]
16. Liu, D.; Maier, A.; Scholze, A.; Rauch, U.; Boltzen, U.; Zhao, Z.; Zhu, Z.; Tepel, M. High glucose enhances transient receptor potential channel canonical type 6-dependent calcium influx in human platelets via phosphatidylinositol 3-kinase-dependent pathway. *Arterioscler. Thromb. Vasc. Biol.* **2008**, *28*, 746–751. [CrossRef] [PubMed]
17. Lizanecz, E.; Bagi, Z.; Pasztor, E.T.; Papp, Z.; Edes, I.; Kedei, N.; Blumberg, P.M.; Toth, A. Phosphorylation-dependent desensitization by anandamide of vanilloid receptor-1 (TRPV1) function in rat skeletal muscle arterioles and in chinese hamster ovary cells expressing TRPV1. *Mol. Pharmacol.* **2006**, *69*, 1015–1023. [PubMed]

18. Toth, A.; Czikora, A.; Pasztor, E.T.; Dienes, B.; Bai, P.; Csernoch, L.; Rutkai, I.; Csato, V.; Manyine, I.S.; Porszasz, R.; et al. Vanilloid receptor-1 (TRPV1) expression and function in the vasculature of the rat. *J. Histochem. Cytochem.* **2014**, *62*, 129–144. [CrossRef] [PubMed]

19. Vennekens, R.; Menigoz, A.; Nilius, B. Trps in the brain. *Rev. Physiol. Biochem. Pharmacol.* **2012**, *163*, 27–64. [PubMed]

20. Morelli, M.B.; Amantini, C.; Liberati, S.; Santoni, M.; Nabissi, M. TRP channels: New potential therapeutic approaches in CNS neuropathies. *CNS Neurol. Disord. Drug Targets* **2013**, *12*, 274–293. [CrossRef] [PubMed]

21. Gao, H.; Miyata, K.; Bhaskaran, M.D.; Derbenev, A.V.; Zsombok, A. Transient receptor potential vanilloid type 1-dependent regulation of liver-related neurons in the paraventricular nucleus of the hypothalamus diminished in the type 1 diabetic mouse. *Diabetes* **2012**, *61*, 1381–1390. [CrossRef] [PubMed]

22. Zsombok, A.; Bhaskaran, M.D.; Gao, H.; Derbenev, A.V.; Smith, B.N. Functional plasticity of central TRPV1 receptors in brainstem dorsal vagal complex circuits of streptozotocin-treated hyperglycemic mice. *J. Neurosci.* **2011**, *31*, 14024–14031. [CrossRef] [PubMed]

23. Nilius, B.; Szallasi, A. Transient receptor potential channels as drug targets: From the science of basic research to the art of medicine. *Pharmacol. Rev.* **2014**, *66*, 676–814. [CrossRef] [PubMed]

24. Suri, A.; Szallasi, A. The emerging role of TRPV1 in diabetes and obesity. *Trends Pharmacol. Sci.* **2008**, *29*, 29–36. [CrossRef] [PubMed]

25. Zsombok, A. Vanilloid receptors—Do they have a role in whole body metabolism? Evidence from TRPV1. *J. Diabetes Its Complicat.* **2013**, *27*, 287–292. [CrossRef] [PubMed]

26. Derbenev, A.V.; Zsombok, A. Potential therapeutic value of TRPV1 and TRPA1 in diabetes mellitus and obesity. *Semin. Immunopathol.* **2016**, *38*, 397–406. [CrossRef] [PubMed]

27. Marshall, N.J.; Liang, L.; Bodkin, J.; Dessapt-Baradez, C.; Nandi, M.; Collot-Teixeira, S.; Smillie, S.J.; Lalgi, K.; Fernandes, E.S.; Gnudi, L.; et al. A role for TRPV1 in influencing the onset of cardiovascular disease in obesity. *Hypertension* **2013**, *61*, 246–252. [CrossRef] [PubMed]

28. Nilius, B.; Appendino, G. Spices: The savory and beneficial science of pungency. *Rev. Physiol. Biochem. Pharmacol.* **2013**, *164*. [CrossRef]

29. Caterina, M.J.; Schumacher, M.A.; Tominaga, M.; Rosen, T.A.; Levine, J.D.; Julius, D. The capsaicin receptor: A heat-activated ion channel in the pain pathway. *Nature* **1997**, *389*, 816–824. [PubMed]

30. Szallasi, A.; Cortright, D.N.; Blum, C.A.; Eid, S.R. The vanilloid receptor TRPV1: 10 years from channel cloning to antagonist proof-of-concept. *Nat. Rev. Drug Discov.* **2007**, *6*, 357–372. [CrossRef] [PubMed]

31. Moran, M.M.; McAlexander, M.A.; Biro, T.; Szallasi, A. Transient receptor potential channels as therapeutic targets. *Nat. Rev. Drug Discov.* **2011**, *10*, 601–620. [CrossRef] [PubMed]

32. Van Der Stelt, M.; Di Marzo, V. Endovanilloids. Putative endogenous ligands of transient receptor potential vanilloid 1 channels. *Eur. J. Biochem.* **2004**, *271*, 1827–1834. [CrossRef] [PubMed]

33. Jordt, S.E.; Julius, D. Molecular basis for species-specific sensitivity to "hot" chili peppers. *Cell* **2002**, *108*, 421–430. [CrossRef]

34. Tominaga, M.; Tominaga, T. Structure and function of TRPV1. *Pflug. Arch.* **2005**, *451*, 143–150. [CrossRef] [PubMed]

35. Rosenbaum, T.; Simon, S.A. TRPV1 receptors and signal transduction. In *TRP Ion Channel Function in Sensory Transduction and Cellular Signaling Cascades*; Liedtke, W.B., Heller, S., Eds.; CRC Press/Taylor & Francis: Boca Raton, FL, USA, 2007.

36. Aranda, F.J.; Villalain, J.; Gomez-Fernandez, J.C. Capsaicin affects the structure and phase organization of phospholipid membranes. *Biochim. Biophys. Acta* **1995**, *1234*, 225–234. [CrossRef]

37. Swain, J.; Kumar Mishra, A. Location, partitioning behavior, and interaction of capsaicin with lipid bilayer membrane: Study using its intrinsic fluorescence. *J. Phys. Chem. B* **2015**, *119*, 12086–12093. [CrossRef] [PubMed]

38. Torrecillas, A.; Schneider, M.; Fernandez-Martinez, A.M.; Ausili, A.; de Godos, A.M.; Corbalan-Garcia, S.; Gomez-Fernandez, J.C. Capsaicin fluidifies the membrane and localizes itself near the lipid-water interface. *ACS Chem. Neurosci.* **2015**, *6*, 1741–1750. [CrossRef] [PubMed]

39. Razavi, R.; Chan, Y.; Afifiyan, F.N.; Liu, X.J.; Wan, X.; Yantha, J.; Tsui, H.; Tang, L.; Tsai, S.; Santamaria, P.; et al. TRPV1+ sensory neurons control beta cell stress and islet inflammation in autoimmune diabetes. *Cell* **2006**, *127*, 1123–1135. [CrossRef] [PubMed]

40. Akiba, Y.; Kato, S.; Katsube, K.; Nakamura, M.; Takeuchi, K.; Ishii, H.; Hibi, T. Transient receptor potential vanilloid subfamily 1 expressed in pancreatic islet beta cells modulates insulin secretion in rats. *Biochem. Biophys. Res. Commun.* **2004**, *321*, 219–225. [CrossRef] [PubMed]

41. Wang, P.; Yan, Z.; Zhong, J.; Chen, J.; Ni, Y.; Li, L.; Ma, L.; Zhao, Z.; Liu, D.; Zhu, Z. Transient receptor potential vanilloid 1 activation enhances gut glucagon-like peptide-1 secretion and improves glucose homeostasis. *Diabetes* **2012**, *61*, 2155–2165. [CrossRef] [PubMed]

42. Zsombok, A.; Jiang, Y.; Gao, H.; Anwar, I.J.; Rezai-Zadeh, K.; Enix, C.L.; Munzberg, H.; Derbenev, A.V. Regulation of leptin receptor-expressing neurons in the brainstem by TRPV1. *Physiol. Rep.* **2014**, *2*, e12160. [CrossRef] [PubMed]

43. Yoshioka, M.; Lim, K.; Kikuzato, S.; Kiyonaga, A.; Tanaka, H.; Shindo, M.; Suzuki, M. Effects of red-pepper diet on the energy metabolism in men. *J. Nutr. Sci. Vitaminol.* **1995**, *41*, 647–656. [CrossRef] [PubMed]

44. Lim, K.; Yoshioka, M.; Kikuzato, S.; Kiyonaga, A.; Tanaka, H.; Shindo, M.; Suzuki, M. Dietary red pepper ingestion increases carbohydrate oxidation at rest and during exercise in runners. *Med. Sci. Sports Exerc.* **1997**, *29*, 355–361. [CrossRef] [PubMed]

45. Yoshioka, M.; St-Pierre, S.; Suzuki, M.; Tremblay, A. Effects of red pepper added to high-fat and high-carbohydrate meals on energy metabolism and substrate utilization in Japanese women. *Br. J. Nutr.* **1998**, *80*, 503–510. [PubMed]

46. Matsumoto, T.; Miyawaki, C.; Ue, H.; Yuasa, T.; Miyatsuji, A.; Moritani, T. Effects of capsaicin-containing yellow curry sauce on sympathetic nervous system activity and diet-induced thermogenesis in lean and obese young women. *J. Nutr. Sci. Vitaminol.* **2000**, *46*, 309–315. [CrossRef] [PubMed]

47. Smeets, A.J.; Westerterp-Plantenga, M.S. The acute effects of a lunch containing capsaicin on energy and substrate utilisation, hormones, and satiety. *Eur. J. Nutr.* **2009**, *48*, 229–234. [CrossRef] [PubMed]

48. Westerterp-Plantenga, M.S.; Smeets, A.; Lejeune, M.P. Sensory and gastrointestinal satiety effects of capsaicin on food intake. *Int. J. Obes.* **2005**, *29*, 682–688. [CrossRef] [PubMed]

49. Yoshioka, M.; Doucet, E.; Drapeau, V.; Dionne, I.; Tremblay, A. Combined effects of red pepper and caffeine consumption on 24 h energy balance in subjects given free access to foods. *Br. J. Nutr.* **2001**, *85*, 203–211. [CrossRef] [PubMed]

50. Ahuja, K.D.; Ball, M.J. Effects of daily ingestion of chilli on serum lipoprotein oxidation in adult men and women. *Br. J. Nutr.* **2006**, *96*, 239–242. [CrossRef]

51. Ahuja, K.D.; Robertson, I.K.; Geraghty, D.P.; Ball, M.J. The effect of 4-week chilli supplementation on metabolic and arterial function in humans. *Eur. J. Clin. Nutr.* **2007**, *61*, 326–333. [CrossRef] [PubMed]

52. Ahuja, K.D.; Robertson, I.K.; Geraghty, D.P.; Ball, M.J. Effects of chili consumption on postprandial glucose, insulin, and energy metabolism. *Am. J. Clin. Nutr.* **2006**, *84*, 63–69. [PubMed]

53. Lejeune, M.P.; Kovacs, E.M.; Westerterp-Plantenga, M.S. Effect of capsaicin on substrate oxidation and weight maintenance after modest body-weight loss in human subjects. *Br. J. Nutr.* **2003**, *90*, 651–659. [CrossRef] [PubMed]

54. Yoshioka, M.; St-Pierre, S.; Drapeau, V.; Dionne, I.; Doucet, E.; Suzuki, M.; Tremblay, A. Effects of red pepper on appetite and energy intake. *Br. J. Nutr.* **1999**, *82*, 115–123. [PubMed]

55. Baskaran, P.; Krishnan, V.; Ren, J.; Thyagarajan, B. Capsaicin induces browning of white adipose tissue and counters obesity by activating TRPV1 dependent mechanism. *Br. J. Pharmacol.* **2016**, *173*, 2369–2389. [CrossRef] [PubMed]

56. Tanaka, H.; Shimaya, A.; Kiso, T.; Kuramochi, T.; Shimokawa, T.; Shibasaki, M. Enhanced insulin secretion and sensitization in diabetic mice on chronic treatment with a transient receptor potential vanilloid 1 antagonist. *Life Sci.* **2011**, *88*, 559–563. [CrossRef] [PubMed]

57. Fredin, M.F.; Kjellstedt, A.; Smith, D.M.; Oakes, N. The novel TRPV1 antagonist, AZV1, improves insulin sensitivity in ob/ob mice. In Proceedings of European Association for the Study of Diabetes 2015, Stockholm, Sweden, 14–18 September 2015.

58. Kim, M.J.; Son, H.J.; Song, S.H.; Jung, M.; Kim, Y.; Rhyu, M.R. The TRPA1 agonist, methyl syringate suppresses food intake and gastric emptying. *PLoS ONE* **2013**, *8*, e71603. [CrossRef] [PubMed]

59. Babes, A.; Fischer, M.J.; Filipovic, M.; Engel, M.A.; Flonta, M.L.; Reeh, P.W. The anti-diabetic drug glibenclamide is an agonist of the transient receptor potential ankyrin 1 (TRPA1) ion channel. *Eur. J. Pharmacol.* **2013**, *704*, 15–22. [CrossRef] [PubMed]

60. Held, K.; Kichko, T.; De Clercq, K.; Klaassen, H.; Van Bree, R.; Vanherck, J.C.; Marchand, A.; Reeh, P.W.; Chaltin, P.; Voets, T.; et al. Activation of TRPM3 by a potent synthetic ligand reveals a role in peptide release. *Proc. Natl. Acad. Sci. USA* **2015**, *112*, E1363–E1372. [CrossRef] [PubMed]

61. Cao, D.S.; Zhong, L.; Hsieh, T.H.; Abooj, M.; Bishnoi, M.; Hughes, L.; Premkumar, L.S. Expression of transient receptor potential ankyrin 1 (TRPA1) and its role in insulin release from rat pancreatic beta cells. *PLoS ONE* **2012**, *7*, e38005. [CrossRef] [PubMed]

62. Uchida, K.; Tominaga, M. TRPM2 modulates insulin secretion in pancreatic beta-cells. *Islets* **2011**, *3*, 209–211. [CrossRef] [PubMed]

63. Uchida, K.; Tominaga, M. The role of TRPM2 in pancreatic beta-cells and the development of diabetes. *Cell Calcium* **2014**, *56*, 332–339. [CrossRef] [PubMed]

64. Mayer, S.I.; Muller, I.; Mannebach, S.; Endo, T.; Thiel, G. Signal transduction of pregnenolone sulfate in insulinoma cells: Activation of Egr-1 expression involving TRPM3, voltage-gated calcium channels, ERK, and ternary complex factors. *J. Biol. Chem.* **2011**, *286*, 10084–10096. [CrossRef] [PubMed]

65. Wagner, T.F.; Loch, S.; Lambert, S.; Straub, I.; Mannebach, S.; Mathar, I.; Dufer, M.; Lis, A.; Flockerzi, V.; Philipp, S.E.; et al. Transient receptor potential M3 channels are ionotropic steroid receptors in pancreatic beta cells. *Nat. Cell Biol.* **2008**, *10*, 1421–1430. [CrossRef] [PubMed]

66. Colsoul, B.; Schraenen, A.; Lemaire, K.; Quintens, R.; Van Lommel, L.; Segal, A.; Owsianik, G.; Talavera, K.; Voets, T.; Margolskee, R.F.; et al. Loss of high-frequency glucose-induced Ca^{2+} oscillations in pancreatic islets correlates with impaired glucose tolerance in $TRPM5^{-}/^{-}$ mice. *Proc. Natl. Acad. Sci. USA* **2010**, *107*, 5208–5213. [CrossRef] [PubMed]

67. Emery, E.C.; Diakogiannaki, E.; Gentry, C.; Psichas, A.; Habib, A.M.; Bevan, S.; Fischer, M.J.; Reimann, F.; Gribble, F.M. Stimulation of GLP-1 secretion downstream of the ligand-gated ion channel TRPA1. *Diabetes* **2015**, *64*, 1202–1210. [CrossRef] [PubMed]

68. Camacho, S.; Michlig, S.; de Senarclens-Bezencon, C.; Meylan, J.; Meystre, J.; Pezzoli, M.; Markram, H.; le Coutre, J. Anti-obesity and anti-hyperglycemic effects of cinnamaldehyde via altered ghrelin secretion and functional impact on food intake and gastric emptying. *Sci. Rep.* **2015**, *5*, 7919. [CrossRef] [PubMed]

69. Jang, H.J.; Kokrashvili, Z.; Theodorakis, M.J.; Carlson, O.D.; Kim, B.J.; Zhou, J.; Kim, H.H.; Xu, X.; Chan, S.L.; Juhaszova, M.; et al. Gut-expressed gustducin and taste receptors regulate secretion of glucagon-like peptide-1. *Proc. Natl. Acad. Sci. USA* **2007**, *104*, 15069–15074. [CrossRef] [PubMed]

70. Kang, J.H.; Goto, T.; Han, I.S.; Kawada, T.; Kim, Y.M.; Yu, R. Dietary capsaicin reduces obesity-induced insulin resistance and hepatic steatosis in obese mice fed a high-fat diet. *Obesity* **2010**, *18*, 780–787. [CrossRef]

71. Baboota, R.K.; Murtaza, N.; Jagtap, S.; Singh, D.P.; Karmase, A.; Kaur, J.; Bhutani, K.K.; Boparai, R.K.; Premkumar, L.S.; Kondepudi, K.K.; et al. Capsaicin-induced transcriptional changes in hypothalamus and alterations in gut microbial count in high fat diet fed mice. *J. Nutr. Biochem.* **2014**, *25*, 893–902. [CrossRef] [PubMed]

72. Kang, J.H.; Tsuyoshi, G.; Le Ngoc, H.; Kim, H.M.; Tu, T.H.; Noh, H.J.; Kim, C.S.; Choe, S.Y.; Kawada, T.; Yoo, H.; et al. Dietary capsaicin attenuates metabolic dysregulation in genetically obese diabetic mice. *J. Med. Food* **2011**, *14*, 310–315. [CrossRef] [PubMed]

73. Khare, P.; Jagtap, S.; Jain, Y.; Baboota, R.K.; Mangal, P.; Boparai, R.K.; Bhutani, K.K.; Sharma, S.S.; Premkumar, L.S.; Kondepudi, K.K.; et al. Cinnamaldehyde supplementation prevents fasting-induced hyperphagia, lipid accumulation, and inflammation in high-fat diet-fed mice. *BioFactors* **2016**, *42*, 201–211. [PubMed]

74. Yoshida, T.; Yoshioka, K.; Wakabayashi, Y.; Nishioka, H.; Kondo, M. Effects of capsaicin and isothiocyanate on thermogenesis of interscapular brown adipose tissue in rats. *J. Nutr. Sci. Vitaminol.* **1988**, *34*, 587–594. [CrossRef] [PubMed]

75. Alim, I.; Teves, L.; Li, R.; Mori, Y.; Tymianski, M. Modulation of NMDAR subunit expression by TRPM2 channels regulates neuronal vulnerability to ischemic cell death. *J. Neurosci.* **2013**, *33*, 17264–17277. [CrossRef] [PubMed]

76. Lee, C.R.; Patel, J.C.; O'Neill, B.; Rice, M.E. Inhibitory and excitatory neuromodulation by hydrogen peroxide: Translating energetics to information. *J. Physiol.* **2015**, *593*, 3431–3446. [CrossRef] [PubMed]

77. Cheung, S.Y.; Huang, Y.; Kwan, H.Y.; Chung, H.Y.; Yao, X. Activation of transient receptor potential vanilloid 3 channel suppresses adipogenesis. *Endocrinology* **2015**, *156*, 2074–2086. [CrossRef] [PubMed]

78. Ye, L.; Kleiner, S.; Wu, J.; Sah, R.; Gupta, R.K.; Banks, A.S.; Cohen, P.; Khandekar, M.J.; Bostrom, P.; Mepani, R.J.; et al. TRPV4 is a regulator of adipose oxidative metabolism, inflammation, and energy homeostasis. *Cell* **2012**, *151*, 96–110. [CrossRef] [PubMed]

79. Liedtke, W.; Choe, Y.; Marti-Renom, M.A.; Bell, A.M.; Denis, C.S.; Sali, A.; Hudspeth, A.J.; Friedman, J.M.; Heller, S. Vanilloid receptor-related osmotically activated channel (VR-OAC), a candidate vertebrate osmoreceptor. *Cell* **2000**, *103*, 525–535. [CrossRef]

80. Yu, Q.; Wang, Y.; Yu, Y.; Li, Y.; Zhao, S.; Chen, Y.; Waqar, A.B.; Fan, J.; Liu, E. Expression of TRPV1 in rabbits and consuming hot pepper affects its body weight. *Mol. Biol. Rep.* **2012**, *39*, 7583–7589. [CrossRef] [PubMed]

81. Szallasi, A.; Blumberg, P.M. [^{3}H]resiniferatoxin binding by the vanilloid receptor: Species-related differences, effects of temperature and sulfhydryl reagents. *Naunyn-Schmiedeberg's Arch. Pharmacol.* **1993**, *347*, 84–91. [CrossRef]

82. Gavva, N.R.; Klionsky, L.; Qu, Y.; Shi, L.; Tamir, R.; Edenson, S.; Zhang, T.J.; Viswanadhan, V.N.; Toth, A.; Pearce, L.V.; et al. Molecular determinants of vanilloid sensitivity in TRPV1. *J. Biol. Chem.* **2004**, *279*, 20283–20295. [CrossRef] [PubMed]

83. Tsui, H.; Razavi, R.; Chan, Y.; Yantha, J.; Dosch, H.M. "Sensing" autoimmunity in type 1 diabetes. *Trends Mol. Med.* **2007**, *13*, 405–413. [CrossRef] [PubMed]

84. Cui, J.; Himms-Hagen, J. Rapid but transient atrophy of brown adipose tissue in capsaicin-desensitized rats. *Am. J. Physiol.* **1992**, *262*, R562–R567. [PubMed]

85. Cui, J.; Zaror-Behrens, G.; Himms-Hagen, J. Capsaicin desensitization induces atrophy of brown adipose tissue in rats. *Am. J. Physiol.* **1990**, *259*, R324–R332. [PubMed]

86. Van de Wall, E.H.; Wielinga, P.Y.; Strubbe, J.H.; van Dijk, G. Neonatal capsaicin causes compensatory adjustments to energy homeostasis in rats. *Physiol. Behav.* **2006**, *89*, 115–121. [CrossRef] [PubMed]

87. Koopmans, S.J.; Leighton, B.; DeFronzo, R.A. Neonatal de-afferentation of capsaicin-sensitive sensory nerves increases in vivo insulin sensitivity in conscious adult rats. *Diabetologia* **1998**, *41*, 813–820. [CrossRef] [PubMed]

88. Motter, A.L.; Ahern, G.P. TRPV1-null mice are protected from diet-induced obesity. *FEBS Lett.* **2008**, *582*, 2257–2262. [CrossRef] [PubMed]

89. Lee, E.; Jung, D.Y.; Kim, J.H.; Patel, P.R.; Hu, X.; Lee, Y.; Azuma, Y.; Wang, H.F.; Tsitsilianos, N.; Shafiq, U.; et al. Transient receptor potential vanilloid type-1 channel regulates diet-induced obesity, insulin resistance, and leptin resistance. *FASEB J.* **2015**, *29*, 3182–3192. [CrossRef] [PubMed]

90. Yue, Z.; Xie, J.; Yu, A.S.; Stock, J.; Du, J.; Yue, L. Role of trp channels in the cardiovascular system. *Am. J. Physiol. Heart Circ. Physiol.* **2015**, *308*, H157–H182. [CrossRef]

91. Pomonis, J.D.; Harrison, J.E.; Mark, L.; Bristol, D.R.; Valenzano, K.J.; Walker, K. N-(4-Tertiarybutylphenyl)-4-(3-cholorphyridin-2-yl)tetrahydropyrazine-1(2H)-carbox-amide (BCTC), a novel, orally effective vanilloid receptor 1 antagonist with analgesic properties: II. In vivo characterization in rat models of inflammatory and neuropathic pain. *J. Pharmacol. Exp. Ther.* **2003**, *306*, 387–393. [PubMed]

92. Valenzano, K.J.; Grant, E.R.; Wu, G.; Hachicha, M.; Schmid, L.; Tafesse, L.; Sun, Q.; Rotshteyn, Y.; Francis, J.; Limberis, J.; et al. N-(4-tertiarybutylphenyl)-4-(3-chloropyridin-2-yl)tetrahydropyrazine-1(2H)-carbox-amide (BCTC), a novel, orally effective vanilloid receptor 1 antagonist with analgesic properties: I. In vitro characterization and pharmacokinetic properties. *J. Pharmacol. Exp. Ther.* **2003**, *306*, 377–386. [CrossRef] [PubMed]

93. Behrendt, H.J.; Germann, T.; Gillen, C.; Hatt, H.; Jostock, R. Characterization of the mouse cold-menthol receptor TRPM8 and vanilloid receptor type-1 VR1 using a fluorometric imaging plate reader (FLIPR) assay. *Br. J. Pharmacol.* **2004**, *141*, 737–745. [CrossRef] [PubMed]

94. Nilius, B.; Owsianik, G.; Voets, T.; Peters, J.A. Transient receptor potential cation channels in disease. *Physiol. Rev.* **2007**, *87*, 165–217. [CrossRef] [PubMed]

95. Zhang, Z.; Zhang, W.; Jung, D.Y.; Ko, H.J.; Lee, Y.; Friedline, R.H.; Lee, E.; Jun, J.; Ma, Z.; Kim, F.; et al. TRPM2 Ca^{2+} channel regulates energy balance and glucose metabolism. *Am. J. Physiol. Endocrinol. Metab.* **2012**, *302*, E807–E816. [CrossRef] [PubMed]

96. Colsoul, B.; Vennekens, R.; Nilius, B. Transient receptor potential cation channels in pancreatic beta cells. *Rev. Physiol. Biochem. Pharmacol.* **2011**, *161*, 87–110. [PubMed]

97. Colsoul, B.; Nilius, B.; Vennekens, R. Transient receptor potential (TRP) cation channels in diabetes. *Curr. Top. Med. Chem.* **2013**, *13*, 258–269. [CrossRef] [PubMed]

98. Togashi, K.; Hara, Y.; Tominaga, T.; Higashi, T.; Konishi, Y.; Mori, Y.; Tominaga, M. TRPM2 activation by cyclic ADP-ribose at body temperature is involved in insulin secretion. *EMBO J.* **2006**, *25*, 1804–1815. [CrossRef] [PubMed]

99. Uchida, K.; Dezaki, K.; Damdindorj, B.; Inada, H.; Shiuchi, T.; Mori, Y.; Yada, T.; Minokoshi, Y.; Tominaga, M. Lack of TRPM2 impaired insulin secretion and glucose metabolisms in mice. *Diabetes* **2011**, *60*, 119–126. [CrossRef] [PubMed]

100. Wagner, T.F.; Drews, A.; Loch, S.; Mohr, F.; Philipp, S.E.; Lambert, S.; Oberwinkler, J. TRPM3 channels provide a regulated influx pathway for zinc in pancreatic beta cells. *Pflug. Arch.* **2010**, *460*, 755–765. [CrossRef] [PubMed]

101. Muller, I.; Rossler, O.G.; Thiel, G. Pregnenolone sulfate activates basic region leucine zipper transcription factors in insulinoma cells: Role of voltage-gated Ca^{2+} channels and transient receptor potential melastatin 3 channels. *Mol. Pharmacol.* **2011**, *80*, 1179–1189. [CrossRef] [PubMed]

102. Marigo, V.; Courville, K.; Hsu, W.H.; Feng, J.M.; Cheng, H. TRPM4 impacts on Ca^{2+} signals during agonist-induced insulin secretion in pancreatic beta-cells. *Mol. Cell. Endocrinol.* **2009**, *299*, 194–203. [CrossRef] [PubMed]

103. Cheng, H.; Beck, A.; Launay, P.; Gross, S.A.; Stokes, A.J.; Kinet, J.P.; Fleig, A.; Penner, R. TRPM4 controls insulin secretion in pancreatic beta-cells. *Cell Calcium* **2007**, *41*, 51–61. [CrossRef] [PubMed]

104. Vennekens, R.; Olausson, J.; Meissner, M.; Bloch, W.; Mathar, I.; Philipp, S.E.; Schmitz, F.; Weissgerber, P.; Nilius, B.; Flockerzi, V.; et al. Increased IgE-dependent mast cell activation and anaphylactic responses in mice lacking the calcium-activated nonselective cation channel TRPM4. *Nat. Immunol.* **2007**, *8*, 312–320. [CrossRef] [PubMed]

105. Nelson, P.L.; Zolochevska, O.; Figueiredo, M.L.; Soliman, A.; Hsu, W.H.; Feng, J.M.; Zhang, H.; Cheng, H. Regulation of Ca^{2+}-entry in pancreatic alpha-cell line by transient receptor potential melastatin 4 plays a vital role in glucagon release. *Mol. Cell. Endocrinol.* **2011**, *335*, 126–134. [CrossRef] [PubMed]

106. Berggren, P.O.; Yang, S.N.; Murakami, M.; Efanov, A.M.; Uhles, S.; Kohler, M.; Moede, T.; Fernstrom, A.; Appelskog, I.B.; Aspinwall, C.A.; et al. Removal of Ca^{2+} channel beta3 subunit enhances Ca^{2+} oscillation frequency and insulin exocytosis. *Cell* **2004**, *119*, 273–284. [CrossRef] [PubMed]

107. Perez, C.A.; Huang, L.; Rong, M.; Kozak, J.A.; Preuss, A.K.; Zhang, H.; Max, M.; Margolskee, R.F. A transient receptor potential channel expressed in taste receptor cells. *Nat. Neurosci.* **2002**, *5*, 1169–1176. [CrossRef] [PubMed]

108. Huang, Y.A.; Roper, S.D. Intracellular Ca^{2+} and TRPM5-mediated membrane depolarization produce ATP secretion from taste receptor cells. *J. Physiol.* **2010**, *588*, 2343–2350. [CrossRef] [PubMed]

109. Palmer, R.K. The pharmacology and signaling of bitter, sweet, and umami taste sensing. *Mol. Interv.* **2007**, *7*, 87–98. [CrossRef] [PubMed]

110. Sprous, D.; Palmer, K.R. The T1R2/T1R3 sweet receptor and TRPM5 ion channel taste targets with therapeutic potential. *Prog. Mol. Biol. Transl. Sci.* **2010**, *91*, 151–208. [PubMed]

111. Palmer, R.K.; Lunn, C.A. TRP channels as targets for therapeutic intervention in obesity: Focus on TRPV1 and TRPM5. *Curr. Top. Med. Chem.* **2013**, *13*, 247–257. [CrossRef] [PubMed]

112. Khan, A.; Safdar, M.; Ali Khan, M.M.; Khattak, K.N.; Anderson, R.A. Cinnamon improves glucose and lipids of people with type 2 diabetes. *Diabetes Care* **2003**, *26*, 3215–3218. [CrossRef] [PubMed]

113. Mang, B.; Wolters, M.; Schmitt, B.; Kelb, K.; Lichtinghagen, R.; Stichtenoth, D.O.; Hahn, A. Effects of a cinnamon extract on plasma glucose, HbA, and serum lipids in diabetes mellitus type 2. *Eur. J. Clin. Investig.* **2006**, *36*, 340–344. [CrossRef] [PubMed]

114. Vanschoonbeek, K.; Thomassen, B.J.; Senden, J.M.; Wodzig, W.K.; van Loon, L.J. Cinnamon supplementation does not improve glycemic control in postmenopausal type 2 diabetes patients. *J. Nutr.* **2006**, *136*, 977–980. [PubMed]

115. Tamura, Y.; Iwasaki, Y.; Narukawa, M.; Watanabe, T. Ingestion of cinnamaldehyde, a TRPA1 agonist, reduces visceral fats in mice fed a high-fat and high-sucrose diet. *J. Nutr. Sci. Vitaminol.* **2012**, *58*, 9–13. [CrossRef] [PubMed]

116. Sartorius, T.; Peter, A.; Schulz, N.; Drescher, A.; Bergheim, I.; Machann, J.; Schick, F.; Siegel-Axel, D.; Schurmann, A.; Weigert, C.; et al. Cinnamon extract improves insulin sensitivity in the brain and lowers liver fat in mouse models of obesity. *PLoS ONE* **2014**, *9*, e92358. [CrossRef] [PubMed]

117. Iwasaki, Y.; Tanabe, M.; Kobata, K.; Watanabe, T. Trpa1 agonists—Allyl isothiocyanate and cinnamaldehyde—Induce adrenaline secretion. *Biosci. Biotechnol. Biochem.* **2008**, *72*, 2608–2614. [CrossRef] [PubMed]

118. Ahn, J.; Lee, H.; Im, S.W.; Jung, C.H.; Ha, T.Y. Allyl isothiocyanate ameliorates insulin resistance through the regulation of mitochondrial function. *J. Nutr. Biochem.* **2014**, *25*, 1026–1034. [CrossRef] [PubMed]

119. Doihara, H.; Nozawa, K.; Kawabata-Shoda, E.; Kojima, R.; Yokoyama, T.; Ito, H. Molecular cloning and characterization of dog TRPA1 and AITC stimulate the gastrointestinal motility through TRPA1 in conscious dogs. *Eur. J. Pharmacol.* **2009**, *617*, 124–129. [CrossRef] [PubMed]

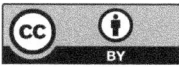

pharmaceuticals

MDPI

Review

Targeting TRPM2 in ROS-Coupled Diseases

Shinichiro Yamamoto and Shunichi Shimizu *

Division of Pharmacology, Faculty of Pharmaceutical Sciences, Teikyo Heisei University, Tokyo 164-8530, Japan;
s.yamamoto@thu.ac.jp
* Correspondence: s.shimizu@thu.ac.jp; Tel.: +81-3-5860-4210; Fax: +81-3-5860-4945

Academic Editors: Arpad Szallasi and Susan M. Huang
Received: 23 May 2016; Accepted: 5 September 2016; Published: 7 September 2016

Abstract: Under pathological conditions such as inflammation and ischemia-reperfusion injury large amounts of reactive oxygen species (ROS) are generated which, in return, contribute to the development and exacerbation of disease. The second member of the transient receptor potential (TRP) melastatin subfamily, TRPM2, is a Ca^{2+}-permeable non-selective cation channel, activated by ROS in an ADP-ribose mediated fashion. In other words, TRPM2 functions as a transducer that converts oxidative stress into Ca^{2+} signaling. There is good evidence that TRPM2 plays an important role in ROS-coupled diseases. For example, in monocytes the influx of Ca^{2+} through TRPM2 activated by ROS contributes to the aggravation of inflammation via chemokine production. In this review, the focus is on TRPM2 as a molecular linker between ROS and Ca^{2+} signaling in ROS-coupled diseases.

Keywords: TRPM2; Ca^{2+} signaling; reactive oxygen species; ROS-coupled diseases

1. Introduction

The physiological concentration of Ca^{2+} in the intracellular compartment ($[Ca^{2+}]_i$) is on the order of 10^{-7} M; this is markedly lower than its extracellular concentration which is in the order of 10^{-3} M [1]. Due to this difference between intracellular and extracellular Ca^{2+} concentrations, Ca^{2+} can function as a second messenger. Recently, a subset of TRP channels has attracted attention because of their permeablity to Ca^{2+}. Indeed, the first *trp* gene was originally discovered in mutant fruit flies with impaired vision due to the lack of a specific Ca^{2+} influx pathway in photoreceptor cells [2]. Subsequently, a large number of TRP channel homologues were identified in vertebrates. As of today, the human TRP channel superfamily has 28 members that are divided into six subfamilies: canonical (C), vanilloid (V), melastatin (M), polycystic kidney disease (P), mucolipin (ML), and ankyrin (A), based on the homology of their protein sequences [3].

Generally speaking, the TRP protein has six putative transmembrane domains and a pore region between the fifth and sixth transmembrane domains. TRP proteins assemble into homo- or heterotetramers in order to form functional channels [4,5]. The TRPC subfamily shows the greatest homology to the *Drosophila* TRP protein. TRPC channels are downstream targets to phospholipase C activation following receptor stimulation [6–9].

The TRPV subfamily (TRPV1 to V6) was named after its founding member, the vanilloid (capsaicin) receptor TRPV1. TRPV channels are polymodal and their activators range from physical and chemical stimuli including heat (TRPV1, TRPV2, TRPV3, and TRPV4) [10–16], through protons (TRPV1) [17] and osmotic stress (TRPV4) [18,19], to capsaicin, the pungent principle in hot peppers (TRPV1) [10]. The TRPM subfamily has eight members. Its best known member is the cold-responsive menthol receptor, TRPM8 [20,21]. The TRPP subfamily includes TRPP1 and TRPP2, which are encoded by the *PKD1* and *PKD2* genes, respectively. *PKD1* and *PKD2* are the genes responsible for autosomal dominant polycystic kidney disease. TRPP1 is thought to interact with TRPP2, which functions as a receptor for mechanical stimuli such as shear stress [22,23].

The TRPML subfamily is composed of TRPML1 and its homologues. A mutation in the *MCOLN1* gene encoding TRPML1 causes mucolipidosis type IV. TRPML1 localizes in lysosomes and late endosomes and is activated by phosphoinositol (3,5)-bisphosphate [24,25].

TRPA1 (named after the large N-terminal domain with 17 predicted ankyrin repeats) is the sole member of the TRPA subfamily [26]. It is activated by irritant compounds such as exhaust fumes and allyl isothiocyanate in mustard oil. The cold activation of TRPA1 remains controversial [27,28]. Interestingly, TRPA1 is activated by both hyper- and hypoxia via oxidative modification of its cysteine residues and the dehydroxylation of the proline residues [29].

Traditionally, reactive oxygen species (ROS) are regarded as non-specific toxins that cause cell and tissue damage [30]. However, recently ROS have been identified as signal-transduction molecules [31]. For example, the oxidative stress-sensitive transcriptional factor Keap1, and the signal-transduction molecule ASK1, are activated by ROS to mediate a number of cellular responses [32,33]. The second member of the TRP melastatin subfamily, TRPM2, is a Ca^{2+}-permeable non-selective cation channel. TRPM2 is expressed broadly in neuronal cells, myocytes, pancreatic β cells, and immune cells such as T lymphocytes, monocytes/macrophages, and neutrophils [34–42]. TRPM2 is activated by oxidative stress including H_2O_2. In other words, TRPM2 functions as a sensor for oxidative stress. Indeed, TRPM2 is more sensitive to ROS than other TRPs including TRPC5, TRPV1 and TRPA1 (which is activated by ROS via oxidative modifications to its cysteine residues).

Large amounts of ROS are generated under pathological conditions that, in turn, contribute to the development and maintenance of various disease states [43]. TRPM2 converts ROS-induced oxidative stress into Ca^{2+} signaling; this Ca^{2+} signaling has been implicated in the aggravation of a number of diseases. In this review, the focus is on TRPM2 as a molecular linker between ROS and Ca^{2+} signaling.

2. TRPM2 Activators and Inhibitors

Among TRP channels TRPM2 is unique in that it contains a NudT9-Homology (NUDT9-H) domain at its cytosolic C-terminal region. Although NUDT9-H shares some homology with NUDT9 ADP-ribose hydrolase, its ADP-ribose hydrolase activity is low. In addition to the full-length TRPM2, several truncated splice variants have been described, including: (1) TRPM2-ΔN (containing a deletion of amino acids 538–557 in the N-terminus); (2) TRPM2-ΔC (deletion of amino acids 1292–1325 in the C-terminus), and (3) TRPM2-S (S for short) that lacks the four C-terminal transmembrane domains, putative Ca^{2+}-permeable pore region, and the entire C terminus [39,41,44].

The activation of TRPM2 is triggered by the binding of ADP-ribose to the NUDT9-H domain [45]. Since the NUDT9-H domain of TRPM2-ΔC is partially missing, TRPM2-ΔC is not activated by ADP-ribose. Nicotinic acid adenine dinucleotide phosphate (NAADP), cADP-ribose, and Ca^{2+} exert synergistic effects on ADP-ribose-induced TRPM2 activation. Moreover, these agents are also capable of activating TRPM2 by themselves [36,46–50].

In neutrophils, resting ADP-ribose levels approach 5 μM [50] which is sufficient to induce the activation of TRPM2 by increasing $[Ca^{2+}]_i$. The IQ-like motif in the calmodulin-binding domain at the N-terminal region, rather than the NUDT9-H domain, is thought to play a pivotal role in the Ca^{2+}-induced activation of TRPM2 [49]. Using inside-out patch recordings, Csanády and colleagues have investigated the direct activation of TRPM2; they found that neither cADP-ribose nor NAADP is able to directly activate TRPM2 [51]. On the other hand, they identified ADP-ribose-2'-phosphate as a direct TRPM2 agonist [52].

Silent information regulator-2 (SIR2), a member of the sirtuin family, is a nicotinamide adenine dinucleotide (NAD^+)-dependent protein deacetylase. SIR2 removes acetyl groups from acetylated substrates, and transfers them to NAD^+. Nicotinamide and O-acetylated-ADP-ribose (OAADPr) are produced as a result of this reaction. OAADPr was reported to activate TRPM2 by binding to the NUDT9-H domain. This implicates SIR2 in TRPM2 regulation [53].

NAD$^+$ was also reported to directly gate TRPM2, although a high concentration (in the mM range) of NAD$^+$ is required for this response [54]. However, purified NAD$^+$ fails to activate TRPM2 [52]. This apparent contradiction was explained by the presence of the NAD$^+$-degradation product ADP-ribose, a known TRPM2 agonist, in the non-purified NAD$^+$ [46,55]. CD38 is an ectoenzyme that catalyzes the production of cADP-ribose and ADP-ribose from its substrate, NAD$^+$ [56]. CD38 is implicated in the activation of TRPM2 via production of cADP-ribose and/or ADP-ribose [38,40,57].

Arguably the most important activator of TRPM2 is oxidative stress induced by ROS, including H$_2$O$_2$ [54]. It has been postulated that the activation of TRPM2 by oxidative stress is triggered via ADP-ribose production. Mitochondria are a major source of ADP-ribose. In mitochondria, ADP-ribose is generated by the oxidative stress-induced hydrolysis of NAD$^+$ [55]. In the nucleus, poly(ADP-ribose) polymerase-1 (PARP-1) plays an important role in repairing DNA damage in response to oxidative stress. The binding of PARP-1 to impaired DNA hydrolyzes NAD$^+$, leading to the production of nicotinamide and ADP-ribose. In turn, ADP-ribose is built into various nuclear proteins, resulting in the activation of DNA repair and stimulation of nuclear factor-mediated transcription [58–61]. Free ADP-ribose is generated following the degradation of poly(ADP-ribose) by poly(ADP-ribose) glycohydrolase (PARG) [61].

Pharmacological [62] or genetic manipulation of PARP-1 [63] blocks H$_2$O$_2$-induced TRPM2 activation. Conversely, H$_2$O$_2$-induced TRPM2 activation is enhanced at body temperature by hydroxyl radical production [64,65]. The hydroxyl radical produced by the reaction of H$_2$O$_2$ with intracellular Fe^{2+} (Fenton reaction) stimulates the PARP-1/PARG pathway, which leads to the activation of TRPM2. The phosphorylation of tyrosine residues in TRPM2 is thought to represent an important mechanism underlying the activation of TRPM2 by H$_2$O$_2$. The phosphorylation/dephosphorylation state is regulated by protein tyrosine phosphatase-L1 [66].

The short splice variant of TRPM2, TRPM2-S, was shown to interact with the full-length TRPM2. The TRPM2-S/full-length TRPM2 complex is not activated by H$_2$O$_2$ [39]. Therefore, TRPM2-S may function as a dominant negative modulator of TRPM2.

A large number of TRPM2 blockers have been reported. Adenosine monophosphate [46] and 8-bromo-ADP-ribose [38] inhibit ADP-ribose-induced TRPM2 activation by preventing the binding of ADP-ribose to the NUDT9-H domain. The antifungal agents clotrimazole and econazole [67], the antipyretic agent flufenamic acid [68], 2-aminoethoxydiphenyl borate (2-APB) [69], *N*-(p-amylcinnamoyl) anthranilic acid (ACA) [70], and curcumin, the active principle in turmeric [71], are TRPM2 channel blockers. PARP inhibitors (e.g., SB750139-B, PJ34, and DPQ) were also reported to prevent the activation of TRPM2 in response to oxidative stress. However, these inhibitors have no effect on ADP-ribose-induced TRPM2 activation.

Iron chelators were shown to attenuate H$_2$O$_2$-induced TRPM2 activation [64]. Surprisingly, the JAK2 inhibitor AG490 was also found to prevent TRPM2 activation by H$_2$O$_2$ [72]. It was, however, suggested that AG490 ameliorates H$_2$O$_2$-induced TRPM2 activation by scavenging hydroxyl radicals rather than inhibiting of JAK2. The AG490-related compounds, AG555 and AG556, exert an even stronger inhibitory effect on H$_2$O$_2$-induced TRPM2 activation than AG490 [73].

3. ROS Production under Pathological Conditions

3.1. Inflammation

Inflammation is a complex biological reaction to injury and/or infection. During inflammation, immune cells are transported from the blood stream into the damaged tissue in an attempt to eliminate the harmful agents and to initiate the process of healing and repair. However, when inflammation becomes chronic, it may exacerbate tissue damage and pose severe health risks.

At the inflamed sites, phagocytes (e.g., macrophages and neutrophils) digest the harmful agents which play an important role in their removal. During phagocytosis, oxygen consumption in the phagocytes is increased. This phenomenon is known as the "respiratory burst": oxygen is utilized for superoxide anion ($\cdot O_2^-$) production by NADPH oxidase [74]. During bacterial phagocytosis, bacteria are engulfed by the plasma membrane, leading to the formation of phagosomes. Then NADPH oxidase activated and the resultant $\cdot O_2^-$ contributes to bacterial killing. NADPH oxidase (NOX) is composed of several isoforms. Seven isoforms, termed as NOX1–5 and DUOX1–2, have been identified as catalytic subunits. These isoforms are localized in the plasma membrane and catalyze electron transport from the electron donor NADPH to oxygen, leading to the production of $\cdot O_2^-$. In phagocytes, NOX2 is strongly expressed and interacts with the membrane protein $p22^{phox}$ [75]. The small G-protein RAC, and the cytosolic proteins $p40^{phox}$, $p47^{phox}$, and $p67^{phox}$ are also known to activate NOX2.

The production of $\cdot O_2^-$ by NOX2 does not occur in a resting state. During phagocytosis, these activators translocate to the plasma membrane and interact with the NOX2/$p22^{phox}$ complex; this, in turn, triggers $\cdot O_2^-$ production following the activation of NOX2 (Figure 1A). In addition, $\cdot O_2^-$ is converted to H_2O_2 by the superoxide dismutase. These ROS contribute to killing bacteria.

Lipopolysaccharide (LPS), found in the outer membrane of Gram-negative bacteria, is a prototypical trigger of sepsis that elicits a strong immune response in animals. The LPS receptor is toll-like receptor-4 (TLR4) which associates with several adaptor molecules such as MyD88 [76]. The activation of TLR4 in response to LPS triggers immune responses including the production of cytokines and ROS accompanied by the activation of NADPH oxidase [77]. Cytokines (e.g., tumor necrosis factor, TNF) are released from immune cells and accumulate at the sites of inflammation. These molecules act in concert to organize the inflammatory network and produce large amount of ROS. The source of ROS appears to be the mitochondria rather than the NADPH oxidase [77–79].

3.2. Ischemia-Reperfusion

Ischemia-reperfusion injury is caused by re-oxygenation during reperfusion following the lack of oxygen during ischemia. Ischemia-reperfusion generates harmful substances that aggravate the tissue injury. This is a major mechanism of tissue damage during stroke and myocardial infarction. The hydroxyl radical scavenger, edaravone, is used as a neuroprotective agent in the management of patients with ischemic brain injury and amyotrophic lateral sclerosis (Lou Gehrig's Disease). During ischemia-reperfusion injury, mitochondria are the major source of ROS. Electrons leaked from the mitochondrial electron transport chain are transferred to molecular oxygen, resulting in the production of $\cdot O_2^-$. The activity of the electron transport chain generates a relatively small amount of $\cdot O_2^-$ under normal conditions, but its production may be greatly magnified by events occurring during ischemia-reperfusion (Figure 1B) [80].

NADPH oxidase also contributes to ROS production during ischemia-reperfusion. NOXs are present in blood vessels [81] where their expression is regulated by the hypoxia-sensitive transcriptional factor, hypoxia-inducible factor-1α (HIF1α) [81]. The expression of NOX isoforms is thus up-regulated by the lack of oxygen during ischemia. Then NOX generates large amounts of ROS during reperfusion (Figure 1B).

During ischemia, a failure in the generation of ATP also occurs concurrently with ATP consumption, leading to the depletion of ATP. ATP is eventually catabolized into hypoxanthine. Xanthine oxidase catalyzes two steps including the formation of xanthine from hypoxanthine, and the formation of uric acid from xanthine. Electrons are also generated in this process and transferred to molecular oxygen, leading to the formation of $\cdot O_2^-$ [82] (Figure 1B). In summary, several factors contribute to ROS production during ischemia-reperfusion.

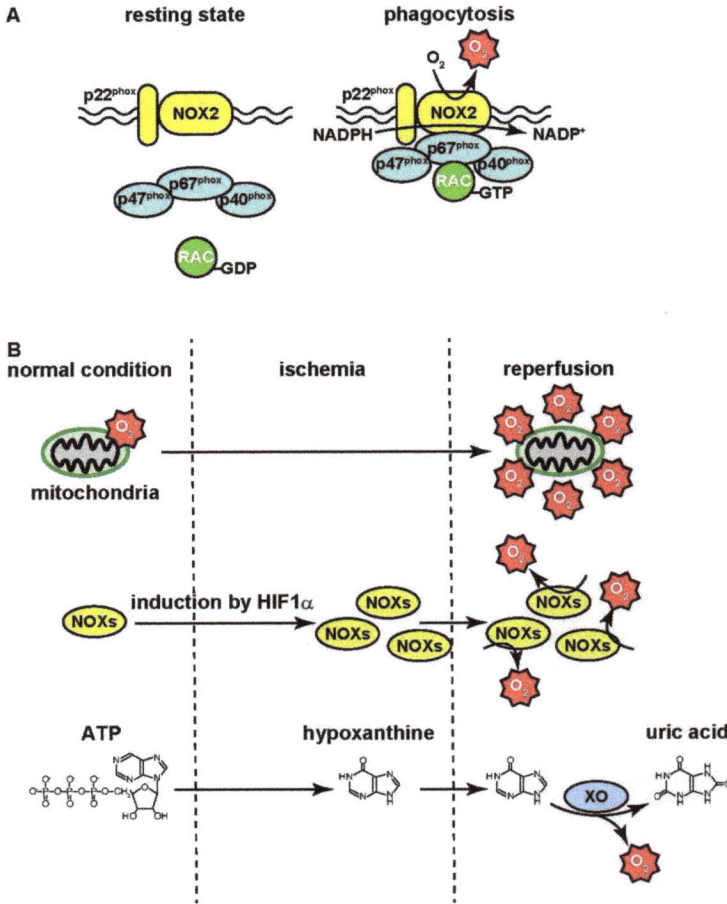

Figure 1. ROS production during inflammation and ischemia-reperfusion. (**A**) In resting state, cytosolic activators such as p40^{phox}, p47^{phox}, p67^{phox} and small G protein RAC do not interact with NOX2-p22^{phox} complex. These activators translocate to the plasma membrane during phagocytosis and interact with the NOX2-p22^{phox} complex. Electrons derived from NADPH are transferred through the complex to molecular oxygen, leading to ˙O$_2^-$ production; (**B**) Oxidative phosphorylation is initiated by electron transport from NADH and/or FADH$_2$ to the electron transport chain in the mitochondrial inner membrane. The electron transport chain is composed of complexes I–IV. Electrons derived from NADH and FADH$_2$ are fed to complex I and complex II, respectively. They are then transferred to complexes in ascending order of the redox potential, which release free energy. Molecular oxygen accepts electrons for the formation of H$_2$O. On the other hand, the electron transport chain uses free energy derived from electron transport to pump H$^+$ out of the matrix, thereby creating proton gradient across the mitochondrial inner membrane. By utilizing energy released by the influx of H$^+$ into the matrix, ADP is phosphorylated, resulting in the generation of ATP. ˙O$_2^-$ is generated by the leakage of electrons from complexes I and III in the electron transport chain. The activity of the electron transport chain generates a relatively small amount of ˙O$_2^-$ under normal conditions, but its production may be greatly magnified by events occurring during ischemia-reperfusion. The expression of NOX isoforms is up-regulated by HIF1α during ischemia, and then NADPH oxidase then generates large amounts of ROS by reoxygenation during reperfusion. During ischemia, ATP is catabolized into hypoxanthine.

4. ROS-Coupled Diseases and TRPM2

4.1. Inflammatory Diseases

4.1.1. TRPM2-Mediated Chemokine Production

TRPM2 contributes to the aggravation of inflammation [40]. In monocytes/macrophages, Ca^{2+} influx through TRPM2 activated by ROS stimulates the production of the chemokine, CXCL2. CXC chemokines, such as macrophage inflammatory protein-2 (CXCL2), exhibit potent neutrophil chemotactic activity [83].

Dextran sulfate sodium (DSS)-induced colitis is a mouse model of human ulcerative colitis. In the colon of DSS-treated wild-type (WT) mice, the expression of CXCL2 was markedly increased in monocytes/macrophages. By contrast, CXCL2 expression was strongly suppressed in the colon of *Trpm2* KO mice following DSS challenge. The number of recruited neutrophils was also significantly reduced in the colon of DSS-treated *Trpm2* KO mice, presumably as a consequence of reduced CXCL2 levels, but their function was intact. No difference was noted in the number of macrophages in the inflamed colon of WT and *Trpm2* KO mice. The bone marrow output of neutrophils was normal, as was their accumulation into the abdominal cavity after intraperitoneal injection of chemokines. Last, DSS-treated *Trpm2* KO mice did not exhibit weight loss and/or ulceration of the colon, suggesting that *Trpm2* KO mice were largely protected from DSS-mediated colitis. Combined, these findings imply that TRPM2-mediated chemokine production in monocytes/macrophages is an important mechanism underlying the progression of DSS-induced ulcerative colitis.

TRPM2-dependent CXCL2 production was also implicated in the carrageenan-induced inflammatory pain and sciatic nerve ligation models [84]. The carrageenan-induced pain model is a widely used and reliable model for inflammatory pain. Sciatic nerve ligation causes neuropathic pain. Both CXCL2 production and neutrophil infiltration were attenuated in *Trpm2* KO mice. By contrast, the recruitment of F4/80-positive macrophages was not altered in the inflamed paw or around the injured sciatic nerve. Importantly, both mechanical allodynia and thermal hyperalgesia were attenuated in *Trpm2* KO mice. Based on these observations one may argue that TRPM2 expressed in macrophages aggravates pronociceptive inflammatory responses to induce inflammatory and neuropathic pain through neuroinflammation-mediated sensitization of the pain-signaling pathway.

TRPM2 in alveolar epithelial cells plays an important role in bleomycin-induced lung injury [85]. Bleomycin is a glycopeptide antibiotic with potent antitumor activity. It is used in the management of squamous cell carcinoma, testicular cancers, and lymphomas. The antitumor activity of bleomycin was attributed to its ability to cause DNA damage in the cancer cells through the production of oxygen radicals. A major dose-limiting side-effect of bleomycin is lung injury. In mice treated with bleomycin, the secretion of CXCL2 from alveolar epithelial cells was attenuated in *Trpm2* KO compared to WT. It was unexpected because alveolar macrophages (which have higher expression of TRPM2 than alveolar epithelial cells) were believed to be the main source of CXCL2 in response to bleomycin. The secretion of CXCL2 from alveolar epithelial cells was essential for neutrophil recruitment and the secretion of inflammatory cytokines including tumor necrosis factor α and interleukin-1β. Taken together, these findings imply that TRPM2-mediated CXCL2 production in alveolar epithelial cells is responsible for the aggravation of bleomycin-induced lung damage.

4.1.2. LPS-Induced Inflammatory Responses and TRPM2

The contribution of TRPM2 to LPS-induced lung inflammation is poorly understood. In vitro, activation by LPS of TRPM2 in monocytes and cultured microglia is involved in the generation of inflammatory cytokines [40,84,86]. By contrast, in vivo studies found no difference between WT and *Trpm2* KO mice in the secretion of inflammatory cytokines and the infiltration of inflammatory cells into the lungs following LPS administration [85,87]. Therefore, other signaling pathways (e.g., TLR4-mediated signaling) rather than Ca^{2+} signaling via TRPM2 may play a pivotal role in LPS-induced lung inflammation in vivo.

Adding to the confusion, recently Di et al suggested a protective anti-inflammatory role for TRPM2 during LPS-induced lung inflammation [88]. In LPS-treated *Trpm2* KO mice lung injury (including cytokine production and the infiltration of inflammatory cells into the lungs) was exacerbated compared to WT animals. In their experimental model, following LPS administration Ca^{2+} influx via TRPM2 was triggered in phagocytes such as neutrophils. The influx of Ca^{2+} depolarized the plasma membrane, contributing to the inhibition of NADPH oxidase. This protective mechanism was absent in the *Trpm2* KO animals. Therefore, *Trpm2* KO phagocytes overproduced ROS, resulting in the exacerbation of LPS-induced lung injury.

4.1.3. Functional Roles of TRPM2 during Infection

TRPM2 may play an important protective role during bacterial infections. For example, the Gram-negative bacterium *Francisella tularensis* (the agent responsible for tularemia) is equipped with an antioxidant system to escape the host immune response. Although *Francisella* is phagocytized by macrophages, it protects itself from ROS-mediated killing by inhibiting the formation of the NADPH oxidase complex [89]. Catalase (that converts H_2O_2 into H_2O and oxygen) also belongs to the antioxidant systems in *Francisella*.

By using a catalase-deficient *F. tularensis* strain, Shakerley et al. suggested that TRPM2 may play a central role in macrophages during bacterial infection [90]. Although macrophages infected with *F. tularensis* showed marginal TRPM2 activation, the influx of Ca^{2+} through TRPM2 was sufficient to induce immune responses such as interleukin-6 (IL-6) production in macrophages infected with catalase-deficient *F. tularensis*. During *Listeria monocytogenes* infection, TRPM2 was found to contribute to innate immunity [91]. In *Trpm2* KO mice infected by *L. monocytogenes*, the production of IL-12 and interferon-γ was diminished. Consequently, *Trpm2* KO mice were more susceptible to *L. monocytogenes* infection.

Formyl-methionyl-leucyl-phenylalanine (fMLP) is a secreted bacterial product that serves as a neutrophil chemotactic factor. fMLP activates CD38 by binding to its receptor. *Cd38*-deficient mice display disturbed Ca^{2+} signaling and neutrophil chemotaxis in response to fMLP [92]. As described above, CD38 is an ectoenzyme that catalyzes the production of cADP-ribose and ADP-ribose from its substrate, NAD^+. fMLP-induced Ca^{2+} influx and neutrophil chemotaxis were significantly suppressed in the *Trpm2*-deficient neutrophils, suggesting that TRPM2 is a molecular entity that links ADP-ribose produced by CD38 to Ca^{2+} signaling [38,40].

4.1.4. NLRP3 Inflammasome and TRPM2

The NOD-like receptor family pyrin domain containing-3 (NLRP3) "inflammasome" is composed of NLRP3, apoptosis-associated speck-like protein (ASC), and caspase-1. NLRP3 associates with the adaptor protein ASC in response to danger-associated stimuli. In order to form an active inflammasome complex, the NLRP3-ASC complex needs to bind caspase-1. This interaction results in the caspase-1-dependent processing of cytoplasmic targets, including the pro-inflammatory cytokines IL-1β and IL-18. Mature cytokines are then released from the cells [93]. The influx of Ca^{2+} via TRPM2 activated by ROS was suggested to participate in the activation of the NLRP3 inflammasome [94].

Particulate substances (e.g., liposomes and urate crystals) induce the production of ROS, partially mediated by the leakage of electrons from the mitochondrial electron transport chain [94,95]. These particulates also initiate a ROS-dependent Ca^{2+} influx via TRPM2; this, in turn, contributes to the secretion of IL-1β, accompanied by NLRP3 inflammasome activation. In *Trpm2*-disrupted macrophages, impaired NLRP3 inflammasome activation and interleukin-1β secretion was observed. Furthermore, *Trpm2* KO mice are resistant to particulate-induced and IL-1β-mediated peritonitis [94].

4.2. Ischemia-Reperfusion Injury

4.2.1. Brain

Ca^{2+} signaling influences a wide array of biological responses, including gene expression, neuronal growth, neurotransmitter release, and, ultimately, cell death. In other words, Ca^{2+} can exert both protective and deleterious effects on neuronal cells [96,97]. TRPM2 is believed to be responsible for the H$_2$O$_2$-induced Ca^{2+} influx that mediates cell death in various tissues [54] including rat cortical neurons [34]. There is good evidence that the influx of Ca^{2+} via TRPM2 contributes to neuronal cell death during ischemia-reperfusion injury both in vitro (oxygen and glucose deprivation, OGD, followed by re-oxygenation) and in vivo (brain ischemia-reperfusion induced by transient middle cerebral artery occlusion, tMCAO). Interestingly, there appears to be a sex-related difference in cell death [98–100]. When both male and female WT and *Trpm2* KO mice were subjected to tMCAO, male *Trpm2* KO mice had smaller infarct volumes than matched WT mice. By contrast, *Trpm2* KO had no protective effect on infarct volumes in female mice. In a second set of experiments, clotrimazole was used as a TRPM2 inhibitor. Clotrimazole reduced infarct volumes in male WT mice subjected to tMCAO. This beneficial effect was absent in *Trpm2* KO mice. Clotrimazole had no effects either on infarct volumes in castrated male mice. However, androgen replacement restored clotrimazole protection in castrated mice. Taken together, these findings suggest that androgen signaling contributes to TRPM2-dependent brain injury during ischemia-reperfusion. One may argue that androgen signaling stimulates PARP-1 which is necessary for the engagement of TRPM2 in ischemic injury in the male brain. However, other mechanisms may also exist because cell death was induced by OGD in neurons isolated from male embryos and cultured in sex steroid-free medium.

There is preliminary evidence that the *N*-methyl-D-aspartate glutamate receptor (NMDA-R) subunit expression pattern is altered in *Trpm2* KO mice [101]. NMDA-R is a heteromer composed of the obligatory GluN1 subunit along with other GluN subunits including GluN2A and GluN2B. An increase in the activity of GluN2A-containing NMDA-R is known to increase the phosphorylation of Extracellular Signal Regulated Kinase-1 (ERK) and AKT, thereby promoting pro-survival mechanisms in the cell. In contrast, an increase in the activity of GluN2B-containing NMDA-R inhibits pro-survival mechanisms [101]. *Trpm2* KO mice subjected to tMCAO showed smaller infarcts than WT mice, and OGD-induced cell death was reduced in hippocampal neurons prepared from *Trpm2* KO embryos. The expression of GluN2B and GluN2A was reduced and increased, respectively, in the hippocampus by the disruption of *Trpm2*. The ERK/AKT pathway was activated in the hippocampus of *Trpm2* KO mice.

As described above, stimulation of the NMDA-R (that contains GluN2A) activates the ERK/AKT pathway that, in turn, promotes pro-survival mechanisms. In the OGD model, the application of known GluN2A antagonists eliminated the neuroprotection in the hippocampal neurons isolated from *Trpm2* KO mouse embryos. This implies that increases in GluN2A by the disruption of *Trpm2* protect neurons from ischemia-reperfusion-induced cell death.

Migration of immune cells including neutrophils from the blood stream into the brain also plays an important role in ischemia-reperfusion brain injury [102]. As mentioned above, the size of the infarct induced by tMCAO was significantly smaller in *Trpm2* KO mice than in WT mice. WT mice transplanted with bone marrow obtained from *Trpm2* KO animals showed significantly smaller brain infract in the tMCAO model than *Trpm2* KO animals reconstituted with bone marrow from WT mice. This experiment supports the pivotal role of TRPM2 expressed in bone marrow-derived immune cells in the pathomechanism of ischemia-reperfusion brain injury.

4.2.2. Heart

Conflicting results have been reported regarding the function of TRPM2 in heart injury during ischemia-reperfusion. Cheung and colleagues reported that TRPM2 protected the heart against ischemia-reperfusion injury [35,103,104]. TRPM2 was expressed in the sarcolemma and transverse tubules of adult cardiomyocytes. After reperfusion following coronary artery occlusion, no significant differences were observed in infarct sizes between WT and *Trpm2* KO mice. The heart function was, however, compromised in *Trpm2* KO mice. ROS levels in left ventricular myocytes were significantly higher in *Trpm2* KO mice than in WT mice after ischemia-reperfusion. The levels of superoxide dismutase and its transcriptional factors, forkhead box transcription factor and HIF, were lower, whereas that of the NADPH oxidase catalytic subunit, NOX4, was higher in *Trpm2* KO mouse hearts subjected to ischemia-reperfusion [35]. In addition, mitochondrial proteins and complex I subunits were down-regulated in *Trpm2* KO mouse heart [103]. These alterations in protein expression triggered by ROS overproduction and mitochondrial dysfunction in *Trpm2* KO mouse heart may be responsible for the heart dysfunction.

Another study, by contrast, found that heart functions were improved in *Trpm2* KO mice, suggesting that a deficiency in TRPM2 protects heart against ischemia-reperfusion injury [105]. Albeit TRPM2 mRNA expression was observed in the heart, its level was markedly lower than that in neutrophils or neurons. Neutrophilic infiltration of the heart after ischemia-reperfusion was reduced in *Trpm2* KO mice. It was speculated that TRPM2 expressed in neutrophils, rather than the heart, is important for ischemia-reperfusion heart injury. Indeed, in isolated hearts infarct sizes were significantly smaller in the heart obtained from *Trpm2* KO mice and perfused with *Trpm2* KO neutrophils compared to *Trpm2* KO hearts perfused with WT neutrophils. Likewise, infarct sizes were significantly larger in the heart of *Trpm2* KO mice carrying WT neutrophils compared to the heart of *Trpm2* KO mice with TRPM2-deficient neutrophils, suggesting that the activation of neutrophil TRPM2 during reperfusion has an important role in the development of myocardial infarction.

By using a cardiac-specific *Trpm2* KO mice, Cheung and colleagues recently reported a functional role for TRPM2 in the heart [104]. Similar to their studies using conventional *Trpm2* KO mice, heart functions after ischemia-reperfusion were aggravated in the cardiac-specific *Trpm2* KO mice. On the other hand, significant differences in infarct sizes were not observed between the WT and cardiac-specific *Trpm2* KO animals. In summary, the role of TRPM2 in cardiac ischemia-reperfusion injury remains controversial.

4.2.3. Kidneys

In the kidneys, TRPM2 is thought to contribute to the aggravation of renal injury and ROS production after ischemia-reperfusion [106]. TRPM2 is expressed in the proximal tubules. The disruption of *Trpm2* protects kidneys against ischemia-reperfusion injury. This involvement of TRPM2 was shown to be linked to the presence of TRPM2 in parenchymal cells rather than hematopoietic cells. Oxidative stress accompanied by the activation of NADPH oxidase was triggered in WT, but in *Trpm2* KO, mouse kidneys subjected to ischemia-reperfusion. Ca^{2+} influx via TRPM2 participated in the activation of RAS-related C3 botulinum toxin substrate-1 (RAC1), an essential factor for the activation of NADPH oxidase.

4.3. Other Diseases and Injuries

4.3.1. Acetaminophen-Induced Liver Injury

Acetaminophen is an antipyretic analgesic drug. Acetaminophen overdose (accidental or intentional) is a well-known cause of potentially fatal liver injury [107,108]. Acetaminophen is mainly metabolized into a non-toxic compound via glucuronidation and a sulfation reaction. On the other hand, a small amount of acetaminophen is converted to the toxic compound, *N*-acetyl-parabenzo-quinoneimine (NAPQI). NAPQI is then metabolized into a non-toxic compound via glutathione conjugation. NAPQI is responsible for acetaminophen-induced liver injury. NAPQI was shown to deplete intracellular glutathione levels, leading to the production of ROS [109]. TRPM2 has been implicated in acetaminophen-induced liver injury [109]. H_2O_2 and acetaminophen induce

Ca^{2+} influx into hepatocytes in a TRPM2-dependent manner. Acetaminophen-induced liver injury is attenuated in *Trpm2* KO mice compared to WT animals.

4.3.2. Radiation-Induced Tissue Damage

Radiation is a mainstay of treatment for head and neck cancer. Unfortunately, it has significant adverse effects on healthy tissues that are in the field of the treatment. For example, xerostomia (dry mouth) is a result of salivary gland damage by radiation. The molecular mechanism of radiation injury is complex including generation of ROS and DNA damage [110]. TRPM2 was reported to exacerbate radiation-induced salivary gland dysfunction [110]. H$_2$O$_2$ and radiation induced the influx of Ca^{2+} in salivary gland acinar cells. This influx was reduced by the disruption of *Trpm2*. The irreversible loss of salivary gland fluid secretion in WT mice subjected to radiation was improved by using free radical scavengers and/or PARP inhibitors.

4.3.3. Alzheimer's Disease

Alzheimer's disease (AD) is a devastating form of progressive dementia of unknown cause and no effective treatment. Therefore, it is an attractive hypothesis that TRPM2 may be involved in neuronal cell death in AD patients [111]. The suggested pathology of AD includes an alteration in the proteolytic processing of the amyloid precursor protein, APP. In addition, amyloid β-peptide (Aβ) is accumulated in the AD brain. Although the molecular defect responsible for AD remain unknown, dysregulation of Ca^{2+} homeostasis is widely believed to be intimately associated with Aβ toxicity [112]. Proposed mechanisms of Aβ neurotoxicity include the production of ROS, as well as excitotoxicity with the intracellular accumulation of Ca^{2+} [113].

Previously, Lustbader *et al* reported that Aβ-binding alcohol dehydrogenase directly interacted with Aβ in the mitochondria of both AD patients and transgenic mice. This interaction promotes the leakage of ROS [114]. A recent study suggested that TRPM2 is involved in Aβ-induced neurotoxicity [112]. APP/PS1 animals are double transgenic mice that express a chimeric mouse/human APP and overproduce Aβ. They are widely used as model of AD. APP/PS1 mice were crossed with *Trpm2* KO animals. Synapse loss and decreased levels of synaptic proteins are early correlates of the severity of AD [112]. The level of the synaptic marker, synaptophysin, in the hippocampus was found to be lower in APP/PS1 mice than in WT mice. Synaptophysin levels in the hippocampus of *Trpm2*-disrupted APP/PS1 mice were similar to those in WT mice. In addition, age-dependent spatial memory deficits in APP/PS1 mice were reversed in *Trpm2*-disrupted APP/PS1 mice. These observations imply an important role for TRPM2 in Aβ-induced neuronal toxicity.

In addition, AD is associated with reductions in cerebral blood flow early in the course of the disease [115]. This Aβ-induced cerebrovascular dysfunction may be mediated by TRPM2 [115]. Indeed, TRPM2 is expressed in brain endothelial cells; in these cells, Aβ stimulated the influx of Ca^{2+} via TRPM2. The Aβ-induced activation of TRPM2 in brain endothelial cells was mediated by ROS derived from the activation of NADPH oxidase. Reduction in cerebral blood flow was induced by the neocortical superfusion of Aβ, and was attenuated by PARP and PARG inhibitors, as well as the disruption of *Trpm2*. Combined, these findings indicate that Aβ-induced TRPM2 activation contributes to endothelial dysfunction.

5. Conclusions

There is increasing evidence that TRPM2 plays an important role in the pathomechanism of ROS-coupled diseases. For example, TRPM2 contributes to aggravation of disease states in which monocytes/macrophages play a pivotal role via cytokine production. In the brain and kidney, TRPM2 is involved in ischemia-reperfusion injury. Moreover, TRPM2 is implicated in innate immunity and the pathobiology of Alzheimer disease.

On the other hand, there are conflicting findings with regard to the function of TRPM2 in myocardial infarction and in LPS-induced lung injury. Non-specific TRPM2 inhibitors (e.g., PARP inhibitors, clotrimazole, and 2-APB) have been shown to attenuate the exacerbation of ROS-coupled diseases. For instance, PARP inhibitors were found to attenuate radiation-induced tissue damage [110], and bleomycin-induced lung injury [85]. Furthermore, clotrimazole attenuated heart [105] and brain damage [98,100] induced by ischemia-reperfusion. 2-APB also exerted protective effects against ischemia-reperfusion-induced brain [102] and kidney [106] damage (Figure 2). These promising results, however, must be confirmed by yet-to-be-synthesized selective TRPM2 antagonists.

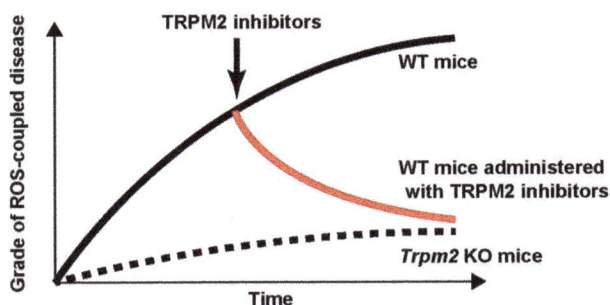

Figure 2. Does administration with TRPM2 inhibitors during ROS-coupled disease development improve the grade of these diseases? Pathological mouse model studies have been performed under *Trpm2*-disrupted conditions, and suggested that *Trpm2* KO mice are protected from ROS-coupled diseases. However, in terms of cure, it is important that the grade of these diseases is improved by the inhibition of TRPM2 during disease development. Therefore, the studies whether the inhibition of TRPM2 during ROS-coupled disease development has curative effects on the diseases should be done in the future.

Acknowledgments: The authors would like to thank Professor Arpad Szallasi in Drexel University College of Medicine for the English language review.

Conflicts of Interest: The authors declare no conflict of interest.

References

1. Clapham, D.E. Calcium signaling. *Cell* **1995**, *80*, 259–268. [CrossRef]
2. Montell, C.; Rubin, G.M. Molecular characterization of the Drosophila trp locus: A putative integral membrane protein required for phototransduction. *Neuron* **1989**, *2*, 1313–1323. [CrossRef]
3. Clapham, D.E. TRP channels as cellular sensors. *Nature* **2003**, *426*, 517–524. [CrossRef] [PubMed]
4. Goel, M.; Sinkins, W.G.; Schilling, W.P. Selective Association of TRPC Channel Subunits in Rat Brain Synaptosomes. *J. Biol. Chem.* **2002**, *277*, 48303–48310. [CrossRef] [PubMed]
5. Hofmann, T.; Schaefer, M.; Schultz, G.; Sudermann, T. Subunit composition of mammalian transient receptor potential channels in living cells. *Proc. Natl. Acad. Sci. USA* **2002**, *99*, 7461–7466. [CrossRef] [PubMed]
6. Zhu, X.; Jiang, M.; Peyton, M.; Boulay, G.; Hurst, R.; Stefani, E.; Birnbaumer, L. trp, a novel mammalian gene family essential for agonist-activated capacitative Ca^{2+} entry. *Cell* **1996**, *85*, 661–671. [CrossRef]
7. Hofmann, T.; Obukhov, A.G.; Schaefer, M.; Harteneck, C.; Gudermann, T.; Schultz, G. Direct activation of human TRPC6 and TRPC3 channels by diacylglycerol. *Nature* **1999**, *397*, 259–263. [PubMed]
8. Okada, T.; Inoue, R.; Yamazaki, K.; Maeda, A.; Kurosaki, T.; Yamakuni, T.; Tanaka, I.; Shimizu, S.; Ikenaka, K.; Imoto, K.; et al. Molecular and functional characterization of a novel mouse transient receptor potential protein homologue TRP7. *J. Biol. Chem.* **1999**, *274*, 27359–27370. [CrossRef] [PubMed]
9. Inoue, R.; Okada, T.; Onoue, H.; Hara, Y.; Shimizu, S.; Naitoh, S.; Ito, Y.; Mori, Y. The transient receptor potential protein homologue TRP6 is the essential component of vascular α_1-adrenoceptor-activated Ca^{2+}-permeable cation channel. *Circ. Res.* **2001**, *88*, 325–332. [CrossRef] [PubMed]
10. Caterina, M.J.; Schumacher, M.A.; Tominaga, M.; Rosen, T.A.; Levine, J.D.; Julius, D. The capsaicin receptor: A heat-activated ion channel in the pain pathway. *Nature* **1997**, *389*, 816–824. [PubMed]

11. Caterina, M.J.; Rosen, T.A.; Tominaga, M.; Brake, A.J.; Julius, D. A capsaicin-receptor homologue with a high threshold for noxious heat. *Nature* **1999**, *398*, 436–441. [PubMed]

12. Güler, A.D.; Lee, H.; Iida, T.; Shimizu, I.; Tominaga, M.; Caterina, M. Heat-evoked activation of the ion channel, TRPV4. *J. Neurosci.* **2002**, *22*, 6408–6414. [PubMed]

13. Peier, A.M.; Reeve, A.J.; Andersson, D.A.; Moqrich, A.; Earley, T.J.; Hergarden, A.C.; Story, G.M.; Colley, S.; Hogenesch, J.B.; McIntyre, P.; et al. A heat-sensitive TRP channel expressed in keratinocytes. *Science* **2002**, *296*, 2046–2049. [CrossRef] [PubMed]

14. Smith, G.D.; Gunthorpe, M.J.; Kelsell, R.E.; Hayes, P.D.; Reilly, P.; Facer, P.; Wright, J.E.; Jerman, J.C.; Walhin, J.P.; Ooi, L.; et al. TRPV3 is a temperature-sensitive vanilloid receptor-like protein. *Nature* **2002**, *418*, 186–190. [CrossRef] [PubMed]

15. Watanabe, H.; Vriens, J.; Suh, S.H.; Benham, C.D.; Droogmans, G.; Nilius, B. Heat-evoked activation of TRPV4 channels in a HEK293 cell expression system and in native mouse aorta endothelial cells. *J. Biol. Chem.* **2002**, *277*, 47044–47051. [CrossRef] [PubMed]

16. Xu, H.; Ramsey, I.S.; Kotecha, S.A.; Moran, M.M.; Chong, J.A.; Lawson, D.; Ge, P.; Lilly, J.; Silos-Santiago, I.; Xie, Y.; et al. TRPV3 is a calcium-permeable temperature-sensitive cation channel. *Nature* **2002**, *418*, 181–186. [CrossRef] [PubMed]

17. Tominaga, M.; Caterina, M.J.; Malmberg, A.B.; Rosen, T.A.; Gilbert, H.; Skinner, K.; Raumann, B.E.; Basbaum, A.I.; Julius, D. The cloned capsaicin receptor integrates multiple pain-producing stimuli. *Neuron* **1998**, *21*, 531–543. [CrossRef]

18. Liedtke, W.; Choe, Y.; Marti-Renom, M.A.; Bell, A.M.; Denis, C.S.; Sali, A.; Hudspeth, A.J.; Friedman, J.M.; Heller, S. Vanilloid receptor-related osmotically activated channel (VR-OAC), a candidate vertebrate osmoreceptor. *Cell* **2000**, *103*, 525–535. [CrossRef]

19. Strotmann, R.; Harteneck, C.; Nunnenmacher, K.; Schultz, G.; Plant, T.D. OTRPC4, a nonselective cation channel that confers sensitivity to extracellular osmolarity. *Nat. Cell Biol.* **2000**, *2*, 695–702. [PubMed]

20. McKemy, D.D.; Neuhausser, W.M.; Julius, D. Identification of a cold receptor reveals a general role for TRP channels in thermosensation. *Nature* **2002**, *416*, 52–58. [CrossRef] [PubMed]

21. Peier, A.M.; Moqrich, A.; Hergarden, A.C.; Reeve, A.J.; Andersson, D.A.; Story, G.M.; Earley, T.J.; Dragoni, I.; McIntyre, P.; Bevan, S.; et al. A TRP channel that senses cold stimuli and menthol. *Cell* **2002**, *108*, 705–715. [CrossRef]

22. Nauli, S.M.; Alenghat, F.J.; Luo, Y.; Williams, E.; Vassilev, P.; Li, X.; Elia, A.E.; Lu, W.; Brown, E.M.; Quinn, S.J.; et al. Polycystins 1 and 2 mediate mechanosensation in the primary cilium of kidney cells. *Nat. Genet.* **2003**, *33*, 129–137. [CrossRef] [PubMed]

23. Mochizuki, T.; Tsuchiya, K.; Nitta, K. Autosomal dominant polycystic kidney disease: Recent advances in pathogenesis and potential therapies. *Clin. Exp. Nephrol.* **2013**, *17*, 317–326. [CrossRef] [PubMed]

24. Jefferies, H.B.; Cooke, F.T.; Jat, P.; Boucheron, C.; Koizumi, T.; Hayakawa, M.; Kaizawa, H.; Ohishi, T.; Workman, P.; Waterfield, M.D.; et al. A selective PIKfyve inhibitor blocks PtdIns(3,5)P_2 production and disrupts endomembrane transport and retroviral budding. *EMBO Rep.* **2008**, *9*, 164–170. [CrossRef] [PubMed]

25. Dong, X.P.; Shen, D.; Wang, X.; Dawson, T.; Li, X.; Zhang, Q.; Cheng, X.; Zhang, Y.; Weisman, L.S.; Delling, M.; et al. PI(3,5)P_2 controls membrane trafficking by direct activation of mucolipin Ca^{2+} release channels in the endolysosome. *Nat. Commun.* **2010**, *1*, 38. [CrossRef] [PubMed]

26. Takahashi, N.; Mizuno, Y.; Kozai, D.; Yamamoto, S.; Kiyonaka, S.; Shibata, T.; Uchida, K.; Mori, Y. Molecular characterization of TRPA1 channel activation by cysteine-reactive inflammatory mediators. *Channels* **2008**, *2*, 287–298. [CrossRef] [PubMed]

27. Macpherson, L.J.; Geierstanger, B.H.; Viswanath, V.; Bandell, M.; Eid, S.R.; Hwang, S.; Patapoutian, A. The pungency of garlic: Activation of TRPA1 and TRPV1 in response to allicin. *Curr. Biol.* **2005**, *15*, 929–934. [CrossRef] [PubMed]

28. Jordt, S.E.; Bautista, D.M.; Chuang, H.H.; McKemy, D.D.; Zygmunt, P.M.; Hogestatt, E.D.; Meng, I.D.; Julius, D. Mustard oils and cannabinoids excite sensory nerve fibres through the TRP channel ANKTM1. *Nature* **2004**, *427*, 260–265. [CrossRef] [PubMed]

29. Takahashi, N.; Kuwaki, T.; Kiyonaka, S.; Numata, T.; Kozai, D.; Mizuno, Y.; Yamamoto, S.; Naito, S.; Knevels, E.; Carmeliet, P.; et al. TRPA1 underlies a sensing mechanism for O_2. *Nat. Chem. Biol.* **2011**, *10*, 701–711. [CrossRef] [PubMed]

30. Henricks, P.A.; Nijkamp, F.P. Reactive oxygen species as mediators in asthma. *Pulm. Pharmacol. Ther.* **2001**, *14*, 409–420. [CrossRef] [PubMed]

31. Dröge, W. Free radicals in the physiological control of cell function. *Physiol. Rev.* **2002**, *82*, 47–95. [CrossRef] [PubMed]

32. Taguchi, K.; Motohashi, H.; Yamamoto, M. Molecular mechanisms of Keap1-Nrf2 pathway in stress response and cancer evolution. *Genes Cells* **2011**, *16*, 123–140. [CrossRef] [PubMed]

33. Soga, M.; Matsuzawa, A.; Ichijo, H. Oxidative stress-induced diseases via the ASK1 signaling pathway. *Int. J. Cell Biol.* **2012**, *2012*. article ID 439587. [CrossRef] [PubMed]

34. Kaneko, S.; Kawakami, S.; Hara, Y.; Wakamori, M.; Itoh, E.; Minami, T.; Takada, Y.; Kume, T.; Katsuki, H.; Mori, Y.; et al. A critical role of TRPM2 in neuronal cell death by hydrogen peroxide. *J. Pharmacol. Sci.* **2006**, *101*, 66–76. [CrossRef] [PubMed]

35. Miller, B.A.; Wang, J.; Hirschler-Laszkiewicz, I.; Gao, E.; Song, J.; Zhang, X.; Koch, W.J.; Madesh, M.; Mallilankaraman, K.; Gu, T.; et al. The second member of transient receptor potential-melastatin channel family protects hearts from ischemia-reperfusion injury. *Am. J. Physiol. Heart Circ. Physiol.* **2013**, *304*, H1010–H1022. [CrossRef] [PubMed]

36. Togashi, K.; Hara, Y.; Tominaga, T.; Higashi, T.; Konishi, Y.; Mori, Y.; Tominaga, M. TRPM2 activation by cyclic ADP-ribose at body temperature is involved in insulin secretion. *EMBO J.* **2006**, *25*, 1804–1815. [CrossRef] [PubMed]

37. Lange, I.; Yamamoto, S.; Partida-Sánchez, S.; Mori, Y.; Fleig, A.; Penner, R. TRPM2 functions as lysosomal Ca^{2+} release channel in β-cells. *Sci. Signal.* **2009**, *71*, ra23. [CrossRef] [PubMed]

38. Partida-Sánchez, S.; Gasser, A.; Fliegert, R.; Siebrands, C.C.; Dammermann, W.; Shi, G.; Mousseau, B.J.; Sumazo-Toledo, A.; Bhagat, H.; Walseth, T.F.; et al. Chemotaxis of mouse bone marrow neutrophils and dendritic cell is controlled by ADP-ribose, the major product generated by the CD38 enzyme reaction. *J. Immunol.* **2007**, *179*, 7827–7839. [CrossRef] [PubMed]

39. Zhang, W.; Chu, X.; Tong, Q.; Cheung, J.Y.; Conrad, K.; Masker, K.; Miller, B.A. A novel TRPM2 isoform inhibits calcium influx and susceptibility to cell death. *J. Biol. Chem.* **2003**, *278*, 16222–16229. [CrossRef] [PubMed]

40. Yamamoto, S.; Shimizu, S.; Kiyonaka, S.; Takahashi, N.; Wajima, T.; Hara, Y.; Negoro, T.; Hiroi, T.; Kiuchi, Y.; Okada, T.; et al. TRPM2-mediated Ca^{2+} influx induces chemokine production in monocytes that aggravates inflammatory neutrophil infiltration. *Nat. Med.* **2008**, *14*, 738–747. [CrossRef] [PubMed]

41. Wehage, E.; Eisfeld, J.; Heiner, I.; Jungling, E.; Zitt, C.; Luckhoff, A. Activation of the cation channel long transient receptor potential channel 2 (LTRPC2) by hydrogen peroxide. A splice variant reveals a mode of activation independent of ADP-ribose. *J. Biol. Chem.* **2002**, *277*, 23150–23156. [CrossRef] [PubMed]

42. Sumoza-Toledo, A.; Lange, I.; Cortado, H.; Bhagat, H.; Mori, Y.; Fleig, A.; Penner, R.; Partida-Sánchez, S. Dendritic cell maturation and chemotaxis is regulated by TRPM2-mediated lysosomal Ca^{2+} release. *FASEB J.* **2011**, *25*, 3529–3542. [CrossRef] [PubMed]

43. Brieger, K.; Schiavone, S.; Miller, F.J.; Krause, K. Reactive oxygen species: From health to disease. *Swiss Med. Wkly.* **2012**, *142*, w13659. [CrossRef] [PubMed]

44. Kühn, F.J.; Lückhoff, A. Sites of the NUDT9-H domain critical for ADP-ribose activation of the cation channel TRPM2. *J. Biol. Chem.* **2004**, *279*, 46431–46437. [CrossRef] [PubMed]

45. Perraud, A.L.; Fleig, A.; Dunn, C.A.; Bagley, L.A.; Launay, P.; Schmitz, C.; Stokes, A.J.; Zhu, Q.; Bessman, M.J.; Penner, R.; et al. ADP-ribose gating of the calcium-permeable LTRPC2 channel revealed by Nudix motif homology. *Nature* **2001**, *411*, 595–599. [CrossRef] [PubMed]

46. Kolisek, M.; Beck, A.; Fleig, A.; Penner, R. Cyclic ADP-ribose and hydrogen peroxide synergize with ADP-ribose in the activation of TRPM2 channels. *Mol. Cell* **2005**, *18*, 61–69. [CrossRef] [PubMed]

47. Starkus, J.; Beck, A.; Fleig, A.; Penner, R. Regulation of TRPM2 by extra- and intracellular calcium. *J. Gen. Physiol.* **2007**, *130*, 427–440. [CrossRef] [PubMed]

48. Lange, I.; Penner, R.; Fleig, A.; Beck, A. Synergistic regulation of endogenous TRPM2 channels by adenine dinucleotides in primary human neutrophils. *Cell Calcium* **2008**, *44*, 604–615. [CrossRef] [PubMed]

49. Du, J.; Xie, J.; Yue, L. Intracellular calcium activates TRPM2 and tis alternative spliced isoforms. *Proc. Natl. Acad. Sci. USA* **2009**, *106*, 7239–7244. [CrossRef] [PubMed]

50. Heiner, I.; Eisfeld, J.; Warnstedt, M.; Radukina, N.; Jüngling, E.; Lückhoff, A. Endogenous ADP-ribose enables calcium-regulated cation currents through TRPM2 channels in neutrophil granulocytes. *Biochem. J.* **2006**, *398*, 225–232. [CrossRef] [PubMed]

51. Tóth, B.; Csanády, L. Identification of direct and indirect effectors of the transient receptor potential melastatin 2 (TRPM2) cation channel. *J. Biol. Chem.* **2010**, *285*, 30091–30102. [CrossRef] [PubMed]

52. Tóth, B.; Iordanov, I.; Csanády, L. Ruling out pyridine dinucleotides as true TRPM2 channel activators reveals novel direct agonist ADP-ribose-2'-phosphate. *J. Gen. Physiol.* **2015**, *145*, 419–430. [CrossRef] [PubMed]

53. Grubisha, O.; Rafty, L.A.; Takanishi, C.L.; Xu, X.; Tong, L.; Perraud, A.L.; Scharenberg, A.M.; Denu, J.M. Metabolite of SIR2 reaction modulates TRPM2 ion channel. *J. Biol. Chem.* **2006**, *281*, 14057–14065. [CrossRef] [PubMed]

54. Hara, Y.; Wakamori, M.; Ishii, M.; Maeno, E.; Nishida, M.; Yoshida, T.; Yamada, H.; Shimizu, S.; Mori, E.; Kudoh, J.; et al. LTRPC2 Ca^{2+}-permeable channel activated by changes in redox status confers susceptibility to cell death. *Mol. Cell* **2002**, *9*, 163–173. [CrossRef]

55. Perraud, A.L.; Takanishi, C.L.; Shen, B.; Kang, S.; Smith, M.K.; Schmitz, C.; Knowles, H.M.; Ferraris, D.; Li, W.; Zhang, J.; et al. Accumulation of free ADP-ribose from mitochondria mediates oxidative stress-induced gating of TRPM2 cation channels. *J. Biol. Chem.* **2005**, *280*, 6138–6148. [CrossRef] [PubMed]

56. Malavasi, F.; Deaglio, S.; Funaro, A.; Ferrero, E.; Horenstein, A.L.; Ortolan, E.; Vaisitti, T.; Aydin, S. Evolution and function of the ADP ribosyl cyclase/CD38 gene family in physiology and pathology. *Physiol. Rev.* **2008**, *88*, 841–886. [CrossRef] [PubMed]

57. Magnone, M.; Bauer, I.; Poggi, A.; Mannino, E.; Sturla, L.; Brini, M.; Zocchi, E.; De Flora, A.; Nencioni, A.; Bruzzone, S. NAD^{+} levels control Ca^{2+} sore replenishment and mitogen-induced increase of cytosolic Ca^{2+} by cyclic ADP-ribose-dependent TRPM2 channel gating in human T lymphocytes. *J. Biol. Chem.* **2012**, *287*, 21067–21081. [CrossRef] [PubMed]

58. Tanuma, S.; Yagi, T.; Johnson, G.S. Endogenous ADP ribosylation of high mobility group proteins 1 and 2 and histone H1 following DNA damage in intact cells. *Arch. Biochem. Biophys.* **1985**, *237*, 38–42. [CrossRef]

59. De Murcia, G.; de Murcia, J.M. Poly(ADP-ribose) polymerase: A molecular nick-sensor. *Trends Biochem. Sci.* **1994**, *19*, 172–176. [CrossRef]

60. Oliver, F.J.; Menissier-de Murcia, J.; Nacci, C.; Decker, P.; Andriantsitohaina, R.; Muller, S.; de la Rubia, G.; Stoclet, J.C.; de Murcia, G. Resistance to endotoxic shock as a consequence of defective NF-κB activation in poly (ADP-ribose) polymerase-1 deficient mice. *EMBO J.* **1999**, *18*, 4446–4454. [CrossRef] [PubMed]

61. Virág, L.; Szabo, C. The therapeutic potential of poly(ADP-ribose) polymerase inhibitors. *Pharmacol. Rev.* **2002**, *54*, 375–429. [CrossRef] [PubMed]

62. Fonfria, E.; Marshall, I.C.; Benham, C.D.; Boyfield, I.; Brown, J.D.; Hill, K.; Hughes, J.P.; Skaper, S.D.; McNulty, S. TRPM2 channel opening in response to oxidative stress is dependent on activation of poly(ADP-ribose) polymerase. *Br. J. Pharmacol.* **2004**, *143*, 186–192. [CrossRef] [PubMed]

63. Buelow, B.; Song, Y.; Andrew, M.; Scharenberg, A.M. The poly(ADP-ribose) polymerase PARP-1 is required for oxidative stress-induced TRPM2 activation in lymphocytes. *J. Biol. Chem.* **2008**, *283*, 24571–24583. [CrossRef] [PubMed]

64. Ishii, M.; Shimizu, S.; Hara, Y.; Hagiwara, T.; Miyazaki, A.; Mori, Y.; Kiuchi, Y. Intracellular-produced hydroxyl radical mediates H_2O_2-induced Ca^{2+} influx and cell death in rat beta-cell line RIN-5F. *Cell Calcium* **2006**, *39*, 487–494. [CrossRef] [PubMed]

65. Shimizu, S.; Yonezawa, R.; Negoro, T.; Yamamoto, S.; Numata, T.; Ishii, M.; Mori, Y.; Toda, T. Sensitization of H_2O_2-induced TRPM2 activation and subsequent interleukin-8 (CXCL8) production by intracellular Fe^{2+} in human monocytic U937 cells. *Int. J. Biochem. Cell Biol.* **2015**, *68*, 119–127. [CrossRef] [PubMed]

66. Zhang, W.; Tong, Q.; Conrad, K.; Wozney, J.; Cheung, J.Y.; Miller, B.A. Regulation of TRP channel TRPM2 by the tyrosine phosphatase PTPL1. *Am. J. Physiol. Cell Physiol.* **2007**, *292*, C1746–C1758. [CrossRef] [PubMed]

67. Hill, K.; McNulty, S.; Randall, A.D. Inhibition of TRPM2 channels by the antifungal agents clotrimazole and econazole. *Naunyn-Schmiedeberg's Arch. Pharmacol.* **2004**, *370*, 227–237. [CrossRef] [PubMed]

68. Hill, K.; Benham, C. D.; McNulty, S.; Randall, A.D. Flufenamic acid is a pH-dependent antagonist of TRPM2 channels. *Neuropharmacology* **2004**, *47*, 450–460. [CrossRef] [PubMed]

69. Togashi, K.; Inada1, H.; Tominaga, M. Inhibition of the transient receptor potential cation channel TRPM2 by 2-aminoethoxydiphenyl borate (2-APB). *Br. J. Pharmacol.* **2008**, *153*, 1324–1330. [CrossRef] [PubMed]

70. Bari, M.R.; Akbar, S.; Eweida, M.; Kühn, F.J.; Gustafsson, A.J.; Lückhoff, A.; Islam, M.S. H_2O_2-induced Ca^{2+} influx and its inhibition by *N*-(p-amylcinnamoyl) anthranilic acid in the beta-cells: Involvement of TRPM2 channels. *J. Cell. Mol. Med.* **2009**, *13*, 3260–3267. [CrossRef] [PubMed]

71. Kheradpezhouh, E.; Barritt, G.J.; Rychkov, G.Y. Curcumin inhibits activation of TRPM2 channels in rat hepatocytes. *Redox Biol.* **2016**, *7*, 1–7. [CrossRef] [PubMed]

72. Shimizu, S.; Yonezawa, R.; Hagiwara, T.; Yoshida, T.; Takahashi, N.; Hamano, S.; Negoro, T.; Toda, T.; Wakamori, M.; Mori, Y.; et al. Inhibitory effects of AG490 on H_2O_2-induced TRPM2-mediated Ca^{2+} entry. *Eur. J. Pharmacol.* **2014**, *742*, 22–30. [CrossRef] [PubMed]

73. Toda, T.; Yamamoto, S.; Yonezawa, R.; Mori, Y.; Shimizu, S. Inhibitory effects of Tyrphostin AG-related compounds on oxidative stress-sensitive transient receptor potential channel activation. *Eur. J. Pharmacol.* **2016**, *786*, 19–28. [CrossRef] [PubMed]

74. Berton, G.; Castaldi, M.A.; Cassatella, M.A.; Nauseef, W.M. Celebrating the 50th anniversary of the seminal discovery that the phagocyte respiratory burst enzyme is an NADPH oxidase. *J. Leukoc. Biol.* **2015**, *97*, 1–2. [CrossRef] [PubMed]

75. Lambeth, J.D. NOX enzymes and the biology of reactive oxygen. *Nat. Rev. Immunol.* **2004**, *4*, 181–189. [CrossRef] [PubMed]

76. Akira, S.; Takeda, K. Toll-like receproe signaling. *Nat. Rev. Immunol.* **2004**, *4*, 499–511. [CrossRef] [PubMed]

77. Kohchi, C.; Inagawa, H.; Nishizawa, T.; Soma, G. ROS and innate immunity. *Anticancer Res.* **2009**, *29*, 817–822. [PubMed]

78. Schwabe, R.F.; Brenner, D.A. Mechanisms of liver injury. I. TNF-α-induced liver injury: Role of IKK, JNK, and ROS pathways. *Am. J. Physiol. Gastrointest. Liver Physiol.* **2006**, *290*, 583–589. [CrossRef] [PubMed]

79. Simon, H.U.; Haj-Yehia, A.; Levi-Schaffer, F. Role of reactive oxygen species (ROS) in apoptosis induction. *Apoptosis* **2000**, *5*, 415–418. [CrossRef] [PubMed]

80. Kalogeris, T.; Bao, Y.; Korthuis, R.J. Mitochondrial reactive oxygen species: A double edged sword in ischemia/reperfusion vs preconditioning. *Redox Biol.* **2014**, *2*, 702–714. [CrossRef] [PubMed]

81. Kleikers, P.W.; Wingler, K.; Hermans, J.J.; Diebold, I.; Altenhöfer, S.; Radermacher, K.A.; Janssen, B.; Görlach, A.; Schmidt, H.H. NADPH oxidases as a source of oxidative stress and molecular target in ischemia/reperfusion injury. *J. Mol. Med.* **2012**, *90*, 1391–1406. [CrossRef] [PubMed]

82. Pacher, P.; Nivorozhkin, A.; Szabó, C. Therapeutic effects of xanthine oxidase inhibitors: Renaissance half a century after the discovery of allopurinol. *Pharmacol. Rev.* **2006**, *58*, 87–114. [CrossRef] [PubMed]

83. Luster, A.D. Chemokines—Chemotactic cytokines that mediate inflammation. *N. Engl. J. Med.* **1998**, *338*, 436–445. [PubMed]

84. Haraguchi, K.; Kawamoto, A.; Isami, K.; Maeda, S.; Kusano, A.; Asakura, K.; Shirakawa, H.; Mori, Y.; Nakagawa, T.; Kaneko, S. TRPM2 contributes to inflammatory and neuropathic pain through the aggravation of pronociceptive inflammatory responses in mice. *J. Neurosci.* **2012**, *32*, 3931–3941. [CrossRef] [PubMed]

85. Yonezawa, R.; Yamamoto, S.; Takenaka, M.; Kage, Y.; Negoro, T.; Toda, T.; Ohbayashi, M.; Numata, T.; Nakano, Y.; Yamamoto, T.; et al. TRPM2 channels in alveolar epithelial cells mediate bleomycin-induced lung inflammation. *Free Radic. Biol.* **2016**, *90*, 101–113. [CrossRef] [PubMed]

86. Wehrhahn, J.; Kraft, R.; Harteneck, C.; Hauschildt, S. Transient receptor potential melastatin 2 is required for lipopolysaccharide-induced cytokine production in human monocytes. *J. Immunol.* **2010**, *184*, 2386–2393. [CrossRef] [PubMed]

87. Hardaker, L.; Bahra, P.; de Billy, B.C.; Freeman, M.; Kupfer, N.; Wyss, D.; Trifilieff, A. The ion channel transient receptor potential melastatin-2 does not play a role in inflammatory mouse models of chronic obstructive pulmonary diseases. *Respir. Res.* **2012**, *13*, 30. [CrossRef] [PubMed]

88. Di, A.; Gao, X.; Qian, F.; Kawamura, T.; Han, J.; Hecquet, C.; Ye, R.D.; Vogel, S.M.; Malik, A.B. The redox-sensitive cation channel TRPM2 modulates phagocyte ROS production and inflammation. *Nat. Immunol.* **2012**, *13*, 29–34. [CrossRef] [PubMed]

89. Mohapatra, N.P.; Soni, S.; Rajaram, M.V.; Dang, P.M.; Reilly, T.J.; El-Benna, J.; Clay, C.D.; Schlesinger, L.S.; Gunn, J.S. *Francisella* acid phosphatases inactivate the NADPH oxidase in human phagocytes. *J. Imunnol.* **2010**, *184*, 5141–5150. [CrossRef] [PubMed]

90. Shakerley, N.L.; Chandrasekaran, A.; Trebak, M.; Miller, B.A.; Melendez, J.A. *Francisella tularensis* catalase restricts immune function by impairing TRPM2 channel activity. *J. Imunnol.* **2016**, *291*, 3871–3881.

91. Knowles, H.; Heizer, J.W.; Li, Y.; Chapman, K.; Ogden, C.A.; Andreasen, K.; Shapland, E.; Kucera, G.; Mogan, J.; Humann, J.; et al. Transient receptor potential melastatin 2 (TRPM2) ion channel is required for innate immunity against *Listeria monocytogenes*. *Proc. Natl. Acad. Sci. USA* **2011**, *108*, 11578–11583. [CrossRef] [PubMed]

92. Partida-Sánchez, S.; Cockayne, D.A.; Monard, S.; Jacobson, E.L.; Oppenheimer, N.; Garvy, B.; Kusser, K.; Goodrich, S.; Howard, M.; Harmsen, A.; et al. Cyclic ADP-ribose production by CD38 regulates intracellular calcium release, extracellular calcium influx and chemotaxis in neutrophils and is required for bacterial clearance in vivo. *Nat. Med.* **2001**, *7*, 1209–1216. [CrossRef] [PubMed]

93. Tschopp, J.; Schroder, K. NLRP3 inflammasome activation: The convergence of multiple signaling pathways on ROS production? *Nat. Rev. Immunol.* **2010**, *10*, 210–215. [CrossRef] [PubMed]

94. Zhong, Z.; Zhai, Y.; Liang, S.; Mori, Y.; Han, R.; Sutterwala, F.S.; Qiao, L. TRPM2 links oxidative stress to NLRP3 inflammasome activation. *Nat. Commun.* **2013**, *4*, 1611. [CrossRef] [PubMed]

95. West, A.P.; Shadel, G.S.; Ghosh, S. Mitochondria in innate immune responses. *Nat. Rev. Immunol.* **2011**, *11*, 389–402. [CrossRef] [PubMed]

96. Chen, Q.; Surmeier, D.J.; Reiner, A. NMDA and non-NMDA receptor-mediated excitotoxicity are potentiated in cultured striatal neurons by prior chronic depolarization. *Exp. Neurol.* **1999**, *159*, 283–296. [CrossRef] [PubMed]

97. Burgoyne, R.D. Neuronal calcium sensor proteins: Generating diversity in neuronal Ca^{2+} signaling. *Nat. Rev. Neurosci.* **2007**, *8*, 182–193. [CrossRef] [PubMed]

98. Jia, J.; Verma, S.; Nakayama, S.; Quillinan, N.; Grafe, M.R.; Hurn, P.D.; Herson, P.S. Sex differences in neuroprotection provided by inhibition of TRPM2 channels following experimental stroke. *J. Cereb. Blood Flow Metab.* **2011**, *31*, 2160–2168. [CrossRef] [PubMed]

99. Verma, S.; Quillinan, N.; Yang, Y.; Nakayama, S.; Cheng, J.; Kelley, M.H.; Herson, P.S. TRPM2 channel activation following in vitro ischemia contributes to male hippocampal cell death. *Neurosci. Lett.* **2012**, *530*, 41–46. [CrossRef] [PubMed]

100. Shimizu, T.; Macey, T.A.; Quillinan, N.; Klawitter, J.; Perraud, A.L.; Traystman, R.J.; Herson, P.S. Androgen and PARP-1 regulation of TRPM2 channels after ischemic injury. *J. Cereb. Blood Flow Metab.* **2013**, *33*, 1549–1555. [CrossRef] [PubMed]

101. Alim, I.; Teves, L.; Li, R.; Mori, Y.; Tymianski, M. Modulation of NMDAR subunit expression by TRPM2 channels regulates neuronal vulnerability of ischemic cell death. *J. Neurosci.* **2013**, *33*, 17264–17277. [CrossRef] [PubMed]

102. Gelderblom, M.; Melzer, N.; Schattling, B.; Gob, E.; Hicking, G.; Arunachalam, P.; Bittner, S.; Ufer, F.; Herrmann, A.M.; Bernreuther, C.; et al. Transient receptor potential melastatin subfamily member 2 cation channel regulates detrimental immune cell invasion in ischemic stroke. *Stroke* **2014**, *45*, 3395–3402. [CrossRef] [PubMed]

103. Miller, B.A.; Hoffman, N.E.; Merali, S.; Zhang, X.Q.; Wang, J.; Rajan, S.; Shanmughapriya, S.; Gao, E.; Barrero, C.A.; Mallilankaraman, K.; et al. TRPM2 cahnnels protect against cardiac ischemia-reperfusion injury. *J. Biol. Chem.* **2014**, *289*, 7615–7629. [CrossRef] [PubMed]

104. Hoffman, N.E.; Miller, B.A.; Wang, J.; Elrod, J.W.; Rajan, S.; Gao, E.; Song, J.; Zhang, X.; Hirschler-Laszkiewicz, I.; Shanmughapriya, S.; et al. Ca^{2+} entry via Trpm2 is essential for cardiac myocyte bioenergetics maintenance. *Am. J. Physiol. Heart Circ. Physiol.* **2015**, *308*, H637–H650. [CrossRef] [PubMed]

105. Hiroi, T.; Wajima, T.; Nrgoro, T.; Ishii, M.; Nakano, Y.; Kiuchi, Y.; Mori, Y.; Shimizu, S. Neutrophil TRPM2 channels are implicated in the exacerbation of myocardial ishchemia/reperfusion injury. *Cardiovasc. Res.* **2013**, *97*, 271–281. [CrossRef] [PubMed]

106. Gao, G.; Wang, W.; Tadagavadi, R.K.; Briley, N.E.; Love, M.I.; Miller, B.A.; Reeves, W.B. TRPM2 mediates ischemic kidney injury and oxidant stress through RAC1. *J. Clin. Investig.* **2014**, *124*, 4989–5001. [CrossRef] [PubMed]

107. Davidson, D.G.; Eastham, W.N. Acute liver necrosis following overdose of paracetamol. *BMJ* **1966**, *2*, 497–499. [CrossRef] [PubMed]

108. Mitchell, J.R.; Jollow, D.J.; Potter, W.Z.; Davis, D.C.; Gillette, J.R.; Brodie, B.B. Acetaminophen-induced hepatic necrosis. I. role of drug metabolism. *J. Pharmacol. Exp. Ther.* **1971**, *187*, 185–194.

109. Kheradpezhouh, E.; Ma, L.; Morphett, A.; Barritt, G.J.; Rychkov, G.Y. TRPM2 channels mediate acetaminophen-induced liver damage. *Proc. Natl. Acad. Sci. USA* **2014**, *111*, 3176–3181. [CrossRef] [PubMed]

110. Liu, X.; Cotrim, A.; Teos, L.; Zheng, C.; Swaim, W.; Mitchell, J.; Mori, Y.; Ambudkar, I. Loss of TRPM2 function protects against irradiation-induced salivary gland dysfunction. *Nat. Commun.* **2013**, *4*, 1515. [CrossRef] [PubMed]

111. Yamamoto, S.; Wajima, T.; Hara, Y.; Nishida, M.; Mori, Y. Transient receptor potential channels in Alzheimer's disease. *Biochim. Biophys. Acta* **2007**, *1772*, 958–967. [CrossRef] [PubMed]

112. Ostapchenko, V.G.; Chen, M.; Guzman, M.S.; Xie, Y.F.; Lavine, N.; Fan, J.; Beraldo, F.H.; Martyn, A.C.; Belrose, J.C.; Mori, Y.; et al. The transient receptor potential melastatin 2 (TRPM2) channel contributes to β-amyloid oligomer-related neurotoxicity and memory impairment. *J. Neurosci.* **2015**, *35*, 15157–15169. [CrossRef] [PubMed]

113. Zuo, L.; Hemmelgarn, B.T.; Chuang, C.; Besr, T.M. The role of oxidative stress-induced epigenetic alterations in amyloid-β production in Alzheimer's disease. *Oxid. Med. Cell. Longev.* **2015**, *2015*, Article ID 604658. [CrossRef] [PubMed]

114. Lustbader, J.W.; Cirilli, M.; Lin, C.; Xu, H.W.; Takuma, K.; Wang, N.; Caspersen, C.; Chen, X.; Pollak, S.; Chaney, M.; et al. ABAD directly links Aβ to mitochondrial toxicity in Alzheimer's disease. *Science* **2004**, *304*, 448–452. [CrossRef] [PubMed]

115. Park, L.; Wang, G.; Moore, J.; Girouard, H.; Zhou, P.; Anrather, J.; Iadecola, C. The key role of transient receptor potential melastatin-2 channels in amyloid-β-induced neurovascular dysfunction. *Nat. Commun.* **2014**, *5*, 5318. [CrossRef] [PubMed]

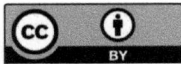

pharmaceuticals

MDPI

Review

Modulation of TRP Channel Activity by Hydroxylation and Its Therapeutic Potential

Yagnesh Nagarajan [1], Grigori Y. Rychkov [2,3] and Daniel J. Peet [1,*

[1] School of Biological Sciences, University of Adelaide, Adelaide 5005, SA, Australia; yagnesh.nagarajan@adelaide.edu.au

[2] School of Medicine, University of Adelaide, Adelaide 5005, SA, Australia; grigori.rychkov@adelaide.edu.au

[3] South Australian Health and Medical Research Institute (SAHMRI), Adelaide 5005, SA, Australia

* Correspondence: daniel.peet@adelaide.edu.au; Tel.: +61-8-8313-5367

Academic Editors: Arpad Szallasi and Susan M. Huang
Received: 30 January 2017; Accepted: 24 March 2017; Published: 27 March 2017

Abstract: Two transient receptor potential (TRP) channels—TRPA1 and TRPV3—are post-translationally hydroxylated, resulting in oxygen-dependent regulation of channel activity. The enzymes responsible are the HIF prolyl hydroxylases (PHDs) and the asparaginyl hydroxylase factor inhibiting HIF (FIH). The PHDs and FIH are well characterized for their hydroxylation of the hypoxic inducible transcription factors (HIFs), mediating their hypoxic regulation. Consequently, these hydroxylases are currently being targeted therapeutically to modulate HIF activity in anemia, inflammation, and ischemic disease. Modulating the HIFs by targeting these hydroxylases may result in both desirable and undesirable effects on TRP channel activity, depending on the physiological context. For the best outcomes, these hydroxylases could be therapeutically targeted in pathologies where activation of both the HIFs and the relevant TRP channels are predicted to independently achieve positive outcomes, such as wound healing and obesity.

Keywords: TRPA1; TRPV3; hydroxylation; PHD; FIH; HIF; oxygen; hypoxia

1. Introduction

The transient receptor potential (TRP) channels are non-selective cation channels broadly expressed in most tissues in the body. TRP channels play a role as cellular sensors which respond to a diverse range of extracellular and intracellular stimuli, including second messengers, chemicals, temperature, redox state, mechanical stimulation, and osmolality [1–4]. Recent research suggests that abnormal activity of some members of the TRP super-family contributes to human pathologies such as cancer, diabetes, lung and liver fibrosis, chronic pain, ischemia-reperfusion injury, pulmonary hypertension, irritable bowel disease, drug toxicity, and others [2,5–9].

TRP channels are formed by homo- or hetero-tetramers of TRP proteins, with each a TRP monomer comprised of six transmembrane domains flanked by intracellular N- and C-terminal domains. Similar to voltage-gated channels, a conserved pore-forming loop between transmembrane domains 5 and 6 in TRP proteins is responsible for cation permeability. Although most TRP channels under physiological conditions conduct more Na^+ than Ca^{2+}, the Ca^{2+} permeability of TRP channels is considered to be important for the maintenance of intracellular Ca^{2+} signaling and homeostasis.

Apart from specific stimuli that gate TRP channels, TRP channel activity can be further controlled by a range of post-translational modifications, including phosphorylation and glycosylation (reviewed in [10]). Two specific TRP channels—TRPA1 and TRPV3—are modified post-translationally by hydroxylation (an oxygen-dependent modification), which mediates a characteristic response to hypoxia [11,12]. The hydroxylases responsible for these modifications have emerged as key therapeutic targets for a range of human diseases due to their direct regulation of the hypoxia-inducible factors

(HIFs, the central transcription factors that mediate the genomic response to hypoxia), with important therapeutic implications for TRP channels.

2. Hydroxylation-Dependent Regulation of Hypoxic Gene Expression

The prolyl hydroxylase containing enzymes (PHDs) and the asparaginyl hydroxylase factor inhibiting HIF (FIH) belong to a conserved family of 2-oxoglutarate-dependent dioxygenases, and act as cellular oxygen sensors [13]. These oxygen-sensing enzymes catalyze the addition of hydroxyl (OH) groups to specific prolyl or asparaginyl residues on target proteins, altering their activity. The three closely related PHD enzymes (PHD1, 2, and 3, also referred to in the literature as EGLN2, 1, and 3) were originally characterized through their oxygen-dependent hydroxylation of two proline residues within the HIFα subunit of the heterodimeric HIF transcription factors. HIFα hydroxylation occurs in normoxia and promotes ubiquitination and rapid proteosomal-mediated degradation (reviewed in [14]). In hypoxia the activity of the PHDs decreases, allowing the HIFα subunits to avoid hydroxylation, ubiquitylation and subsequent degradation, and consequently the stabilized HIFα mediates robust gene induction in response to hypoxia (Figure 1). Thus, the PHDs act as the essential oxygen sensors in this pathway and are the primary regulators of the HIF-driven genomic response to hypoxia. FIH was subsequently characterized as a related hydroxylase that hydroxylates a single asparaginyl residue in a transactivation domain of the HIFα subunit, resulting in transcriptional repression in hypoxia (reviewed in [15]). As with the PHDs, hypoxia results in the loss of efficient oxygen-dependent hydroxylation, and alleviates the transcriptional repression, contributing to increased hypoxic gene induction mediated by the HIFs. However, the role of FIH in modulating oxygen-dependent gene regulation via the HIFs is modest compared to the PHDs, and its physiological importance less well characterized.

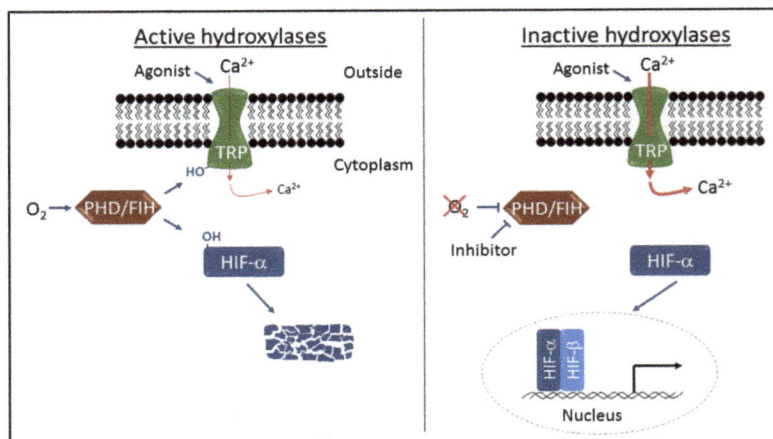

Figure 1. Schematic representation of transient receptor potential (TRP) channel and hypoxia-inducible factor (HIF) regulation by the prolyl hydroxylase containing enzymes (PHD) and asparaginyl hydroxylase factor inhibiting HIF (FIH) hydroxylases. Oxygen-dependent hydroxylation (-OH) of TRPA1 and TRPV3 channels inhibits cation entry through activated channels, and hydroxylation of HIFα proteins leads to proteolytic degradation and transcriptional repression. Inhibition of hydroxylase activity by hypoxia or specific inhibitors leads to increased cation entry and robust HIF-dependent gene activation.

The PHDs and FIH also have a number of substrates in addition to the HIF proteins, although the physiological consequence of hydroxylation on these substrates has not been well established. Other substrates for the PHDs include pyruvate kinase M2, RNA polymerase II, erythropoietin receptor, eukaryotic elongation factor 2, and beta(2)-adrenergic receptor [16]. FIH has been shown to hydroxylate a number of proteins containing ankyrin repeat domains (ARDs), although in most cases there is no obvious effect on the function of the hydroxylated substrate [17]. However, two more recently identified ARD substrates and one non-ARD substrate show some hydroxylation-dependent changes in activity [11,18,19].

3. Hydroxylation-Dependent Regulation of TRP Channel Activity

TRPA1 is activated by a range of chemical agonists (both endogenous and exogenous), mechanical stimulation, and cold temperature (reviewed in [20]). It has been implicated in a number of pathologies, including acute inflammation and cartilage degeneration in osteoarthritis [21], urinary bladder pain in cystitis [22], neuropathic and inflammatory pain, migraine, and familial episodic pain syndrome [23,24]. Takahashi and colleagues reported that TRPA1 is also sensitive to changes in oxygen, undergoing oxygen-dependent hydroxylation on a single proline residue within the ARD by the PHDs in normoxia [12]. Their data supported hydroxylation-dependent inhibition of channel activity that was rapidly reversed in hypoxia, when the oxygen-sensing PHDs have greatly diminished activity, leading to an increase in activity of the unmodified channel. Furthermore, they demonstrated that TRPA1 channels also respond to oxygen through the oxidation in hyperoxia of specific cysteine residues located within the seventeenth ARD (Cys 633 and Cys 856). A recent study proposes a role for TRPA1 hydroxylation in the hypoxic ventilator response [25]. In addition, this oxygen-dependent hydroxylation has been implicated in mediating the response to cold temperature through the production of reactive oxygen species [26]. Of interest, TRPA1 also responds to ischemia in oligodendrocytes, mediating Ca^{2+} entry and subsequent damage to myelin, although the role of hydroxylation in this response has not been explored [27].

TRPV3 was originally characterized as a warm temperature sensing channel [28–30], and is also activated by endogenous and exogenous chemical ligands. It plays roles in the maintenance of epidermal barrier function, hair growth, and nociception, and has been implicated in pathologies associated with dermatitis, pruritus, inflammation, ischemia, and wound healing [31,32]. The TRPV3 channel has also been shown to be hydroxylated, but on a single asparaginyl residue within the ARD, by FIH [11]. In common with the PHD-mediated hydroxylation of TRPA1, FIH-dependent hydroxylation of TRPV3 in normoxia inhibits channel activity, but is rapidly reversed in hypoxia, leading to increased hypoxic TRPV3 activity (Figure 1).

In the case of both TRPA1 and TRPV3, the mechanism by which hydroxylation modulates channel activity has not been determined. For example, hydroxylation may influence the physical structure of the channels and consequently influence gating, or may affect agonist binding, multimerisation with other TRP channels, or the recruitment of accessory proteins that modulate function. In addition, while the evidence for TRPA1 and TRPV3 hydroxylation is strong, as with other non-HIF substrates, the physiological role for these hydroxylation events remains poorly defined.

Whether other TRP channels are regulated by hydroxylation, mediated by the PHDs, FIH, or other hydroxylases remains unclear. In addition to TRPA1 and TRPV3, it has also been reported that peptides from the ARD of TRPV4 can be hydroxylated in vitro by FIH [33]. We have investigated the hydroxylation of nine other TRP channels predicted using bioinformatics to be substrates of FIH (TRPC1, C3, C4, C5, C6, V2, V5, V6), but found no evidence for hydroxylation using in vitro hydroxylation assays (unpublished data). Furthermore, other than TRPA1, none of the nine other TRP channels analyzed by Takahashi et al. displayed hypoxic induction, including TRPV3. However, it is important to note that these experiments were performed in 10% oxygen, which is relatively mild hypoxia and unlikely to influence FIH-mediated hydroxylation [12,34]. A recent report of interest implicated mouse TRPC2 in sensing low oxygen within olfactory epithelium [35]. While it is unclear whether this response involves hydroxylation (and TRPC2 is only a pseudogene in humans), it does support the hypothesis that other TRP channels may also be regulated in a similar manner to TRPA1 and TRPV3. The formation of heterotetramers with other channels may also cause the modification of one channel to influence the activity of another. For example, TRPV3 is known to form functional heterotetramers with TRPV1 [29,36], hence regulation of TRPV3 via hydroxylation may indirectly influence the activity of a TRPV1/V3 heterotetramer where V1 is activated.

Although the body of literature on TRP-hydroxylation is clearly very limited and more research is required to ascertain the physiological relevance, these studies establish that the oxygen-dependent hydroxylation of at least two members of the TRP superfamily confers hypoxic responsiveness to these channels. These findings have important implications regarding the potential for novel therapeutic manipulation of the activity of these specific TRP channels via altered hydroxylation, either directly or as a consequence of the therapeutic targeting of the PHDs and FIH to regulate other substrates.

4. Therapeutic Targeting of PHDs and FIH to Activate HIF

Given that hypoxia contributes to the pathophysiology of most major diseases, including myocardial and cerebral ischemia, vascular disease, and cancer, it is not surprising that therapeutic manipulation of the ubiquitous HIF pathway has become a highly sought after goal. The PHDs and FIH are attractive therapeutic targets, as they are well characterized functionally and structurally [37–40], can be expressed recombinantly [41,42], and inhibition results in HIF activation, with the PHDs of particular interest as the primary regulators of the HIFs [43]. However, specificity is an important issue when targeting PHDs or FIH in human pathologies, given the large family of related 2-oxoglutarate-dependent oxygenases, the hundreds of target genes directly regulated by the HIFs that influence diverse biological processes including erythropoiesis, angiogenesis, metabolism, cell migration and survival, and the other less well characterized substrates of the PHDs and FIH, including the TRP channels.

To date, numerous PHD inhibitors have been developed, with a number in pre-clinical and clinical trials (reviewed in [43]). The initial focus has been on the treatment of anemia, as erythropoietin is a direct target gene of HIF, with two PHD inhibitors currently in Phase 3 clinical trials showing considerable promise. Additional clinical and preclinical trials have also targeted ischemia and inflammation, with other pathologies also under investigation. Specificity for different HIF-mediated outcomes is achieved through the use of inhibitors that display selectivity for one or more of the PHDs (the three different PHDs show some specificity for different HIFα proteins, and consequently regulate distinct target gene responses), as well as distinct delivery and treatment regimes. Little is known regarding the consequence of these treatments on non-HIF targets of the PHDs, including TRPA1.

Preliminary screens have also been performed to identify specific inhibitors of FIH [44,45], but given the modest effects on HIF activity mediated by FIH, it has not been a focus of pharmaceutical research. However, one potential advantage of targeting FIH is that additional specificity may be achieved compared with the PHDs, as FIH only influences the expression of a discrete subset of HIF target genes, and shows some specificity for different HIF isoforms [34,46].

5. Therapeutic Targeting of PHDs and FIH to Modulate TRP Channel Activity

Therapeutic manipulation of the PHDs and FIH is likely to modulate the activity of TRPA1 and TRPV3, respectively. Importantly, inhibition of hydroxylase activity—which has been the focus of therapeutic manipulation to achieve HIF activation—has the potential to increase TRPA1 and TRPV3 activity through abrogation of hydroxylation. However, given the key role of the hydroxylases— specifically the PHDs—in regulating the ubiquitously expressed HIFs, specificity is likely to be a major issue. Importantly, while specific inhibitors of the PHDs and FIH should theoretically also modulate TRPA1 and TRPV3 activity, respectively, through altered hydroxylation, this needs to be determined experimentally. This characterization should include inhibitors that show specificity for each of the hydroxylases, including those currently in clinical trials, and their consequence on both hydroxylation and activity. In the case of both TRPA1 and TRPV3, loss of hydroxylation does not appear to independently activate the channels, but rather the limited data are consistent with an increase in the activity of an already active channel. Hence therapeutic targeting of the PHDs or FIH might only modulate the activity of an already active channel. Physiologically, this would depend on the presence of endogenous chemical agonists, mechanical stimuli, or temperature to activate the channels.

The knowledge that TRPA1 is also regulated by PHD-mediated hydroxylation should also inform the current clinical and preclinical trials using PHD inhibitors to activate the HIFs. For example, a number of pre-clinical studies have targeted inflammation in mouse models of colitis with mostly positive outcomes [43]. However, in similar models of colitis, TRPA1 channels are shown to contribute to disease pathology [47], with TRPA1 antagonists being designed and trialed for treatment of inflammation and pain [48]. Consequently, the activation of TRPA1 achieved with PHD inhibitors is likely to promote rather than inhibit disease pathology and associated pain.

Targeting TRPV3 activity via FIH should be more specific, given the modest role for FIH in HIF regulation and the apparent lack of an effect of hydroxylation on the activity of most characterized ARD substrates [17]. However, this is complicated by the metabolic phenotype of FIH null mice, which are viable and display hypermetabolism, hyperventilation, lowered body mass and adiposity, resistance to weight gain when fed a high fat diet, and insulin hypersensitivity. This phenotype is not readily explained by the known roles for FIH in regulating the HIFs or other characterized ARD substrates, and supports the existence of one or more additional substrates involved in controlling metabolism [49].

A more prudent strategy to therapeutically target the PHDs or FIH to modulate TRP channel activity would focus on pathologies where activation of both the HIFs and the relevant TRP channels are predicted to independently achieve positive outcomes. For example, both TRPV3 and HIF have been implicated in wound healing [50,51], hence the therapeutic inhibition of FIH may promote wound healing through two independent pathways, via activation of both HIF and TRPV3. The targeted deletion of FIH in mice and mice treated with activators of TRPV3 channels both display similar metabolic effects, including decreased adiposity and resistance to weight gain on a high fat diet [49,52]. So, the therapeutic inhibition of FIH in the context of obesity or diabetes may also result in beneficial outcomes through two independent pathways.

6. Conclusions

The recent identification of hydroxylation-mediated changes in TRPA1 and TRPV3 channel activity—although based on a limited number of highly focused studies—has expanded our understanding of the role of channel post-translational modifications, and the oxygen-dependent modulation of these channels. It has also uncovered new therapeutic strategies to modulate the activity of these specific channels by targeting the PHDs and FIH, while identifying potential TRP channel-mediated side effects as a consequence of targeting these hydroxylases to therapeutically regulate HIF activity.

Acknowledgments: This work was supported by a grant from the Australian Research Council (DP150102860).

Author Contributions: Yagnesh Nagarajan, Grigori Y. Rychkov and Daniel J. Peet all contributed to the planning and writing of this manuscript.

Conflicts of Interest: The authors declare no conflict of interest.

References

1. Brierley, S.M.; Hughes, P.A.; Page, A.J.; Kwan, K.Y.; Martin, C.M.; O'Donnell, T.A.; Cooper, N.J.; Harrington, A.M.; Adam, B.; Liebregts, T.; et al. The ion channel TRPA1 is required for normal mechanosensation and is modulated by algesic stimuli. *Gastroenterology* **2009**, *137*, 2084–2095. [CrossRef] [PubMed]

2. Darby, W.G.; Grace, M.S.; Baratchi, S.; McIntyre, P. Modulation of TRPV4 by diverse mechanisms. *Int. J. Biochem. Cell Biol.* **2016**, *78*, 217–228. [CrossRef] [PubMed]

3. Ogawa, N.; Kurokawa, T.; Mori, Y. Sensing of redox status by TRP channels. *Cell Calcium* **2016**, *60*, 115–122. [CrossRef] [PubMed]

4. Vrenken, K.S.; Jalink, K.; van Leeuwen, F.N.; Middelbeek, J. Beyond ion-conduction: Channel-dependent and -independent roles of TRP channels during development and tissue homeostasis. *Biochim. Biophys. Acta* **2016**, *1863*, 1436–1446. [CrossRef] [PubMed]

5. Dai, Y. TRPs and pain. *Semin. Immunopathol.* **2016**, *38*, 277–291. [CrossRef] [PubMed]

6. De Logu, F.; Patacchini, R.; Fontana, G.; Geppetti, P. TRP functions in the broncho-pulmonary system. *Semin. Immunopathol.* **2016**, *38*, 321–329. [CrossRef] [PubMed]

7. Derbenev, A.V.; Zsombok, A. Potential therapeutic value of TRPV1 and TRPA1 in diabetes mellitus and obesity. *Semin. Immunopathol.* **2016**, *38*, 397–406. [CrossRef] [PubMed]

8. Shapovalov, G.; Ritaine, A.; Skryma, R.; Prevarskaya, N. Role of TRP ion channels in cancer and tumorigenesis. *Semin. Immunopathol.* **2016**, *38*, 357–369. [CrossRef] [PubMed]

9. Xu, T.; Wu, B.M.; Yao, H.W.; Meng, X.M.; Huang, C.; Ni, M.M.; Li, J. Novel insights into TRPM7 function in fibrotic diseases: A potential therapeutic target. *J. Cell. Physiol.* **2015**, *230*, 1163–1169. [PubMed]

10. Voolstra, O.; Huber, A. Post-translational modifications of TRP channels. *Cells* **2014**, *3*, 258–287. [CrossRef] [PubMed]

11. Karttunen, S.; Duffield, M.; Scrimgeour, N.R.; Squires, L.; Lim, W.L.; Dallas, M.L.; Scragg, J.L.; Chicher, J.; Dave, K.A.; Whitelaw, M.L.; et al. Oxygen-dependent hydroxylation by FIH regulates the TRPV3 ion channel. *J. Cell Sci.* **2015**, *128*, 225–231. [CrossRef] [PubMed]

12. Takahashi, N.; Kuwaki, T.; Kiyonaka, S.; Numata, T.; Kozai, D.; Mizuno, Y.; Yamamoto, S.; Naito, S.; Knevels, E.; Carmeliet, P.; et al. TRPA1 underlies a sensing mechanism for O_2. *Nat. Chem. Biol.* **2011**, *7*, 701–711. [CrossRef] [PubMed]

13. Loenarz, C.; Schofield, C.J. Physiological and biochemical aspects of hydroxylations and demethylations catalyzed by human 2-oxoglutarate oxygenases. *Trends Biochem. Sci.* **2011**, *36*, 7–18. [CrossRef] [PubMed]

14. Kaelin, W.G., Jr.; Ratcliffe, P.J. Oxygen sensing by metazoans: The central role of the HIF hydroxylase pathway. *Mol. Cell* **2008**, *30*, 393–402. [CrossRef] [PubMed]

15. Peet, D.; Linke, S. Regulation of HIF: Asparaginyl hydroxylation. *Novartis Found. Symp.* **2006**, *272*, 37–49. [PubMed]

16. Nguyen, T.L.; Duran, R.V. Prolyl hydroxylase domain enzymes and their role in cell signaling and cancer metabolism. *Int. J. Biochem. Cell Biol.* **2016**, *80*, 71–80. [CrossRef] [PubMed]

17. Cockman, M.E.; Webb, J.D.; Ratcliffe, P.J. FIH-dependent asparaginyl hydroxylation of ankyrin repeat domain-containing proteins. *Ann. N. Y. Acad. Sci.* **2009**, *1177*, 9–18. [CrossRef] [PubMed]

18. Janke, K.; Brockmeier, U.; Kuhlmann, K.; Eisenacher, M.; Nolde, J.; Meyer, H.E.; Mairbaurl, H.; Metzen, E. Factor inhibiting HIF-1 (FIH-1) modulates protein interactions of apoptosis-stimulating p53 binding protein 2 (ASPP2). *J. Cell Sci.* **2013**, *126*, 2629–2640. [CrossRef] [PubMed]

19. Scholz, C.C.; Rodriguez, J.; Pickel, C.; Burr, S.; Fabrizio, J.A.; Nolan, K.A.; Spielmann, P.; Cavadas, M.A.; Crifo, B.; Halligan, D.N.; et al. FIH regulates cellular metabolism through hydroxylation of the deubiquitinase OTUB1. *PLoS Biol.* **2016**, *14*, e1002347. [CrossRef] [PubMed]

20. Laursen, W.J.; Bagriantsev, S.N.; Gracheva, E.O. TRPA1 channels: Chemical and temperature sensitivity. *Curr. Top. Membr.* **2014**, *74*, 89–112. [PubMed]

21. Moilanen, L.J.; Hamalainen, M.; Nummenmaa, E.; Ilmarinen, P.; Vuolteenaho, K.; Nieminen, R.M.; Lehtimaki, L.; Moilanen, E. Monosodium iodoacetate-induced inflammation and joint pain are reduced in trpa1 deficient mice-potential role of TRPA1 in osteoarthritis. *Osteoarthr. Cartil.* **2015**, *23*, 2017–2026. [CrossRef] [PubMed]

22. DeBerry, J.J.; Schwartz, E.S.; Davis, B.M. TRPA1 mediates bladder hyperalgesia in a mouse model of cystitis. *Pain* **2014**, *155*, 1280–1287. [CrossRef] [PubMed]

23. Kremeyer, B.; Lopera, F.; Cox, J.J.; Momin, A.; Rugiero, F.; Marsh, S.; Woods, C.G.; Jones, N.G.; Paterson, K.J.; Fricker, F.R.; et al. A gain-of-function mutation in TRPA1 causes familial episodic pain syndrome. *Neuron* **2010**, *66*, 671–680. [CrossRef] [PubMed]

24. Nassini, R.; Materazzi, S.; Benemei, S.; Geppetti, P. The TRPA1 channel in inflammatory and neuropathic pain and migraine. *Rev. Physiol. Biochem. Pharmacol.* **2014**, *167*, 1–43. [PubMed]

25. Pokorski, M.; Takeda, K.; Sato, Y.; Okada, Y. The hypoxic ventilatory response and TRPA1 antagonism in conscious mice. *Acta Physiol.* **2014**, *210*, 928–938. [CrossRef] [PubMed]

26. Miyake, T.; Nakamura, S.; Zhao, M.; So, K.; Inoue, K.; Numata, T.; Takahashi, N.; Shirakawa, H.; Mori, Y.; Nakagawa, T.; et al. Cold sensitivity of TRPA1 is unveiled by the prolyl hydroxylation blockade-induced sensitization to ROS. *Nat. Commun.* **2016**, *7*, 12840. [CrossRef] [PubMed]

27. Hamilton, N.B.; Kolodziejczyk, K.; Kougioumtzidou, E.; Attwell, D. Proton-gated Ca(2+)-permeable TRP channels damage myelin in conditions mimicking ischaemia. *Nature* **2016**, *529*, 523–527. [CrossRef] [PubMed]

28. Peier, A.M.; Reeve, A.J.; Andersson, D.A.; Moqrich, A.; Earley, T.J.; Hergarden, A.C.; Story, G.M.; Colley, S.; Hogenesch, J.B.; McIntyre, P.; et al. A heat-sensitive TRP channel expressed in keratinocytes. *Science* **2002**, *296*, 2046–2049. [CrossRef] [PubMed]

29. Smith, G.D.; Gunthorpe, M.J.; Kelsell, R.E.; Hayes, P.D.; Reilly, P.; Facer, P.; Wright, J.E.; Jerman, J.C.; Walhin, J.P.; Ooi, L.; et al. TRPV3 is a temperature-sensitive vanilloid receptor-like protein. *Nature* **2002**, *418*, 186–190. [CrossRef] [PubMed]

30. Xu, H.; Ramsey, I.S.; Kotecha, S.A.; Moran, M.M.; Chong, J.A.; Lawson, D.; Ge, P.; Lilly, J.; Silos-Santiago, I.; Xie, Y.; et al. TRPV3 is a calcium-permeable temperature-sensitive cation channel. *Nature* **2002**, *418*, 181–186. [CrossRef] [PubMed]

31. Broad, L.M.; Mogg, A.J.; Eberle, E.; Tolley, M.; Li, D.L.; Knopp, K.L. TRPV3 in drug development. *Pharmaceuticals* **2016**, *9*, 55. [CrossRef] [PubMed]

32. Luo, J.; Hu, H. Thermally activated TRPV3 channels. *Curr. Top. Membr.* **2014**, *74*, 325–364. [PubMed]

33. Yang, M.; Chowdhury, R.; Ge, W.; Hamed, R.B.; McDonough, M.A.; Claridge, T.D.; Kessler, B.M.; Cockman, M.E.; Ratcliffe, P.J.; Schofield, C.J. Factor-inhibiting hypoxia-inducible factor (FIH) catalyses the post-translational hydroxylation of histidinyl residues within ankyrin repeat domains. *FEBS J.* **2011**, *278*, 1086–1097. [CrossRef] [PubMed]

34. Bracken, C.P.; Fedele, A.O.; Linke, S.; Balrak, W.; Lisy, K.; Whitelaw, M.L.; Peet, D.J. Cell-specific regulation of hypoxia-inducible factor (HIF)-1alpha and HIF-2alpha stabilization and transactivation in a graded oxygen environment. *J. Biol. Chem.* **2006**, *281*, 22575–22585. [CrossRef] [PubMed]

35. Bleymehl, K.; Perez-Gomez, A.; Omura, M.; Moreno-Perez, A.; Macias, D.; Bai, Z.; Johnson, R.S.; Leinders-Zufall, T.; Zufall, F.; Mombaerts, P. A sensor for low environmental oxygen in the mouse main olfactory epithelium. *Neuron* **2016**, *92*, 1196–1203. [CrossRef] [PubMed]

36. Cheng, W.; Yang, F.; Liu, S.; Colton, C.K.; Wang, C.; Cui, Y.; Cao, X.; Zhu, M.X.; Sun, C.; Wang, K.; et al. Heteromeric heat-sensitive transient receptor potential channels exhibit distinct temperature and chemical response. *J. Biol. Chem.* **2012**, *287*, 7279–7288. [CrossRef] [PubMed]

37. Dann, C.E., 3rd; Bruick, R.K.; Deisenhofer, J. Structure of factor-inhibiting hypoxia-inducible factor 1: An asparaginyl hydroxylase involved in the hypoxic response pathway. *Proc. Natl. Acad. Sci. USA* **2002**, *99*, 15351–15356. [CrossRef] [PubMed]

38. Elkins, J.M.; Hewitson, K.S.; McNeill, L.A.; Seibel, J.F.; Schlemminger, I.; Pugh, C.W.; Ratcliffe, P.J.; Schofield, C.J. Structure of factor-inhibiting hypoxia-inducible factor (HIF) reveals mechanism of oxidative modification of HIF-1 alpha. *J. Biol. Chem.* **2003**, *278*, 1802–1806. [CrossRef] [PubMed]

39. Lee, C.; Kim, S.J.; Jeong, D.G.; Lee, S.M.; Ryu, S.E. Structure of human FIH-1 reveals a unique active site pocket and interaction sites for HIF-1 and von hippel-lindau. *J. Biol. Chem.* **2003**, *278*, 7558–7563. [CrossRef] [PubMed]

40. McDonough, M.A.; Li, V.; Flashman, E.; Chowdhury, R.; Mohr, C.; Lienard, B.M.; Zondlo, J.; Oldham, N.J.; Clifton, I.J.; Lewis, J.; et al. Cellular oxygen sensing: Crystal structure of hypoxia-inducible factor prolyl hydroxylase (PHD2). *Proc. Natl. Acad. Sci. USA* **2006**, *103*, 9814–9819. [CrossRef] [PubMed]

41. Hewitson, K.S.; Schofield, C.J.; Ratcliffe, P.J. Hypoxia-inducible factor prolyl-hydroxylase: Purification and assays of PHD2. *Methods Enzymol.* **2007**, *435*, 25–42. [PubMed]

42. Linke, S.; Hampton-Smith, R.J.; Peet, D.J. Characterization of ankyrin repeat-containing proteins as substrates of the asparaginyl hydroxylase factor inhibiting hypoxia-inducible transcription factor. *Methods Enzymol.* **2007**, *435*, 61–85. [PubMed]

43. Chan, M.C.; Holt-Martyn, J.P.; Schofield, C.J.; Ratcliffe, P.J. Pharmacological targeting of the HIF hydroxylases—A new field in medicine development. *Mol. Asp. Med.* **2016**, *47–48*, 54–75. [CrossRef] [PubMed]

44. Flagg, S.C.; Martin, C.B.; Taabazuing, C.Y.; Holmes, B.E.; Knapp, M.J. Screening chelating inhibitors of HIF-prolyl hydroxylase domain 2 (PHD2) and factor inhibiting hif (FIH). *J. Inorg. Biochem.* **2012**, *113*, 25–30. [CrossRef] [PubMed]

45. McDonough, M.A.; McNeill, L.A.; Tilliet, M.; Papamicael, C.A.; Chen, Q.Y.; Banerji, B.; Hewitson, K.S.; Schofield, C.J. Selective inhibition of factor inhibiting hypoxia-inducible factor. *J. Am. Chem. Soc.* **2005**, *127*, 7680–7681. [CrossRef] [PubMed]

46. Dayan, F.; Roux, D.; Brahimi-Horn, M.C.; Pouyssegur, J.; Mazure, N.M. The oxygen sensor factor-inhibiting hypoxia-inducible factor-1 controls expression of distinct genes through the bifunctional transcriptional character of hypoxia-inducible factor-1alpha. *Cancer Res.* **2006**, *66*, 3688–3698. [CrossRef] [PubMed]

47. Engel, M.A.; Leffler, A.; Niedermirtl, F.; Babes, A.; Zimmermann, K.; Filipovic, M.R.; Izydorczyk, I.; Eberhardt, M.; Kichko, T.I.; Mueller-Tribbensee, S.M.; et al. TRPA1 and substance p mediate colitis in mice. *Gastroenterology* **2011**, *141*, 1346–1358. [CrossRef] [PubMed]

48. Kaneko, Y.; Szallasi, A. Transient receptor potential (TRP) channels: A clinical perspective. *Br. J. Pharmacol.* **2014**, *171*, 2474–2507. [PubMed]

49. Zhang, N.; Fu, Z.; Linke, S.; Chicher, J.; Gorman, J.J.; Visk, D.; Haddad, G.G.; Poellinger, L.; Peet, D.J.; Powell, F.; et al. The asparaginyl hydroxylase factor inhibiting HIF-1alpha is an essential regulator of metabolism. *Cell Metab.* **2010**, *11*, 364–378. [CrossRef] [PubMed]

50. Aijima, R.; Wang, B.; Takao, T.; Mihara, H.; Kashio, M.; Ohsaki, Y.; Zhang, J.Q.; Mizuno, A.; Suzuki, M.; Yamashita, Y.; et al. The thermosensitive TRPV3 channel contributes to rapid wound healing in oral epithelia. *FASEB J.* **2015**, *29*, 182–192. [CrossRef] [PubMed]

51. Hong, W.X.; Hu, M.S.; Esquivel, M.; Liang, G.Y.; Rennert, R.C.; McArdle, A.; Paik, K.J.; Duscher, D.; Gurtner, G.C.; Lorenz, H.P.; et al. The role of hypoxia-inducible factor in wound healing. *Adv. Wound Care* **2014**, *3*, 390–399. [CrossRef] [PubMed]

52. Cheung, S.Y.; Huang, Y.; Kwan, H.Y.; Chung, H.Y.; Yao, X. Activation of transient receptor potential vanilloid 3 channel suppresses adipogenesis. *Endocrinology* **2015**, *156*, 2074–2086. [CrossRef] [PubMed]

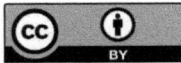

MDPI AG

St. Alban-Anlage 66

4052 Basel, Switzerland

Tel. +41 61 683 77 34

Fax +41 61 302 89 18

http://www.mdpi.com

Pharmaceuticals Editorial Office

E-mail: pharmaceuticals@mdpi.com

http://www.mdpi.com/journal/pharmaceuticals

www.ingramcontent.com/pod-product-compliance
Lightning Source LLC
Chambersburg PA
CBHW051729210326
41597CB00032B/5654